Strategic Capital Planning for Healthcare Organizations

**An Executive Guide to
Capital Planning, Debt Management,
Derivatives, Fixed-Income Investing
and Mergers & Aquisitions**

Christopher T. Payne

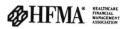

HFMA® HEALTHCARE FINANCIAL MANAGEMENT ASSOCIATION

A HEALTHCARE 2000 PUBLICATION

PROBUS PUBLISHING

Chicago, Illinois
Cambridge, England

A **2000** *PUBLICATION*

Portions of this book were adapted, with permission from *Hospital Capital Formation: Strategies and Tactics for the 1990s,* published by American Hospital Publishing, Inc., copyright 1991.

ISBN 1-55738-615-3

Printed in the United States of America

BB

CTV

1 2 3 4 5 6 7 8 9 0

***To Ginger**
a beautiful person both inside and out,
and fortunately for me,
my wife*

*and while I'm at it. . . ,
to our beautiful daughters
Katie and **Kristy***

(because I may never do this again!)

Table of Contents

List of Figures

Preface

In 1990, I was asked to write a chapter entitled "Hospital Debt Management" for the book *Hospital Capital Formation: Strategies and Tactics for the 1990s,* which was published by American Hospital Publishing in 1991. After the book and chapter were well received, Probus Publishing approached me to expand the concepts presented in that chapter into this book.

The object of this text is to acquaint readers with the many factors and pitfalls involved in effective capital planning for healthcare institutions. It was written to give more casual readers an overview of the process of planning for and issuing debt, while providing a fair amount of detail to more serious readers who desire to learn more about the specifics of the process. It may also serve as a reference tool for healthcare personnel when specific decisions relating to the topics covered must be made. It is hoped that the end result will be better educated healthcare professionals who can make well informed decisions about capital planning and issuing debt, resulting in their ability to access the capital markets at lower cost.

Running a healthcare organization is a full-time job . . . and then some. The healthcare industry is constantly evolving, and healthcare professionals must expand their efforts to cope with the changes confronting them and to anticipate the trends that will dominate the industry in the future. Similarly, methods of financing healthcare organizations are constantly evolving, and it is a full-time job for the professionals who finance them to keep up with the latest developments that may be useful to these organizations.

This book was written primarily for healthcare professionals, to help them make more informed decisions about capital planning and acquisition for their organizations. It can also serve as a springboard for investment bankers, commercial bankers, lawyers, accountants, consultants, and other professionals who are new to the healthcare finance industry, as well as for students who hope to embark on careers that will involve healthcare finance.

Any healthcare professional who undertakes the development of a capital plan, and the implementation of the financings resulting from the plan, will rely upon finance professionals for advice on the process. In some cases, the advice comes from the investment bankers retained to sell bonds. In other cases, advice may come from lawyers or accountants. In many cases, advice is sought from professional financial advisors who specialize in this service. The point to be made is that this process is not part of the normal day-to-day activity of healthcare professionals. Some outside party, or parties, inevitably end up serving as financial advisor and providing advice on the process, regardless of whether they are specifically hired to fill that role, or are serving primarily in another role on the financing team.

The key objective of the healthcare professional, therefore, is to discriminate between advice that is self-serving to the party giving financial recommendations, and advice that will lead to the best possible capital planning for the organization. While no book can give a healthcare professional the experience of a full-time financial advisor, this book can impart the information necessary to determine whether or not they are being well served by the professionals they have chosen to work with in the financing process. The phrase "buyer beware" is very appropriate in the healthcare finance industry. Representatives of healthcare organizations are asked to make decisions that can save, or cost, their institutions millions of dollars. Poor capital planning decisions are becoming increasingly devastating as margins in the healthcare industry continue to be squeezed. Margins are also being squeezed in the municipal finance industry, to the point where any borrower is well advised to realize that advice received from a party that stands to benefit from any particular outcome may not always be in the best interest of the borrower. The information in this book can help healthcare organizations retain the best professionals to assist in the financing process and provide enough knowledge to trustees and management of the organization to help them keep their hired professionals on their toes and responsive to the needs of the organization.

A note on style: Key terms that are used fairly regularly in the industry are printed in *italics* where they are defined or explained. Of course, italics may occasionally be used for emphasis as well. Jargon-type terms are printed in quotation marks (" ").

▍ Acknowledgments

Thanks to my associates at Ponder & Co., Bob Gottschalk and Josh Nemzoff, for contributing chapters on their specific areas of expertise. Their efforts resulted in far more knowledgeable, informative, and useful discussions on these topics than if I had tried to cover them myself. Thanks to Julian Head and Michele DuBose for editorial assistance, and Terry Shirey and his team for helping me think through some of the more technical examples presented. Thanks also to the rating agencies that supplied the information contained in Appendix A, and the municipal bond insurance companies that supplied the information contained in Appendix B. Finally, thanks to the other principals at Ponder & Co., for allowing me the time to complete this work.

1 An Introduction to Capital Planning

The healthcare industry in America has faced a tremendous amount of uncertainty and change during recent years, and this trend shows no sign of letting up in the near future. A shakeout has begun and lines are being drawn between the winners and the losers, i.e., those organizations that will continue to provide healthcare services while maintaining their corporate identities versus those that either will be forced out of business or forced to merge their corporate identities into stronger organizations. Healthcare organizations that insist on maintaining the status-quo, and running their operations in the traditional manner, may be in for a very unpleasant surprise. Those organizations that look to the future, by planning and evolving to meet expected changes head on, have a far greater likelihood of being the survivors in an industry whose number of distinct individual providers is certain to diminish.

More than ever before, healthcare organizations are discovering the value of planning as management attempts to cope with an ever-changing environment. Therefore, the management and trustees of healthcare organizations across America are searching for answers to questions such as:

- What business are we truly in?

- What services do we need to provide to fulfill our mission?

- How can we provide those services at a level of profitability that will allow us to stay in business?

- What physical plant and equipment will we need to provide the services that we determine are necessary to fulfill our mission and to survive?

- What will our business be five years from now?

- How can we best conduct that business?

- What do we have to do now to be in the position we want to be in five years from now?

The answers to these and many other questions are typically accumulated in a *strategic plan* for the organization. Strategic planning deals with the business changes that must be made for an organization to perform as well as possible, given certain expectations for the environment within which that organization will be operating in the future. A good *capital plan* develops a systematic approach for acquiring the physical assets necessary to carry out the strategic plan. Where the strategic plan deals with basic business strategy and more global issues, the focus of a capital plan should be to identify the sources of capital available to the organization, and in which priority they should be utilized. The capital plan should complement and evolve out of the strategic plan, which has little chance of being successfully implemented without a sound capital plan to back it up. *Strategic capital planning,* therefore, is the process of developing a sound capital plan to maximize the likelihood of success of the organization's strategic plan.

Assets are funded with capital. The term "capital" is generally considered to refer to the combined total of long-term debt plus fund balance (equity) of an organization. The not-for-profit version of equity is called fund balance, but it represents the same thing that equity, or stock, represents to a for-profit company: investment. In the not-for-profit healthcare industry, investment is built up through donations and the excess of revenues over expenses (surplus) that accumulates during a period of time. For-profit healthcare organizations have the ability to sell shares of stock to build investment (equity), in addition to generating profits and receiving donations. However, few hospitals have the ability to generate enough capital through earnings and donations to fund all the necessary asset acquisitions to remain competitive in the industry. As a result, most hospitals have turned to debt to fund some of their capital needs.

There is a grave misconception among many that a not-for-profit healthcare organization is not supposed to generate any excess of revenues over expenses, or "profits." After all, they are "not-for-profit" organizations. This philosophy has been one of the leading causes of failure of not-for-profit hospitals. It is also one of the primary reasons that the amount of debt issued by not-for-profit healthcare organizations has grown so considerably.

For example, take the case of a hospital built 30 years ago for a cost of $10 million. Most likely, that hospital depreciated the building over the 30 years and may have built up a depreciation reserve of $10 million. The problem is, the building now needs to be completely renovated or replaced, and the cost is going to be more like $50 to $70 million. The hospital should have been accumulating additional reserves at a pace at least equal to the rate of inflation. To do so, the hospital would have had to generate an excess of revenues over expenses to fund this reserve. In addition, reserves should have been built to provide capital for new technology as well as a cushion to cover expenses during periods of transition imposed by the market or the government. All healthcare organizations must generate a surplus, or profit, if they are to survive. At a minimum, not-for-profit healthcare organizations should earn a surplus equal to a return on assets commensurate with the rate of inflation, plus enough to reserve for new technology, new business strategies, and for working capital during periods of adjustment.

Working capital, as opposed to capital, generally is considered to be the excess of current assets over current liabilities on a balance sheet. It represents the amount of short-term assets that an organization has on hand to fund future expenses. Working capital is used to fund current operating expenses of a business, whereas capital is used to finance physical assets.

Capital planning involves the systematic management of liabilities and fund balance (equity) to acquire the necessary assets for an organization to carry out its strategic plan. Any strategic plan can fail if there is no proper capital planning to allow it to be fulfilled. Neither plan can succeed without the other unless the organization has capital to waste, a practice that has become fatal in the healthcare industry.

The capital plan is best prepared with the assistance of a qualified financial advisor, i.e., someone experienced in the specialized field of healthcare finance and with no vested interest in the final outcome of the plan. Running a healthcare organization is a full-time job, as is keeping up with the changes in the financing alternatives available to healthcare organizations. No single individual can perform both jobs at the same time to their full potential. Managers of a healthcare institution may have been through several financings during their careers, and have a good feel for the overall process, but it is impossible for them to remain current as to the state of the art in the finance industry unless they devote their full attention to it. Likewise, a good healthcare financial advisor works full time at keeping up with the developments in healthcare finance. As a result, it is unlikely that a financial advisor could run a hospital as well as a full-time hospital administrator. Together, however, a good financial advisor and management can put together a capital plan that serves the organization well.

■ Alternative Sources of Capital and Their Relative Costs

The capital plan should begin with an evaluation of the alternative forms of capital that are available to the organization. The stronger the financial condition of the organization, the more alternative sources of capital will be available, and at a lower cost. A generally accepted premise is that it is best to use the cheapest (least expensive) capital available to fund a project. The cheaper the capital used to fund a project, the lower the break-even point for that project becomes, which leads to greater profitability.

There are four categories of capital that should be investigated by most healthcare organizations. The first is an evaluation of the funds that have been generated internally by the organization, namely *cash reserves*. A second source of capital is *donations* (philanthropy), although this source has become less important as the capital needs of healthcare organizations have grown faster than the ability or willingness of the public to fund them on a continuing basis. A third potential source of capital is *external equity*, where investors actually participate with an ownership interest. For-profit healthcare organizations are easily able to take advantage of this source of capital, while not-for-profit organizations must be very careful on how they make use of equity so they do not jeopardize their tax-exempt status. The fourth source of capital available is *debt*. It is important for a healthcare organization to be able to discriminate between these sources of capital, especially in terms of cost, in order to be able to generate the most cost-effective capital plan.

Debt

Debt issued on behalf of not-for-profit healthcare organizations can be taxable or tax-exempt. That is, the interest paid to bondholders (investors) can be taxable income or tax-exempt income. The key distinction between taxable and tax-exempt debt is that borrowers pay lower interest rates on tax-exempt debt than on taxable debt with comparable terms. This is because investors demand a higher interest rate to make up for the added tax liability on the interest received on taxable debt. As a result, tax-exempt debt usually should be a cheaper source of capital than comparable taxable debt. In addition, in many states, debt that is exempt from federal income taxes is also exempt from state income taxes, making it that much more attractive.

Internally Generated Funds and Philanthropy

The cost of utilizing capital generated internally or through philanthropy represents an opportunity cost incurred if these funds are spent on projects rather than retained and invested for the future. Not-for-profit healthcare organizations have the ability to borrow capital for specific projects in the tax-exempt markets while retaining and investing their own cash reserves at higher rates in the taxable markets for later use. As a result, the overall cost of a project may be higher if internal funds are used and the investment opportunity is lost. Although this opportunity cost never shows up on an income statement, it represents a real economic loss.

This is a very important concept. *Properly structured tax-exempt debt can be a cheaper source of capital than a healthcare organization's own cash reserves.* In this case, "properly structured" means tax-exempt debt that is issued efficiently and with terms that are favorable to the borrowing organization, resulting in the lowest possible cost.

It is important to emphasize that the proceeds of tax-exempt debt must be used to fund the projects for which the bonds are issued, and may not be invested and used to hedge bonds or earn profits. The cash that may be invested is the healthcare organization's own cash reserves, which are not bond proceeds. Proceeds of taxable debt may be used in any way a healthcare organization chooses, but it is unlikely that it could consistently invest its cash at a rate of return higher than the interest rate paid on its taxable debt. Because of this, taxable debt is usually a more expensive form of capital than a healthcare organization's cash reserves.

Equity Offerings

The equity markets generally require a rate of return that is greater than the return on taxable debt. This is because equity carries more risk, in that debtholders (creditors) get paid prior to equity shareholders in the event of a bankruptcy. This means that the use of equity to fund a project typically will cost a healthcare organization more than using debt or its own cash reserves. The additional cost may be warranted if other benefits are generated through the use of equity, such as firming up relationships with doctors or risk sharing. Of course the primary advantage of outside equity is the freedom from a contractual obligation to repay the amount invested or to generate any set return for the investor. The use of equity also may allow a healthcare organization to tap a larger pool of capital, resulting in the ability to fund more projects, albeit at a higher cost.

The use of equity by not-for-profit healthcare organizations has become increasingly difficult as more and more scrutiny is being placed on interactions with for-profit entities. As a result, funding a project with outside equity may not only result in utilizing more expensive capital, but it may end up causing complications relative to the tax-exempt status of the organization if it is not done very carefully. As government regulations become increasingly burdensome to not-for-profit healthcare organizations, there may be increasing incentive for these organizations to give up their not-for-profit status and turn to the less restrictive but more expensive taxable capital markets.

Summary of Alternative Sources of Capital

Properly structured tax-exempt debt usually is the least expensive form of capital available to not-for-profit healthcare organizations. Consequently, they should use tax-exempt debt whenever possible and maintain their cash reserves for projects that are ineligible for financing with tax-exempt debt, or for future projects when tax-exempt debt may no longer be available. Taxable debt and equity are relatively more expensive forms of capital and should be used only on a temporary basis, or when tax-exempt debt is not available and cash reserves are down to the minimum required for operations. The relative costs of these alternative sources of capital are depicted in Figure 1–1.

Aggressive strategic plans for healthcare organizations frequently require tapping into several of these sources of capital. A good capital plan should identify the realistic quantities of capital available in each of these categories, as well as the relative cost of each. While management should be well equipped to ascertain the availability of internally generated capital and donations, the organization's financial advisor should perform a debt capacity analysis as a preliminary step in forming the capital plan.

Figure 1–1   Relative Costs of Capital

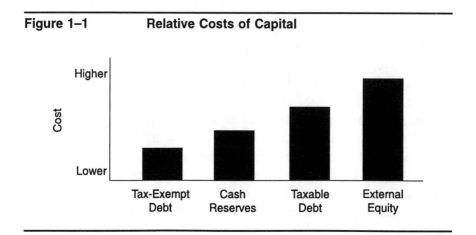

▌ Debt Capacity Analysis

A *debt capacity analysis* typically takes the form of a comparison of the various financial ratios of a healthcare organization as they compare to the published ratios (by various rating agencies) for comparable organizations. The ratios fall into several categories, including financial performance (profitability), debt service coverage, liquidity, capitalization (leverage), and utilization. Figure 1-2 shows some of the ratios typically used for this type of comparison.

The analysis generally begins by computing the appropriate ratios for the healthcare organization before any new debt is issued to verify the stability of any rating of the organization's outstanding debt. Rating agencies can only update outstanding ratings every so often, and the purpose of this first step is to reconfirm any existing ratings, or to estimate a rating if none exists.

The second step in a debt capacity analysis is to recalculate the ratios assuming various levels of additional indebtedness, until an estimation can be obtained as to the amount of debt that might result in a downgrade of the organization's rating if that debt were issued.

The process of obtaining a rating involves much more than a simple comparison of financial ratios. It includes an analysis of the effectiveness of management; the organization's service area and competition; how the borrower is coping with the growing managed-care environment; and many other aspects that can affect the overall creditworthiness of a healthcare organization. This rating process is covered in more detail in Chapter 9. The purpose of this financial ratio comparison in a debt capacity analysis is to highlight the likely effect on any existing ratings if additional debt is incurred by the healthcare organization, ignoring the other variables that go into the rating process.

Debt capacity analysis usually becomes the most important element of the capital plan for several reasons. First, as previously explained, tax-exempt debt should be a cheaper source of capital for a healthcare organization than other sources, including its own internal cash. Second, internal cash reserves are limited, and can best be used on projects that are not eligible for tax-exempt financing. Third, philanthropy has not kept up with the capital needs of most healthcare organizations. Fourth, external equity capital is not only more expensive than other forms of capital for an organization, but it also may result in prob-

Figure 1–2   Typical Ratios Used in a Debt Capacity Analysis

Ratio	Computation
Profitability Ratios Operating Margin (%)	$$\dfrac{\text{operating revenue} - \text{operating expenses}}{\text{operating revenue}}$$
Excess Margin (%)	$$\dfrac{\text{operating income} + \text{non-operating income}}{\text{operating revenue} + \text{non-operating revenue}}$$
Coverage Ratios Annual Debt Service Coverage (×)	$$\dfrac{\text{net income} + \text{depreciation expense} + \text{interest expense}}{\text{principal payments} + \text{interest expense}}$$
Maximum Annual Debt Service Coverage (×)	$$\dfrac{\text{net income} + \text{depreciation expense} + \text{interest expense}}{\text{maximum annual debt service}}$$
Liquidity Ratios Current Ratio (×)	$$\dfrac{\text{current assets}}{\text{current liabilities}}$$
Days Cash on Hand	$$\dfrac{\text{unrestricted cash and investments} \times 365}{\text{operating expenses} - \text{depreciation and amortization expenses}}$$
Cushion Ratio (×)	$$\dfrac{\text{unrestricted cash and investments}}{\text{maximum annual debt service}}$$
Capitalization (Leverage) Ratios Debt to Capitalization (%)	$$\dfrac{\text{outstanding debt}}{\text{outstanding debt} + \text{unrestricted fund balance}}$$
Capital Expense (%)	$$\dfrac{\text{interest expense} + \text{depreciation and amortization expenses}}{\text{operating expenses}}$$
Utilization Ratios Outpatient (%)	$$\dfrac{\text{gross outpatient revenue}}{\text{gross patient revenue}}$$

Other (e.g., # beds in service, length of stay, occupancy (%), #FTE's/occupied bed)

Figure 1–2   **Typical Ratios Used in a Debt Capacity Analysis (continued)**

Ratio	Computation
Miscellaneous Ratios Days Accounts Receivable	$\dfrac{\text{net patient accounts receivable} \times 365}{\text{net patient revenue}}$
Average Payment Period (days)	$\dfrac{\text{current liabilities} \times 365}{\text{operating expenses} - \text{depreciation and amortization expenses}}$
Average Age of Plant (years)	$\dfrac{\text{accumulated depreciation}}{\text{depreciation expense}}$

lems with a not-for-profit healthcare organization maintaining its tax-exempt status. For these reasons, as well as others, debt has become the primary source of capital used to implement the capital programs dictated by strategic plans for the not-for-profit healthcare industry.

Many not-for-profit healthcare organizations tend to make as much use as possible of tax-exempt debt, while for-profit healthcare organizations fund capital projects with internal funds, taxable debt, and external equity. Once a debt capacity analysis has been developed and the overall level of desirable debt has been determined, the capital plan should continue to evaluate and recommend the basic structure of the debt to be issued.

2 Debt

Debt is the general term used to describe a variety of obligations to repay borrowed money. Debt is usually evidenced by instruments such as bonds, notes, and mortgages. In each case, a lender or group of lenders allows a borrower the use of a specified amount of money, which is the *principal* amount of the loan, in return for a rental fee for use of that money, known as *interest*. Both principal and interest must be paid to the lender at specified times pursuant to the terms and conditions of the loan. The required payments of principal and interest are referred to as *debt service*. The required payments of principal and interest for any given year are referred to as *annual debt service*. The sum of all debt service payments is referred to as the *total debt service* under the obligation.

Historically, healthcare organizations have used debt as a primary source of funds for acquiring capital assets, and bond issues have been the primary source of debt. In the early days of healthcare bond financings, each new bond issue looked quite similar to the last one. Legal *covenants*, which are restrictions on the borrower's operations aimed at protecting the lender's ability to collect on the loan, were virtually standard from one deal to the next. Those were the days of the "plain vanilla" bond issue.

Today, healthcare organizations can choose from a large menu of debt options. Each of these options can be tailored to the individual needs of the organization; in other words, today's healthcare debt can be custom designed to make the best use of the debt markets. A good capital plan for a healthcare organization will review many different aspects of debt, with the ultimate goal being to recommend a debt structure that is best suited to the borrower.

▌ Taxable versus Tax-Exempt Debt

Once a healthcare organization has determined that it will use debt to finance all or a portion of its capital projects, it must determine whether taxable or tax-exempt debt is more appropriate. For every form of tax-exempt debt there is a comparable version of taxable debt that can be used if the ability to access tax-exempt debt is not available or desirable to the borrower.

Although tax-exempt debt usually is a less expensive means of long-term financing, federal law severely restricts its use, making it unavailable for a variety of projects. The Tax Reform Act of 1986 specifies, with very few exceptions, that any project that directly or indirectly benefits any person or entity other than a tax-exempt entity cannot be financed with tax-exempt debt. Examples of projects that normally cannot be financed with tax-exempt debt under current tax law, referred to as "bad money" projects, include physicians' office buildings, parking garages used by people visiting doctor's offices, athletic facilities used for purposes other than rehabilitation, or any joint venture with individuals or for-profit corporations. As such, for-profit healthcare organizations currently are prevented from using tax-exempt debt, and not-for-profit healthcare organizations are prevented from using tax-exempt debt for any projects that involve virtually any direct benefit to individuals or for-profit entities.

While current tax law generally prohibits the use of the proceeds of a tax-exempt bond issue to provide space or equipment primarily for the benefit of independent physicians, a trend has recently begun in the healthcare industry that involves not-for-profit healthcare organizations acquiring physician practices and employing the physicians. The practice of employing physicians may have benefits that satisfy certain strategic plan goals of not-for-profit healthcare organizations. If structured properly, it is possible for a healthcare organization to use tax-exempt bonds to fund the acquisition of the physical assets of physician practices. Competent bond counsel should be consulted when transactions of this type are being negotiated because tax law generally restricts the use of tax-exempt bond proceeds to the acquisition of hard assets, and not goodwill or other intangibles.

For interest on debt to be exempt from federal income tax, the debt must be issued by a state or a political subdivision of a state, such as a county or city. Some states (and some state subdivisions) have legislatively established agencies, known as *authorities,* to issue tax-exempt bonds for specific public purposes such as housing, education, and healthcare. Private not-for-profit healthcare organizations must use a conduit issuer to make their bonds tax-exempt. A *conduit issuer,* such as an authority, a city, or a county, issues tax-exempt bonds on behalf of a borrower and lends the proceeds of the bond issue to that borrower. The availability of tax-exempt conduit issuers varies by state. Some states severely limit the number of entities that can issue bonds for private not-for-profit healthcare organizations. Public healthcare institutions, which are owned by a city, county, hospital district, authority, or other political subdivision, may be able to issue their own tax-exempt bonds without the need for a conduit issuer.

Federal tax law imposes a key drawback to tax-exempt debt: it must always be tied to a specific project or purpose. Taxable debt carries no such restriction and can be issued for any purpose, which may change at any time without the borrower having to redeem (pay off) the debt. As a result, taxable debt and equity offer a degree of flexibility that is not available with the proceeds of tax-exempt bonds. A not-for-profit healthcare organization can greatly offset this drawback by financing more eligible projects with tax-exempt debt and building and maintaining its own cash reserves for later use on projects not eligible for tax-exempt financing.

In summary, there are many forms of tax-exempt debt, and generally there are corresponding forms of taxable debt that can be used by for-profit healthcare organizations or by not-for-profit healthcare organizations that do not have access to tax-exempt debt. No special issuer is required for taxable debt, so any healthcare organization able to incur debt can issue its own taxable debt.

■ Revenue Bonds versus GO Bonds

Most private healthcare organizations issue revenue bonds as opposed to general obligation bonds. *Revenue bonds* depend on the revenue stream generated by the borrower to provide for their repayment. *General obligation bonds (GO bonds)* have the backing of a governmental body empowered to raise taxes to provide for the payment of the bonds. Generally, revenue bonds are considered somewhat less creditworthy than GO bonds and tend to carry lower credit ratings from the rating agencies. Lower ratings result in higher interest rates due to a perceived greater risk of default. Public healthcare organizations may have the ability to issue GO bonds. It is unusual for a private healthcare organization to be able to issue debt that is backed by the general obligation of any taxing entity.

■ Fixed Rate versus Variable Rate Debt

When the interest rate on a debt instrument is set to maturity, the debt is said to have a fixed interest rate and is referred to as *fixed rate debt*. If the interest rate changes prior to maturity, it is *variable rate debt,* which is also referred to as *floating rate debt*. Both fixed and variable rate financings have their appropriate uses by healthcare organizations.

Fixed Rate Debt

The primary advantage of fixed rate debt is that the interest cost is a known factor throughout the life of the debt. The primary disadvantage is that fixed rate debt generally costs more than variable rate debt, in terms of issuance costs as well as interest rates at the time of issuance. At any point in time, current fixed interest rates typically will be higher than current variable interest rates. If variable interest rates rise and remain relatively higher throughout the life of the debt, the fixed rate may prove to be the less expensive option in the long run. Conversely, if interest rates fall or remain relatively constant throughout the life of the debt, the variable rate option will prove to be relatively cheaper. Fixed rate debt generally is most appropriate for funding projects where the borrowing organization does not have cash reserves to offset the risk of variable rates. It should be used when long-term rates are relatively low and acceptable to the borrower.

Variable Rate Debt

Variable rate tax-exempt debt became popular in 1981, when interest rates were reaching all time highs. The Bond Buyer Revenue Bond Index reached 14.24% in September 1981. Some organizations, not wanting to lock into such high long-term fixed rates, chose to implement interim financings until long-term rates returned to acceptable levels. The intent was to refinance this interim debt at long-term fixed interest rates once they fell to acceptable levels.

The first of these interim financings were fixed rate, with maturities of three to five years, and backed by letters of credit from major banks. The term of the bonds matched the term of the letter of credit, and the rating on the bonds was determined by the rating held by the bank. They were issued as *balloon* (or *bullet*) *debt,* meaning that there was no amortization of principal other than a single payment at the final maturity. In the event that there was no permanent financing implemented to refinance these bond issues, the bank would be obligated to convert its letter of credit to a term loan, and the borrower would be required to pay off the debt according to the terms of the term loan.

After several of these fixed rate short-term notes were issued, investment bankers realized that borrowers could save money by issuing these short-term bond issues on a variable rate basis rather than at fixed rates. A bond that paid interest based on a fixed rate for five years was likely to pay a higher interest rate than a bond that paid interest on a variable rate basis that changed weekly. A new financing vehicle was created to provide variable interest exposure to the borrowers for these interim financings. *Variable rate demand bonds (VRDBs),* sometimes referred to as *variable rate demand obligations (VRDOs)* or *lower floaters,* became the most common vehicle for these interim financings.

▪ Evolution of Variable Rate Demand Bonds

As they were first developed in 1981, VRDBs had three- to five-year maturities. The interest rate changed every seven days, and the bondholders had the right to *put* (which means the right to sell) these bonds to the trustee, at *par* (face value), on seven days' notice. This put feature is what allowed these bonds to sell at seven-day interest rates rather than three- to five-year rates. An underwriting firm served as a *remarketing agent* to resell the bonds if they were ever put. A letter of credit secured the bonds to provide cash to buy them back from a bondholder if they were ever put and the remarketing agent was unable to resell them. The use of a letter of credit allowed the VRDBs to obtain the ratings of the bank rather than the ratings of the borrower.

The letter of credit provided both credit strength as well as liquidity. In other words, the letter of credit could be drawn upon to make regularly scheduled interest payments in the event the underlying borrower was not able to do so, in addition to providing the liquidity needed in the event that the bonds were put and the remarketing agent was unable to resell them. Purchasers of these bonds generally required a AA/Aa ("double A") rating, or better, to purchase them. This limited the number of banks that could enter this new market to provide these letters of credit.

Another popular feature of VRDBs was that they could be *called* (paid off) on short notice, usually 30 days or less. This feature made them particularly attractive for interim financings, in that three- to five-year fixed rate bonds rarely could be called prior to maturity.

The interest resetting mechanism for VRDBs initially was pegged to an index. The most common form of index used initially was the most current auction rate for 90-day Treasury bills. For example, the interest rate on the bond might be reset weekly at 67 percent of the most recent 90-day Treasury bill auction rate. Some of these bonds were also priced off of the prime rates of some of the major banks that provided the letters of credit, as well as off of the London Interbank Offered Rate, or LIBOR (pronounced "lie bore"), an interest rate commonly used in international financings and for short-term loans between international banks. Because each of these indexes is derived from taxable markets, a percentage of the index was used to compensate for the tax-exempt nature of the bonds. Eventually, some tax-exempt indexes were created, allowing the bonds to float relative to the tax-exempt market rather than the taxable market.

The use of indexes as pricing mechanisms eventually gave way to using the remarketing agent as a *pricing agent,* with a rate determined by that agent for each pricing period. The rate set by the pricing agent was to be the lowest interest rate that would cause all the bonds to be sold on that day if they actually were for sale. This allowed the pricing of the bonds to reflect more closely what the remarketing agent felt was the true market for the bonds each week.

As time passed, and healthcare borrowers became accustomed to the low interest rates that VRDBs provided, they began to question the desirability of refinancing with fixed rate bonds. This new attitude led to an evolution of VRDBs that made them more suitable for permanent financing. VRDBs were improved by lengthening the final maturity and adding a conversion feature. The final maturity on most VRDBs stretched out to 30 and even 40 years. The concept was to issue the bonds for as long as possible because they could always be paid off on short notice if the borrower ever chose to do so. The borrower could make use of the relatively cheap capital for as long as possible with no downside risk or cost. The conversion feature allowed healthcare organizations to convert the bonds to a fixed interest rate whenever they chose to do so, without issuing new bonds.

These changes were developed for two main reasons. First, Congress was threatening to eliminate the use of tax-exempt debt by private healthcare organizations. This might have prevented a healthcare organization that had implemented an interim financing from obtaining long-term, permanent financing when interest rates fell. The conversion feature reduced the risk that a borrower would be prevented from obtaining fixed rate debt in the future. Second, many healthcare organizations found that the interest rates of VRDBs were so attractive that they were in no hurry to refinance them with fixed rate debt. As long-term rates came down, the rates on VRDBs got even lower, which made it desirable to leave VRDBs outstanding longer than originally anticipated. For example, a borrower in 1981 might have been in a situation where the fixed rate on a long-term financing would have been in the range of 14.0%. The interest rate on seven-day VRDBs was around 9.0% at that time. In later years, when long-term fixed rates dropped in the neighborhood of 9.0%, the rates on VRDBs were around 5.0%. Every time a borrower looks at converting or refinancing variable rate debt with fixed-rate debt, there is an immediate and significant increase in interest cost. As a result, many variable rate financings were never refinanced with fixed rate debt, or were not converted until long-term fixed rates hit their record lows in 1992 and 1993.

Variable Rate Demand Bonds Today

Variable rate demand bonds continue to provide the ability to access long-term debt at short-term rates, with the opportunity to lock in a fixed rate later. Most versions of VRDBs provide additional flexibility, such as a *multi-mode* format where a seven-day repricing feature is only one alternative. Repricing can occur daily, weekly, monthly, quarterly, semiannually, annually, or at any other interval the borrower chooses. Some VRDBs include a *commercial paper mode,* which allows different bonds within one series to be priced for different periods. This mimics the performance of *commercial paper,* where bonds are sold at fixed rates for differing short-term maturities ranging from one day to 270 days, and then "rolled over," or reissued for additional short-term periods. The net effect of a commercial paper program is similar to a VRDB. The difference is that with commercial paper, the bond actually matures on each roll-over date and is reissued for the next period. With a VRDB, the bond does not mature until the final maturity, but is repriced periodically.

Another desirable feature that may be included in a VRDB issue is the ability for each bond to be in a different mode. This means that some of the bonds could be repriced on a weekly basis, some on a quarterly basis, some in the commercial paper mode, and any conceivable combination of all the different modes. This will allow the greatest possible amount of flexibility for the borrower in adjusting its bond issue to capitalize on anticipated interest rate environments.

When structuring a VRDB issue, a healthcare organization and its financial advisor should determine which of the various possible modes are desirable for the borrower and whether or not it is worth including all of them. The inclusion of more modes means lengthier and more complicated documents. Some issuers and bond counsel may not be familiar with all the various modes, and may need some education.

While the ability to convert the variable rate bonds into long-term fixed rate bonds has become standard in virtually all VRDB issues, the majority of these issues have not provided for the ability to create serial bonds (bonds with short maturities) at the time the bonds are converted. If a VRDB issue is converted to long-term fixed rate bonds with a single-term bond, then all the bonds will pay the highest possible interest rate upon conversion. (The concept and benefits of serial bonds versus term bonds is covered in more detail later in this chapter.) If the borrower is able to designate certain bonds to be paid off in years one, two, three, etc., after conversion to fixed rates, the interest coupon on these serialized maturities will be less than if they are all priced for 20- or 30-year maturities. The ability to serialize the bonds upon conversion can result in significant savings for the borrower. It may be preferable for healthcare organizations with outstanding VRDB issues that do not contain this serialization feature to refund the bonds with a new fixed rate issue rather than convert the existing bonds. A new issue would allow the use of serial bonds, thereby lowering the interest cost to the borrower.

As previously mentioned, the primary market for commercial paper or VRDBs requires that provisions be made for both credit and liquidity on these types of instruments. The *credit* evaluation is based upon the ability of the borrower, or some credit enhancer, to make the required payments of principal and interest when they become due. Generally, the most favorable interest rates on these types of instruments are only available to borrowers that either have a rating of AA/Aa on their own, or with the help of credit enhancement through a *credit facility*. A credit facility usually is obtained through the use of a letter of credit or bond insurance. There is a market for VRDBs rated in the A or A1/A+ categories, but at higher interest rates.

A *liquidity facility,* on the other hand, provides comfort to bondholders that funds will be available in the event the VRDBs are put and the remarketing agent is not able to remarket them. Similarly, commercial paper programs require liquidity facilities because the intent is to remarket the commercial paper as it comes due. The liquidity facility provides funds to pay off the maturing paper in the event new paper is not able to be sold.

VRDBs generally have dual ratings. This means they have a long-term rating to describe the overall credit (the likelihood of timely payment of principal and interest), and a short-term rating reflecting the strength of the liquidity facility to purchase the bonds in the event they are not remarketed. Ratings are discussed in greater detail in Chapter 9. Credit facilities are discussed in Chapter 10.

VRDBs Without External Credit or Liquidity Facilities

While it is necessary for a borrower to provide comfort to bondholders as to both credit and liquidity on a VRDB issue, very strong organizations may be able to meet the necessary requirements with their own resources. While the greater portion of the market for VRDBs requires a rating of AA/Aa or AAA/Aaa, a fair market exists for issues rated A1/A+ or even A. This means a healthcare organization that maintains an A rating or better on its *senior debt*—or that which is not subordinate to any other debt—does not necessarily need any form of credit enhancement. A healthcare organization with a rating of A– or less on its senior debt probably would be well advised to obtain credit enhancement of some sort to increase the rating on the bonds to AA/Aa or better.

Purchasers of VRDBs generally also require a short-term rating, reflecting the liquidity on the bonds, in one of the two highest rating categories. The short-term liquidity rating is intended to be a measure as to the likelihood that funds will be available to make payment on the VRDBs in the event they are put and the remarketing agent is unable to find other purchasers to buy the bonds at the time the put is exercised. In order to obtain this sort of rating, the rating agencies must be satisfied that funds will be available from a reasonable source, on the day of the put. They generally also require that notification of the need for the funds not be necessary until the day of the put. In other words, these funds must be available on same-day notice.

This liquidity feature can be provided through a letter of credit or a line of credit from a bank. As the cost of these facilities from banks is increasing, more and more healthcare organizations are looking into providing their own liquidity. To do this, they must have sufficient liquid assets to cover the entire amount of the bond issue, plus the maximum amount of interest that can come due at any point in time. In calculating this interest requirement, the rating agencies generally require that the calculation be made using the maximum allowable rate on the bonds, for the maximum number of days between interest payments, plus a few days extra cushion. The nature of the liquid securities must also be taken into account to determine the potential for market fluctuations affecting their value. In most cases, it is likely that the agencies will require that the total exposure of any put be covered with some cushion in the value of the portfolio of the securities to allow for market fluctuations. As previously mentioned, it is also required that the funds be available on the same day that notice is given that they are required. This means the only allowable investments for these funds will be securities that can be liquidated, and cash received, on the same day they are offered for sale.

While more and more healthcare organizations are investigating the option of providing their own liquidity for VRDBs, the decision is frequently made that the required investment constraints for the securities are too severe, and will cost the organization more than maintaining a bank facility. As the cost of bank facilities continues to increase, more organizations are expected to evaluate the option of providing their own liquidity.

Another form of variable rate debt, called Dutch auction bonds, does not have a put feature at all. As a result, the borrower is not required to provide any liquidity facility because bondholders expect to be able to sell their bonds at the periodic Dutch auctions. The pricing for these bonds is also determined by the auctions. This type of variable rate debt is a viable alternative for organizations that do not want the requirement of providing liquidity on variable rate bond issues. Dutch auction bonds are discussed in much greater detail in Chapter 13.

■ Appropriate Uses of Variable Rate Debt

Variable rate debt is most appropriate in two situations: first, when long-term interest rates are at unacceptable levels, and it is desirable to avoid locking into a long-term fixed rate until rates drop; and second, when a healthcare organization has sufficient cash reserves that will, in effect, offset the risk of the variable rates.

If a healthcare organization issues fixed rate debt while maintaining significant cash reserves, and rates decline in the future, it may find itself in a situation where its cash reserves are earning a lower rate than what is being paid on the debt. The healthcare organization typically will invest its cash reserves at short- to intermediate-term maturities to maintain liquidity and avoid market risk. The rate on its fixed rate debt would be set for as many as 30 years, or more. Consequently, when interest rates drop, the healthcare organization may not be able to invest at the desired shorter maturities and still earn enough return (or yield) to equal or exceed the rate it is paying on its tax-exempt bonds. In this case, the cost of capital for the fixed rate debt would be higher than the cost of using the cash reserves.

This risk can be avoided by issuing VRDBs instead of long-term, fixed rate bonds. When VRDBs are issued, the cost of the debt moves in tandem with changes in the return on any cash reserves invested in the short-term markets. The healthcare organization should be able to invest its cash reserves at rates higher than the rates on the VRDBs, thereby generating a net gain in income. This is true even if rates increase significantly, because the net gain comes from the spread between income earned on the taxable investments and the interest cost of the tax-exempt bonds, rather than from the absolute level of the interest rates.

It is important to point out that the cash reserves must not be tied to a tax-exempt issue in any way lest they be considered to be an invested sinking fund. An *invested sinking fund* is a cash reserve that can be reasonably expected to be used to pay debt service on the tax-exempt bonds. The determination that the cash reserves are an invested sinking fund would result in a *yield restriction,* which is a limitation placed on the yield that can be earned on the cash reserves, eliminating part of the advantage of such a program. Strategies of this type can be extremely beneficial to healthcare organizations, but tax counsel should be consulted to avoid any potential conflicts with tax law.

■ Benefits of Variable Rate Debt and Cash Reserves

Using VRDBs to finance projects while a healthcare organization maintains cash reserves has several significant benefits. The first is the considerable flexibility that the cash reserves provide to the healthcare organization. There are no restrictions on these reserves, other than those self-imposed by the organization itself. These reserves can be used to fund projects that are not eligible for tax-exempt financing. They also may be retained and invested for use on future projects. The healthcare organization retains total control of these reserves, which results in a greater ability to take advantage of future opportunities for expansion or acquisitions when its competition may not be able to do so. Cash reserves provide a not-for-profit healthcare organization with capital that has flexible uses, comparable to the flexibility of taxable debt and equity used by for-profit healthcare organizations, but at a lower cost.

A second benefit is that the market and the rating agencies place a strong emphasis on the liquidity of healthcare organizations. A healthcare organization with significant cash reserves is more likely to be perceived as being successful, well run, and able to withstand swings in the business environment. In other words, a healthcare organization with $50 million in debt and $60 million in cash reserves is likely to be perceived as being stronger than a healthcare organization with no debt and $10 million in cash reserves.

Third, it should be possible to invest the cash reserves at a return that is greater than the cost of the VRDBs until the reserves are used. This results in a lower overall cost of capital for the borrower than if its own cash reserves were spent on the project.

A fourth benefit is that the VRDBs can be converted to a fixed rate when the healthcare organization decides to spend the cash reserves that are serving to offset the risk of the variable rates. This ability to convert to a fixed rate might prove to be valuable if Congress ever eliminates the ability of healthcare organizations to issue new tax-exempt debt, or if the healthcare organization has a significant capital need that is not eligible for tax-exempt financing. In either case, a healthcare organization might choose to use its cash reserves to fund projects rather than use the more expensive alternative of taxable debt, and find it beneficial to convert its VRDBs to fixed interest rates.

A fifth benefit is that the VRDBs can be paid off at par, with no prepayment penalty, on short (30 days or less) notice. This ability to call on short notice removes any risk of not being able to pay off the bonds whenever the healthcare organization decides it wants to.

All these benefits make VRDBs an attractive vehicle for a healthcare organization to warehouse (store up) tax-exempt debt while it is able to do so. With all the turmoil in the healthcare industry, an organization that is able to attract capital today may not be able to do so in the future for various reasons. Many organizations are choosing to obtain as much capital from the debt markets as possible, and VRDBs allow them to do so in a way that reduces their overall cost of capital at the same time, without incurring any additional risk.

▌ Long-Term versus Short-Term Maturities

A generally accepted premise in the business world is that assets should match liabilities; that is, long-term assets should be funded with long-term debt, and short-term assets should be funded with short-term debt.

An exception to this rule may be taken in the case of tax-exempt debt because long-term, fixed rate, tax-exempt debt generally contains provisions that allow it to be called (paid off) in 10 years or less, and long-term VRDBs can be called in 30 days or less. As a result, it is sometimes prudent to stretch the maturity of tax-exempt debt as long as possible. This gives a healthcare organization the ability to make efficient use of the cheaper capital to fund additional projects in the future, with cash generated through the depreciation of the original assets, even if the ability to issue new tax-exempt debt is eliminated. If the healthcare organization chooses, it can always pay off the debt on a call date if it is no longer beneficial. Current tax law limits the ability to stretch the maturity of tax-exempt debt by requiring that the average maturity of a tax-exempt bond issue not exceed 120 percent of the useful life of the project being financed. The average life of a 30-year bond issue, with level debt service, is usually in the range of 18 to 20 years. This means the average life of the project financed with such a bond issue must be at least 14 to 16 years. If the average life of the project is less than this, then the maturities of the bond issue will have to be shortened to comply with this rule.

∎ Serial Bonds and Term Bonds

Long-term bond issues are usually structured like a home mortgage, with a growing amount of principal maturing each year and a decreasing amount of interest due each year, so that the net effect to the borrower is level payments. This is referred to as having *level debt service,* and is depicted in Figure 2-1. A long-term fixed rate bond issue usually consists of two types of bonds: serial bonds and term bonds. Serial bonds typically mature each year, creating a succession of principal payments to bondholders by the borrower. Term bonds mature on a given date several years from the date the bonds are issued, and the borrower typically makes periodic payments into a separate fund known as a *sinking fund* to provide for their repayment. With some types of debt instruments, sinking funds accumulate money over a period of time and then pay off the instrument. In a tax-exempt bond issue, the sinking fund will usually accumulate funds for one year, and then make a partial call on the next maturing term bond and redeem that amount of bonds. As a result, sinking funds in a tax-exempt bond issue typically are cleaned

Figure 2–1   Level Debt Service Amortization

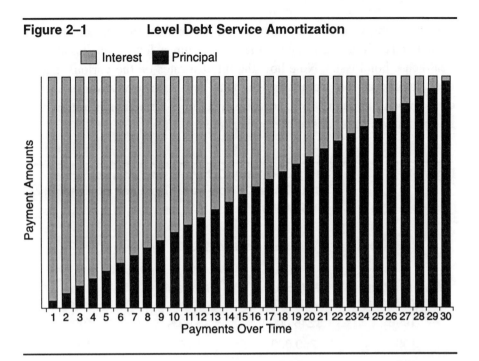

out once a year and do not accumulate for longer than that. The typical healthcare organization long-term bond issue includes several serial maturities and one or more term maturities. Usually, the shorter the maturity of the bond, the lower the interest rate. By using serial bonds in the early years of a bond issue, the overall interest cost is reduced.

Ideally, a healthcare organization would issue serial bonds for each year of the entire bond issue, thereby keeping its interest rates as low as possible. Unfortunately, there usually are no buyers for the middle maturities, such as 13 to 20 years. As a result, a typical long-term structure might include serial bonds maturing each year for as many as 10 to 15 years, and then one or more term bonds maturing in 25 or 30 years, or both. In the early years, the principal component of the borrower's loan payment goes to pay off the maturing serial bonds. After the final serial bond has been paid off, the next year's principal payment will go into a sinking fund and will be used to redeem, or call, a portion of the next maturing term bond.

More than one term bond might be used when the additional term maturity can be sold at a lower interest rate than the final maturity. This usually happens when an investor needs bonds with a particular maturity and is willing to accept an interest rate lower than the rate on the final term bonds. Figure 2-2 shows the scale from a long-term, tax-exempt healthcare bond issue. Note how the interest rates on the various maturities increase as the maturities lengthen. This borrower saved a significant amount in interest expense by including serial bonds rather than issuing only term bonds at the higher interest rates.

Figure 2–2	Sample Maturity Schedule and Interest Scale for a 30-Year, Fixed-Rate, Tax-Exempt Healthcare Bond Issue

Issue Size $22,275,000

Maturity Date (February 15)	Principal Amount	Interest Rate	Price
1996	$245,000	5.90%	100%
1997	260,000	6.00	100
1998	275,000	6.10	100
1999	290,000	6.20	100
2000	310,000	6.30	100
2001	330,000	6.40	100
2002	350,000	6.50	100
2003	375,000	6.60	100
2004	400,000	6.70	100
2005	425,000	6.80	100
2006	455,000	6.90	100
2007	485,000	6.95	100
2008	520,000	7.00	100
2009	555,000	7.05	100
2010	595,000	7.05	99.75

$4,165,00 7 1/8% Term Bonds Due February 15, 2015, Price 99%

$12,240,000 7.20% Term Bonds Due February 15, 2025, Yield 7.30% (plus accrued interest from October 1, 1995)

■ Amortization Alternatives

The capital plan should consider alternative amortization schedules for a bond issue to determine which will be most beneficial for the borrower. *Amortization* means the schedule of when principal and interest payments (debt service payments) are due on the debt. Most bond issues are structured using level debt service, as described above, making the regular payments relatively equal on that particular series of debt for the borrower. When a bond issue is structured with level debt service, most of the repayment in early years goes towards interest, with the amount being applied to principal increasing over the years until final maturity. A graphical representation of a debt issue with level debt service is depicted in Figure 2-1.

Another alternative for structuring the amortization on a bond issue is *level principal amortization.* In this situation, the amount of principal paid on the bonds is constant throughout the life of the bond issue. As a result, the total payments made by the borrower will decline over the life of the bond issue as depicted in Figure 2-3, assuming the interest rate is fixed. This is because the amount of interest owed each year will decrease as the amount of principal outstanding decreases. This form of

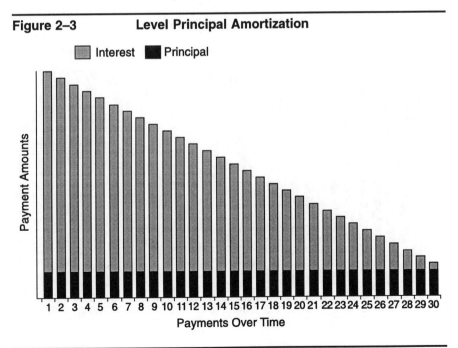

Figure 2–3   Level Principal Amortization

Interest   Principal

Payment Amounts

Payments Over Time

amortization is used occasionally in the healthcare industry, but not very often.

A third amortization structure that can be used in a bond issue is referred to as a *wrap-around amortization* structure. This technique is used frequently by borrowers that have outstanding debt and wish to wrap the amortization of the new debt around that of the existing debt so when the total payments for all debt are combined, it will result in level debt service. Figure 2-4 depicts a graphical representation of a situation where a borrower has outstanding debt and wraps the amortization of a new issue around that debt to effectuate level debt service on its total debt obligations.

A fourth amortization technique that is used frequently by healthcare organizations creates a hole, or window, in the amortization schedule to provide for some anticipated debt in the future. This technique was used frequently in the 1980s in a form referred to as a *window refunding,* where a refunding issue would amortize in the later maturities of the bond issue, thereby incurring a higher interest cost while creating room for a new money issue in the early years at a lower interest cost. As is described in Chapter 12 on refundings, the actual interest

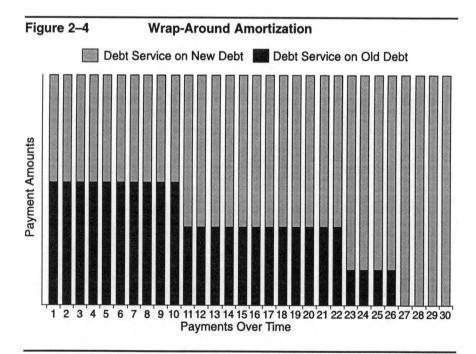

Figure 2–4   Wrap-Around Amortization

rate paid on a refunding issue is not as important as the interest rate paid on a new money issue. The Tax Reform Act of 1986 severely limited the ability to use the window refunding technique, but there are certain situations where a similar approach may be desirable and allowable under tax law. Figure 2-5 depicts a window amortization.

A final amortization structure that is frequently used is a *balloon amortization*. In this situation there is little, if any, reduction in principal for a period of time, and then a large amount of principal is paid all at once. Conceivably, a balloon structure could be devised so that there is a small amount of principal reduction for a period of time, then a large payment (the balloon), and then smaller payments again for a period of time. In most cases, however, the balloon comes at the final maturity of a debt obligation. The concept of a balloon merely means that a payment that is significantly larger than the other payments is made at one time during the life of the debt. The most extreme example of a balloon amortization is where there is no amortization of principal until the final maturity of the debt, at which time it is paid in its entirety. This is referred to as a *bullet amortization*. Figures 2-6 and 2-7 depict graphical representations of a balloon amortization and a bullet amortization, respectively.

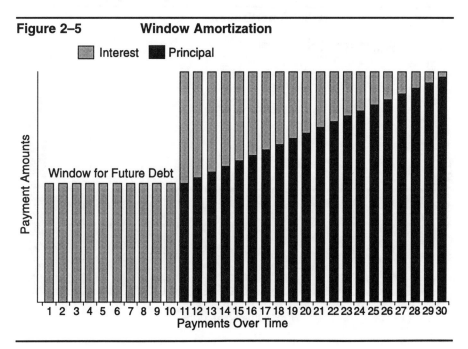

Figure 2–5   **Window Amortization**

Interest   Principal

Payment Amounts

Window for Future Debt

1 2 3 4 5 6 7 8 9 10 11 12 13 14 15 16 17 18 19 20 21 22 23 24 25 26 27 28 29 30
Payments Over Time

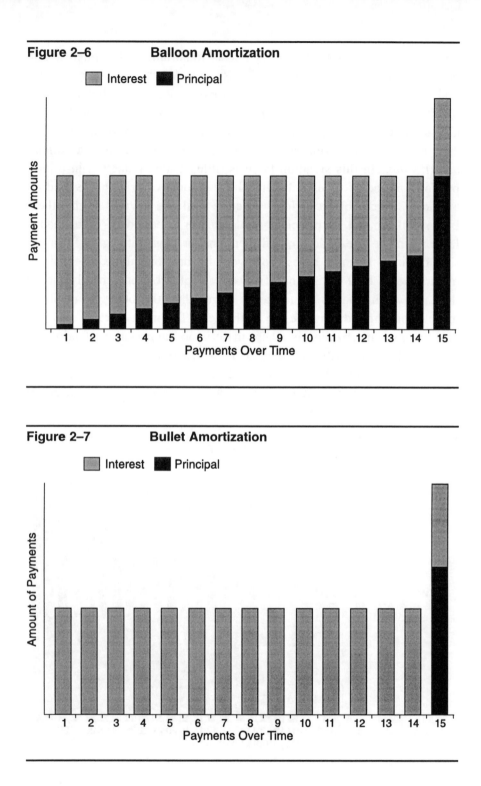

Figure 2–6   Balloon Amortization

Interest   Principal

Payment Amounts

Payments Over Time

Figure 2–7   Bullet Amortization

Interest   Principal

Amount of Payments

Payments Over Time

■ Financing Working Capital

Working capital is generally defined as the excess of current assets over current liabilities, but many people consider working capital to be cash available to be used for the operations of a business. There has been a growing emphasis on working capital financings during recent years as Medicare and Medicaid payments have declined and slowed down. Healthcare organizations without sufficient liquidity have found themselves running short of working capital to carry on normal operations. Most of the working capital financing programs that have been developed to meet this need are funded with taxable debt. As a result, they tend to be more expensive than tax-exempt alternatives.

Some states allow tax-exempt financings for working capital. Federal tax law does not specifically preclude tax-exempt financing of working capital, but it does place fairly severe restrictions on the ability to do so, including limiting the useful life of working capital. This presents a problem because, as discussed earlier, federal tax law requires that the average life of a tax-exempt bond issue cannot exceed 120 percent of the useful life of the assets financed. If working capital has a short useful life, then it becomes difficult to finance on its own.

Healthcare organizations have several options for financing working capital under current tax law. First, the taxable programs being offered may provide a reasonable alternative if no tax-exempt funds are available. Second, a limited amount of working capital could be included in a regular tax-exempt financing where the useful life of the capital projects being financed is sufficient to include a certain amount of working capital at a short, or zero useful life. Any financing in which the proceeds are used to fund a significant "bricks-and-mortar" project with a long useful life should be able to accommodate a certain amount of zero-life project (working capital). The key factor here is whether the tax-exempt issuer has the statutory authority to issue debt for working capital, and whether or not the borrower can comply with the other restrictions imposed by tax law, which may prove to be more restrictive than the useful life rules.

The best alternative for any not-for-profit healthcare organization is to finance more eligible capital projects with tax-exempt debt than it otherwise might, and save its cash to build working capital. A healthcare organization following this approach is far less likely to develop a working capital shortfall and less likely to be forced to use the more expensive taxable financing programs.

▌ Pooled Financing Programs

Many organizations do not have capital needs great enough at one point in time to warrant a tax-exempt bond issue because of the front-end costs of issuing bonds. To help the healthcare organizations with smaller needs, pooled financing programs were introduced to the industry in 1981 as a means of providing less expensive tax-exempt financing for smaller loans. The concept was simple. A large, and therefore, more cost-effective, tax-exempt bond issue would be implemented and the proceeds lent to several individual healthcare organizations, with each borrower obligated only for its proportionate share of these front-end or issuance costs. The system worked well because the primary obstacle to issuing bonds in smaller amounts was the high issuance cost. The only benefit that a pool can offer is economies of scale. If a healthcare organization has a need for roughly $5 to $7 million or more, most pools will offer little benefit compared with a stand-alone financing for that organization.

Some issuers were required by state law to issue only *dedicated pools,* where the individual borrowers were committed and ready to draw funds at the time the bonds were issued. This is a cumbersome process due to the timing problems of coordinating several different healthcare organizations at one time.

A much easier structure to implement was a *blind pool,* where bonds were issued based on a demand survey, and individual borrowers were not committed to borrow from the pool until they formally applied for funds. The pools usually had three years to make loans. The blind pool system worked well because bonds could be issued based on timing considerations of the issuer and the market, rather than the entire group of borrowers. Tax laws in effect prior to the Tax Reform Act of 1986 allowed the proceeds of tax-exempt bond issues to be invested at an unlimited yield during the three-year temporary period. This allowed the blind pools to earn enough interest income to cover the issuance costs if no loans were made.

The 1986 tax law requires earnings on bond proceeds above the bond yield to be rebated to the U.S. Government, so blind pools are very difficult to implement today, unless there is another source of revenue to cover the issuance costs of the bonds. Dedicated pools, though still possible under the tax law, continue to be very cumbersome to implement.

Many of these pooled financings issued prior to 1986 contained *recycling provisions*. This means funds that are paid down on loans can be re-lent to other borrowers. Because of this, healthcare organizations that have small borrowing needs should check on the availability of pre-1986 pools in their states. Making use of the recycled funds from these pools is not only a very economical way to finance small loans, but there is the added benefit that pre-1986 tax law applies. This can be particularly beneficial for organizations that have a need to finance projects that cannot be financed with proceeds of bond issues subject to the 1986 tax law. Prior tax law was significantly more liberal on the types of projects that could be financed or, more to the point, the amount of proceeds of a bond issue that can be spent on "bad money" projects. The Tax Reform Act of 1986 limits the amount of bad money in a bond issue to 5 percent of the total issue. Tax law prior to 1986 allowed up to 25 percent of the proceeds of a bond issue to be used on projects that normally were not eligible to be financed with tax-exempt bonds. This ability to finance some projects that cannot be financed with a new bond issue makes loans from recycled tax-exempt pool financings issued prior to 1986 very attractive for some healthcare organizations.

3 Debt Management Strategies and a Case Study

The final step in putting together a good strategic capital plan for a healthcare organization is the careful development of alternative financing strategies and a final recommendation as to which strategy is most appropriate to pursue. Most healthcare organizations are able to take advantage of a number of strategies to maximize the benefits of the debt markets. Successful use of these strategies can increase profitability and make a healthcare organization more competitive. For-profit organizations are limited to taxable financings, which do not offer the same potential as tax-exempt financings. As a result, for-profit healthcare organizations must use an appropriate balance of taxable debt and equity for their capital formation.

Any discussion of debt management strategies for not-for-profit healthcare organizations should include a section on the *A* word: arbitrage. Tax law frowns upon any structure that uses the proceeds of tax-exempt bonds to produce arbitrage. It is important to note that there is nothing inherently evil about arbitrage. It is only considered bad when it is associated with tax-exempt bond proceeds. To better understand arbitrage, it may be helpful to put it in a broader context.

In the generic sense, *arbitrage* is the purchasing of an asset in one market, with the immediate resale in another market at a higher price.

By definition, it is a riskless transaction and serves the function of stabilizing the relationship between different markets.

For example, in the realm of foreign exchange, traders practice arbitrage and make significant profits while stabilizing the relationship between the exchange rates of various currencies. To illustrate this example, assume the hypothetical situation depicted in Figure 3-1 occurs, where one British pound (£1) can be traded for two American dollars ($2.00), and five French francs can be traded for one American dollar ($1.00). If it is also true, at a given point in time, that £1 could buy 11 francs, then a potential for arbitrage exists. Foreign exchange traders would quickly use American dollars to purchase British pounds, and then use the pounds to purchase French francs, which then could be

---

Figure 3–1　　　　**Arbitrage in the Foreign Currency Markets**

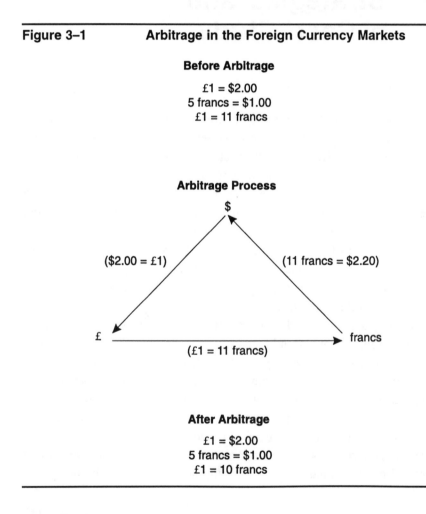

Before Arbitrage

£1 = $2.00
5 francs = $1.00
£1 = 11 francs

Arbitrage Process

$

($2.00 = £1)　　　　(11 francs = $2.20)

£　　　　　　　　　　　　　　　　　francs
(£1 = 11 francs)

After Arbitrage

£1 = $2.00
5 francs = $1.00
£1 = 10 francs

---

converted back to American dollars at a profit. Two dollars would purchase £1, which would purchase 11 francs, which could be converted back to $2.20. When hundreds of millions of pounds are used to purchase French francs, the demand for the franc will cause its price to rise to a point where a trader will only be able to purchase 10 francs for £1, thus bringing the relationship among the three currencies into equilibrium, and removing any profit incentive for further trading. The transaction is risk free to the foreign exchange traders, as long as they do not hold any position in any one currency relative to the others.

The above example has little to do with the realm of healthcare finance, other than to demonstrate that in the rest of the world, arbitrage is not considered to be a bad thing. While there is little opportunity for a healthcare organization to take advantage of arbitrage solely in the taxable markets, there is significant opportunity to do so between the tax-exempt and taxable markets. Any organization that has the ability to borrow money in the tax-exempt market and to invest other money in the taxable market has the opportunity to engage in a legal form of arbitrage. However, the tax laws have become very strict regarding the ability of organizations to do so. Were it not for these restrictions, not-for-profit healthcare organizations would be well advised to borrow billions of dollars in the tax-exempt market, and then turn around and invest them in the taxable market at higher interest rates. However, tax law virtually has eliminated the ability of healthcare organizations to borrow money in the tax-exempt market and invest the bond proceeds in the taxable market at a profit.

A healthcare organization also must be cautious about any funds of its own that it invests when it has an outstanding tax-exempt bond issue. As mentioned in Chapter 2, one of the provisions in the tax law dictates that any moneys that may reasonably be expected to be used to repay tax-exempt bonds, including the borrower's own funds, may be deemed to be an *invested sinking fund,* and may not be used to derive arbitrage profits. Invested sinking funds are yield restricted, meaning they cannot be invested at interest rates higher than the yield on the bonds they are expected to pay down. Because of this, it is important for healthcare organizations to keep a clear distinction as to the expected use of various reserves that it maintains, so that those reserves may not be deemed to be invested sinking funds.

Fortunately, the tax law recognizes that healthcare organizations must maintain certain cash reserves, and that not all such reserves could reasonably be expected to repay outstanding tax-exempt bonds. Healthcare organizations should consult with their financial advisers, and bond counsel, to develop strategies for the appropriate use of tax-exempt debt while maintaining appropriate cash reserves. Technically, this does not result in a form of arbitrage under tax law, because the moneys that are invested are not derived from the proceeds of any tax-exempt bond issue, but the result to the healthcare organization is the same.

▌ Debt Management Strategies

The following strategies can be useful for not-for-profit healthcare organizations:

1. Tax-exempt debt is the least expensive form of capital available to not-for-profit healthcare organizations. If structured properly, it is cheaper than the organization's own cash. As a result, it is advisable for not-for-profit organizations to finance more projects that are eligible for tax-exempt financing than they otherwise might, and save their own cash for use on projects that are not eligible for tax-exempt funding. This approach does not necessarily result in a healthcare organization incurring any more debt than it otherwise would in the long run, but it does result in more of the organization's debt being incurred on a tax-exempt basis, and a lower overall cost of capital

2. Taxable debt and equity are more expensive forms of capital than tax-exempt debt or a healthcare organization's cash reserves. They should be used only on a temporary basis, or when tax-exempt debt is not available and cash reserves are down to the minimum desirable levels.

3. Because tax-exempt debt always must be tied to a specific project, not-for-profit healthcare organizations should build cash reserves to add flexibility to their balance sheets and accumulate capital that can be used for any purpose. By building these reserves and issuing tax-exempt debt to fund eligible projects on which the reserves would have otherwise been spent, a not-for-profit healthcare organi-

zation can regain the flexibility it needs to apply its capital to those projects where it can generate the greatest return, whether or not those projects could have been financed with tax-exempt debt.

4. Tax law limits the ability of not-for-profit healthcare organizations to reimburse themselves with the proceeds of a tax-exempt bond issue for projects on which they have already spent their own cash. Because of these limitations, every not-for-profit healthcare organization that anticipates seeking reimbursement from a future tax-exempt bond issue should make sure that the intent is clearly expressed in the minutes of the board meeting when the appropriate capital expenditures are approved, and that all necessary procedures are followed to comply with tax law. It is wise to obtain advice on the required procedures from the bond counsel firm that the organization expects to use on its bond issue. Any healthcare organization's efforts may be wasted if bond counsel is not satisfied with the procedures employed to "grandfather" reimbursement.

5. Variable rate tax-exempt debt is most appropriate to fund projects on an interim basis when long-term rates are unacceptably high, or when a borrower has sufficient cash reserves to offset the risk of swings in the market. As the cost of the debt rises, so should the return on the reserves. This virtually eliminates the risk of variable rates.

6. Financially sound not-for-profit healthcare organizations should not have to borrow for working capital in the taxable markets. Instead, they should be able to build cash reserves for working capital by funding all eligible capital projects with tax-exempt debt. Healthcare organizations in some states can use tax-exempt debt to finance a limited amount of working capital as part of a larger issue including capital projects.

7. Not-for-profit healthcare organizations with regular capital needs and sufficient cash reserves should routinely issue VRDBs to fund new projects and only issue fixed rate debt when the long-term market is very favorable. This strategy removes the healthcare organization from the trap of being forced to lock into unfavorable long-term rates just because there is a current need to issue debt. Instead, the organization can take more control of its destiny by

enjoying the lower interest cost of VRDBs until the long-term market is more favorable. In this way, the healthcare organization keeps its overall cost of capital to a minimum by taking advantage of favorable long-term rates when they occur, and converting blocks of its variable rate debt to fixed rate.

8. Healthcare organizations should explore the use of competitive sales when evaluating financing alternatives. If an organization is working with an experienced financial advisor, there should be no harm in delaying the decision of whether to use a competitive sale until late in the process. An underwriting firm can always be brought in at the last minute if the decision is made to use a negotiated sale, and its fees will be lower if its representatives have not had to spend time structuring and documenting the deal. This option is discussed in detail in Chapter 8.

Not-for-profit healthcare organizations that make appropriate use of these strategies will gain an advantage over those that do not. These strategies can allow an organization to exert more control over the debt markets, resulting in a lower cost of capital and greater access to capital.

The healthcare industry is facing increasingly difficult situations as the cost of healthcare rises and the ability to generate revenue is further hindered. Tax-exempt debt is one way that society has bestowed a benefit to not-for-profit healthcare organizations in return for their service to the public. Not-for-profit healthcare organizations that do not take the greatest advantage of the ability to use tax-exempt debt place themselves at a competitive disadvantage to other healthcare organizations that do. For-profit healthcare organizations do not have the advantage of tax-exempt debt, but that makes it all the more important that they manage their debt carefully and efficiently. In the long run, it will be the healthcare organizations that manage their debt and other capital resources most effectively that will continue to thrive under adverse conditions. The following case study illustrates one example of how this can be done. A few new concepts and terms are introduced here that are explained further in ensuing chapters.

■ Case Study

The fictitiously named Charitable Health System (CHS) was formed in 1984. It owned seven private not-for-profit healthcare institutions in four states. Some of the facilities were profitable and some were not. The CHS trustees felt that the weaker institutions were important to the overall mission of CHS because they were located in inner cities and served the poor in those areas. Overall, CHS was profitable and set a goal of a 5 percent to 7 percent operating margin on net revenues and total income of 8 percent to 10 percent of net revenues.

When CHS became a system, some of the institutions had their own debt issues outstanding. Although CHS knew it needed $20 million in financing for capital projects in 1985, it was not sure how to coordinate the various institutions or what type of debt was appropriate. Underwriters were constantly calling on CHS, each with a different idea as to what debt structure made sense.

In June of 1985, CHS retained an experienced independent financial advisory firm to assist in developing a capital plan and in the selection of an investment banker. The financial advisor developed a capital plan that called for two different financings. The first was to be a fixed-rate issue of roughly $36 million to refund the outstanding debt of the various healthcare institutions under a new master trust indenture with an obligated group.

The second issue was to be a VRDB issue of about $70 million. The proceeds of this multi-mode VRDB issue were to reimburse CHS for prior projects that had been temporarily funded with the various institutions' cash reserves, and to fund anticipated capital expenditures for the next three years. Because the capital plan called for a VRDB issue, that narrowed the field of potential underwriters.

The trustees of CHS adopted this capital plan for several reasons:

1. It consolidated the credit into what turned out to be a healthcare system whose senior debt was rated A1/A+ on the basis of the combined credit strength of all the various healthcare institutions that were owned by CHS.

2. The master trust indenture provided a single source of covenants to govern this debt and all future debt.

3. The existing debt would be refinanced at savings in the case of high-to-low refundings, and at no additional cost in the case of the low-to-high refundings by structuring the escrows properly.

4. By the time the proceeds of the VRDB issue were spent, CHS would have built up cash reserves equal to $100 million, so there was no risk on the variable rate nature of the VRDB issue.

5. The cash reserves would serve as an internal bank within the system to fund projects that were not eligible for tax-exempt financing. Until they were needed, the cash reserves could be invested to earn 1.0 percent to 3.0 percent over the total cost on the VRDB issue, thereby allowing CHS to maintain its overall profitability objective with smaller rate increases.

6. CHS would be able to convert the VRDB issue into fixed rate bonds by either making use of the conversion feature or refunding the VRDB issue when it became necessary to spend the cash reserves, thereby remaining free of variable rate risk.

7. This capital plan would allow CHS to manage the debt markets rather than being forced to accept whatever fixed rates were available in the market when CHS needed capital in the future. This advantage was provided by the cash reserves and the ability to issue more VRDB debt in the future. Whenever the long-term market was not favorable, CHS would issue VRDBs to fund projects. When the long-term fixed rate market was favorable, CHS would convert some of the VRDBs to fixed rate bonds. There would be no need for CHS to be stuck with unfavorable long-term fixed interest rates again.

8. A final reason this plan was attractive was that Congress was revising the tax laws in 1985, and there was a threat that the new laws might prohibit the ability of 501(c)(3) (a form of private not-for-profit) healthcare organizations to use tax-exempt debt. The $100 million in cash reserves would provide CHS with a low-cost "war chest" that would allow it to continue to take advantage of business opportunities that might not be practical if they had to be funded with taxable debt or equity. This could prove to be a tremendous competitive advantage in the future.

As it turned out, the Tax Reform Act of 1986 did not prohibit CHS from continuing to issue tax-exempt debt. By the end of 1989, it had roughly $100 million of fixed rate bonds outstanding, $100 million of VRDBs outstanding, and $150 million in cash reserves. In late 1989, long-term rates were in the low 7 percent range, and CHS decided to convert about $65 million of its VRDBs to fixed rate status if it could be done at 7.5 percent or less. This was so that debt incurred during the next several years could be issued on a variable rate basis, and CHS could ignore unfavorable long-term interest rates when it needed capital.

The working group prepared for a conversion in January of 1990, and interest rates moved above 7.5 percent. CHS held firm to its threshold and waited until rates came back to 7.5 percent in August to convert its bonds. By using this approach, the overall cost of CHS capital was less than 8.0 percent on all its debt. (Some of the 1985 fixed rate debt remained outstanding, raising the average interest rate above 7.5 percent.) Had CHS issued fixed rate bonds each time it needed capital, the average cost on its debt would have been 100 to 150 basis points (1.0 percent to 1.5 percent) higher.

As the years went by, CHS took advantage of the tax-exempt markets as much as possible, and worked with its financial advisor to make use of the most appropriate investment banking firms for each different type of financing. It began making use of derivative products in 1992 to achieve a lower interest cost on its fixed rate financings. During 1992 and 1993 CHS advance refunded virtually all its outstanding fixed rate debt using derivative financing structures. This brought its average cost of capital to around 6.0 percent.

In evaluating the various derivative products to issue, CHS chose to use those that offered no additional risk, or those that offered only a slight risk that CHS felt was identifiable and reasonable. CHS did not issue any derivative products that it felt contained potential risks that were either unidentifiable or unacceptable. To this end, it made use of combined Dutch auction and inverse floater financings, as well as embedded swap products that contained swap periods of seven years or less. It did not make use of embedded swap bonds that use swaps of longer than 10 years. (These derivative products are explained in detail in Chapter 13.) As interest rates rose in 1994 and later, CHS again began to make more use of variable rate debt to keep its cost of capital as low as possible while continuing to build and invest its cash reserves, which offset the interest rate exposure on the variable rate debt.

When there was a need to develop medical office buildings (MOBs), CHS made use of a couple of alternative ways to finance them. In states that had pre-1986 tax-exempt pools with recycling provisions, CHS made use of the allowable "bad money" portions of the pools to finance MOBs. In other states, CHS used its cash reserves that had been built up by financing more eligible projects with tax-exempt bonds. CHS centralized the cash management for all its facilities and used these funds as a sort of bank to lend funds to any facilities that had projects that were not eligible for tax-exempt financing. These strategies allowed CHS to fund all its capital needs without the use of taxable debt, although taxable debt was used on occasion on a temporary basis.

During the 1990s, CHS entered into numerous merger and acquisition arrangements, and continues to mold itself to remain competitive in a changing healthcare environment. CHS continues to seek opportunities to finance projects with variable rate debt and to maintain and increase its own cash reserves. This strategy continues to increase CHS's overall profitability and provides levels of liquidity that continue to give it a very strong credit presentation in the markets. The significant liquidity that CHS was able to build, coupled with a strong profitability and willingness to adapt its operations and overall corporate structure to accommodate the changing environment, has made CHS a very strong healthcare provider, and maintained its ability to carry out its healthcare mission.

The CHS case is an example of a healthcare organization that has taken control of its capital base and taken advantage of the opportunities that exist in the debt markets. As a result, it has a lower cost of capital than many of its competitors and an extremely liquid balance sheet. This liquidity and strong operating performance have allowed it to retain its A1/A+ rating and to maintain a good reputation in the market, both of which will enhance its ability to obtain more capital from the debt markets in the future.

The experience of CHS demonstrates the benefits of strategic capital planning for a healthcare organization. Many terms and concepts were introduced in this chapter, most of which will be discussed in the chapters that follow.

4 Typical Characteristics of Healthcare Bonds

When representatives of a healthcare organization go to a bank to borrow money, they sign a note to evidence the obligation to repay the debt with interest. The note will detail the terms and conditions under which the debt obligation must be repaid. If the terms and conditions tend to be lengthy, they are often contained in a separate loan agreement. When an institution borrows from the "market," the document evidencing the obligation usually is some sort of bond. A bond form contains some detail on the relevant terms and conditions of the obligation, but the complete detail is contained in supporting documentation that typically is held by a bond trustee. The bond is what is held by the bondholder or depository as the primary evidence of the debt.

Another distinction of a bond versus a note from a bank or other lender is that bonds typically are drawn up before the actual lender is known. In other words, a bond issue usually is put together, and then the bonds are sold after the documentation is either fully completed or mostly completed. In some cases, the bonds are *publicly offered,* which means that they are offered to many potential purchasers. In other cases, bonds are sold in *private offerings,* in which case a limited number of potential bondholders are given the option to purchase the bonds. In the event that the bonds are being sold as a private placement, the purchaser(s) of the bonds is (are) frequently given the ability to make final comments on the documentation to customize the bonds—provided the borrower agrees. Purchasers of bonds in a public offering typically are not given the chance to comment on the bond documentation, other than in details that are finalized during pricing such as call provisions, interest rates, or the amount of original issue discount.

Bonds may be fixed rate or variable rate, long-term or short-term, secured or unsecured, or contain any of the characteristics described in previous chapters. Bonds may be either taxable or tax-exempt, meaning that the interest paid to a bondholder will be either taxable or tax-exempt to that bondholder. Every bond has a set maturity, and interest and principal are payable to the bondholder according to the terms spelled out in the bond documentation.

Bonds are usually *dated* as of a certain date. The *dated date* is most commonly the first day of a month, although it is not unusual to see bonds dated as of the 15th of a month. The dated date usually is a date prior to the closing date of the bond issue, and represents the date from which interest will accrue. On the day the bond issue is *closed,* all the documents have been (or will be) executed, and usually the borrower receives the bond proceeds and the purchaser of the bonds receives the bonds. The day on which bonds are released to the purchaser is referred to as the *delivery date* of the bonds. While it is most typical for the closing date and the delivery date to coincide, it is possible to close in escrow where the delivery of the bonds and the release of cash to the borrower happen after some period of time or after some event occurs.

On the day of closing, the purchasers of the bonds will pay what is called *accrued interest* in addition to the purchase price (par value less any original issue discount or plus any original issue premium) of the bonds. This is because the borrower will be required to pay interest according to the schedule on the bonds from, and including, the dated date on the bonds. The accrued interest represents the amount of interest that will be paid on the bonds from the dated date until the closing date. The net effect is that the purchaser of the bonds pays up the accrued interest at closing and then those funds are returned to the bondholder at the first interest payment date. In some types of bond issues, especially VRDB issues, it is common to have the bonds dated as of the date of closing so that the bondholder will not have to pay any accrued interest when the bonds are purchased.

■ Average Life

The *average life* of a bond issue is a weighted average of the period of time that the debt will be outstanding. This calculation takes into account the principal amount of each maturity as it becomes due. Because there is a large amount of principal outstanding in the early years of a bond issue with level debt service and a small amount of principal outstanding in the last few years, the average life of a bond issue set up with level debt service is usually a little more than half of the actual life. For example, the average life of a 30-year bond issue with level debt service typically will be in the range of 17 to 19 years. If the principal amortization of a bond issue is weighted more heavily in the later years, the average life lengthens. Similarly, if the amortization is weighted more in the early years, the average life of the issue is reduced. The average life of a bond issue can be calculated either from the delivery date, which is the date that the borrower delivers the bonds and receives the cash (usually the day of closing), or it may be calculated from the dated date of the bonds, which is usually earlier than the closing date.

■ Calculating Interest Cost

There are several different ways that the interest cost on a bond issue can be calculated. Some of them take into account more factors that affect the actual yield paid by the borrower than others. It is important that the same methodology in calculating interest cost be used when comparing the cost of different bond issues. Otherwise, the result is an apples-to-oranges comparison.

Average Coupon

The term "coupon" stems from the days when the majority of bonds were issued in the form of *bearer bonds,* meaning the bonds were not registered and could be cashed in by whomever presented them at the appropriate time and place. Bearer bonds had a series of coupons that were printed as part of the bonds themselves, and represented the interest payments to be made on the bonds. The coupons were "clipped" and cashed in for interest payments when they were due. Because the interest payments on any bond are determined by the interest rate or formula agreed upon when they are sold, each interest coupon reflected the interest rate that would be paid on the par amount of its bond. The term "coupon" has stuck even though bearer bonds are no longer allowed for tax-exempt bond issues. They must now be *registered,* which means that the trustee keeps a record of the owners of all the bonds, and sends interest payments to the registered owners when they are paid. Registered bonds do not actually have coupons, but it is common to refer to the stated interest rate on a bond as its *coupon* even if it is registered.

In a fixed rate bond issue, it is normal for the issue to contain serial maturities of bonds and term bonds. Each maturity of the serial bonds will mature on a different date, and will be sold at a different interest rate, or coupon. The *average coupon* of a bond issue is a weighted average of all the stated interest rates (coupons) of the various maturities in the bond issue. It represents the average of all the various interest rates paid by the borrower, and is determined by dividing the interest amount paid over the entire life of the bond issue by the total number of bond years. *Bond years* are computed by multiplying the principal amount of a maturity by the number of years until it matures. The average coupon calculation does not take into account the actual yields on the bonds at the time of the initial offering because it does not take into account any original issue discount or premium, which determines the actual purchase price for the bonds. The average coupon is strictly a weighted average of the coupon rates on all of the outstanding bonds.

Net Interest Cost

The *net interest cost (NIC)* of a bond issue is a more accurate calculation of the average interest cost for a borrower because it takes into account the underwriter's discount and any original issue discount or premium when it is calculated. The NIC equals the total amount of interest that will be paid on the bond issue, plus the bond discount (fee) paid to the underwriter, plus any original issue discount, less any premium, all divided by the number of bond years.

True Interest Cost

The calculation of the *true interest cost (TIC)* of a bond issue is similar to the calculation of the NIC, but is slightly more accurate in describing the true yield of the issue because it also accounts for any credit enhancement fee as well as the time value of money. The TIC is the present value of a bond issue's stream of payments (both principal and interest) discounted to the net amount received by the borrower at the time the bonds are issued.

Arbitrage Yield

The *arbitrage yield* is the maximum yield at which the proceeds of a tax-exempt bond issue may be invested, in most cases, without conflicting with the arbitrage provisions in the tax law. This calculation is sometimes referred to as the *bond yield* or the *gross yield*. The calculation for the arbitrage yield is similar to that of the TIC, except that it excludes the underwriter's discount, thereby making it slightly lower. Current tax law requires that bonds issued under a common plan of finance and within a fairly narrow time frame all be blended together for this calculation. It also requires, in most cases, that any earnings on the majority of bond proceeds be rebated to the U.S. Treasury to the extent that they exceed this yield.

All-In True Interest Cost

The *all-in true interest cost* is similar to the TIC, but is even more accurate in that it also takes into account all the borrower's costs of issuance when it is calculated.

∎ Call Features

When a borrower retains the ability to pay off a debt prior to maturity, that debt is said to be *callable*. Most bank debt is callable at any time, but most fixed rate bonds have some restrictions on the ability of the borrower to call them. Most variable rate bond issues are callable at any time, upon notice to the trustee of 30 days or less, because the bond-holder is receiving a short-term rate and is treating the bond like a short-term security.

There are two basic types of call provisions commonly contained in healthcare bond issues. The first is an *optional call* provision that allows the borrower to prepay bonds at its discretion alone. The second type is referred to as an *extraordinary call* provision, which allows the borrower the option of paying off the bonds prior to maturity under certain extraordinary circumstances. Extraordinary calls are generally allowed on healthcare bonds if there has been a significant amount of damage to the facility of the borrower and the borrower elects not to repair the facility with insurance proceeds. Many bonds issued by Catholic health organizations contain what is referred to as the *Catholic call,* which is an extraordinary call feature that gives the borrower the right to pay off the bonds if any change in law or government regulations requires the institution to perform certain procedures that are contrary to the Catholic faith.

In a typical long-term, tax-exempt, fixed rate bond issue, the term bonds will not be callable solely at the option of the borrower for roughly 10 years. It is then common for these bond issues to include a *premium* (prepayment fee) at the first call date that reduces in subsequent years until the bonds can be called at par (face value). For example, the most common format seen in tax-exempt healthcare bond issues is for any term bonds with maturities of 20 to 30 years to be non-callable by the borrower for a period of 10 years, other than under any extraordinary call provisions. It is common for a premium equal to 2 percent of the face amount of the bond to be paid to the bondholder if the bonds are called anytime during the 11th year. This would typically be followed by a premium of 1 percent if the bonds are called in the 12th year, and the bonds can be called at par thereafter.

While this format reflects the typical standard in the current markets, some long-term bond issues are sold that are callable after year five, generally at some premium higher than 2 percent. As with the 10-year call, the premium will reduce over several years until the bonds can be called at par. Bonds that are callable in less than 10 years typically are sold in the retail market, as institutional buyers currently tend to insist upon the 10-year call protection. Bonds that mature in less than 10 years typically are non-callable, but occasionally may contain optional call provisions as well, with a scale of declining premiums similar to the longer term bonds.

The ability to call bonds prior to maturity solely at the option of the borrower is considered to be a benefit to the borrower, and a detriment to the bondholder. Because of this, including optional call provisions in the bond issue generally results in a higher interest rate than if the bonds are not callable at all. For example, if a typical healthcare bond issue could be sold with a 30-year maturity at 7.0 percent, with the customary optional call provisions of 102 percent after year 10, that same bond issue might be able to be sold at 6.95 percent if there were no option to call the bonds. Likewise, that same bond issue might sell at an interest rate of 7.10 percent if there were provisions included that allowed the bonds to be called at the option of the borrower after year five at 105 percent. There may be certain situations where a healthcare institution chooses to take advantage of a lower interest rate by eliminating optional call provisions in its bond issue. These considerations should be evaluated very carefully by the borrower and its financial advisor to determine the advisability of deviating from the standard call provisions that the market is accustomed to seeing.

While it is customary for optional call provisions to be set up so that the bonds are redeemed when they are called, it may be advisable to structure optional call provisions where the borrower is not required to redeem the bonds, and retains the right to remarket the bonds. The bonds would be callable according to the normal optional call schedule, but they would remain outstanding and would be resold at current market rates to new purchasers. This structure is not common, but it could prove to be valuable to the borrower if the ability to issue tax-exempt debt is ever lost.

For example, assume a borrower issued fixed rate tax-exempt bonds 10 years ago, at an average coupon of 10.0 percent. The bonds are now callable at 102 percent. If the current interest rate at which the bonds could now be refunded is 7.0 percent, the borrower could call the bonds, pay the 2 percent premium, and resell the bonds at a large enough premium for them to yield 7.0 percent to the new bondholders. The result to the borrower is the same as if the bonds had been current refunded at 7.0 percent, but no new bonds were issued. This option may have questionable value as long as tax-exempt bonds can be issued to implement current refundings of other tax-exempt bonds, but could preserve the borrower's ability to enjoy the benefit of a current refunding even if new tax-exempt bonds cannot be issued.

Detachable Call Options

Another interesting variation on optional call provisions is to structure the options so that the borrower has the ability to sell them if it ever chooses to give up the right to exercise them. This structure is referred to as *detachable call options.*

Under normal optional call provisions, the borrower is the only party that can call the bonds. This limits the usefulness of the options to the situation where the borrower wants to pay off or refund the debt. If the borrower decides that it will never exercise the option to call the bonds, there is no way to earn back the added cost (in terms of higher interest rates) of including the optional call provisions in the bond issue when the bonds were issued rather than issuing non-callable bonds.

Detachable call options can give the borrower some added flexibility—in concept at least. Rather than never making use of the call options, the borrower has at least two additional courses of action. First, the borrower could sell the options to the bondholders, thereby making the bonds non-callable. The price for the options would depend on the current interest rate environment relative to the one that existed when the bonds were originally sold. Any remaining call protection also would affect the price. For example, the call options would be worth more if current interest rates were significantly lower than the coupon rates on the bonds and the call protection period (10 years) was coming to an end.

Alternatively, in a lower interest rate environment, the borrower could sell the call options to another party who wants to own the bonds. The price for the options should reflect the current lower interest rates and would be comparable to the savings that the borrower could receive by implementing a current refunding of the bonds (i.e., issuing new bonds at the current lower interest rates to pay off the old bonds).

A number of bond issues have included language to allow detachable call options, but an opinion from bond counsel is required at the time the option to sell is exercised. The viability of using this feature will be dependent on the tax laws at the time it is exercised, and the Internal Revenue Service has issued some rulings that have limited their use. As a result, no one can guaranty that detachable call options will provide any significant benefit to a borrower in the future, but they may be worth investigating.

∎ Price Volatility

When a bond is issued at par, the purchaser of the bond pays the face value of the bond and receives interest paid at the coupon rate designated on the bond. For example, if a bond has a face value of $5,000, and pays an interest rate of 5.0 percent, the purchaser would pay $5,000 for the bond and would receive $250 per year in interest until the bond matures and the principal is repaid. On a fixed rate bond, the coupon is fixed for the life of the bond. In this example, the coupon rate is 5.0 percent, which actually means that the bondholder will receive $250 per year in interest regardless of the price paid for the bond. The coupon rate on a bond equals the return that a bondholder will receive only if the bondholder pays the face amount (par value) for the bond. The actual return to the bondholder will be determined by the price paid for the bond.

To continue the example, assume that the interest rate demanded for bonds similar to the one being held by a bondholder has now increased to 10.0 percent. Since the annual payment of $250 is fixed on the bond, the value of the bond will have reduced to the neighborhood of $2,500, because $250 per annum represents a 10.0 percent return on $2,500. This example negates the effect of principal on the price of the bond, and the actual volatility of the bond would not be this great, but it demonstrates why the price of a fixed rate bond does vary with changes in market interest rates. Likewise, if the market for similar bonds reduces to 2.5 percent, the value of this bond would almost double, and it might be sold for roughly $10,000.

The longer the maturity of the bond, the more the volatility in its price because the less effect the actual repayment of principal will have is relative to the stream of interest payments. For this reason, the values of shorter term bonds are less volatile than those of longer term bonds, and they generally are deemed to be more conservative investments.

▮ Original Issue Discount

When bonds are offered at a price below face value (par) at the time of issuance, they are said to contain an *original issue discount (OID)*. An OID can range from a very small amount, such as .25 percent, to a deep discount of 5 percent to 50 percent or more. The bonds with the greatest OID are zero coupon bonds, where no interest is paid until the final maturity. Original issue discount bonds are sought by many institutional investors. On a typical long-term fixed rate healthcare financing, institutional investors might be willing to buy the term bonds at a yield that is 10 to 20 basis points (.10 percent to .20 percent) lower if an OID is offered, compared to term bonds offered at par. An OID usually has little effect on the retail market.

A disadvantage to the borrower of bonds issued with an OID is that the yield paid on the bonds will be greater if the bonds are called prior to maturity, because they will be paid off at par or at a premium. The borrower only gets the benefit of the lower coupon for the number of years until the bonds are called, rather than until the final maturity. Because of this, the likelihood of a call prior to maturity should be evaluated before a healthcare organization decides to use a significant OID on its bonds. Similarly, a healthcare organization should determine whether its bonds are likely to be sold in the retail market or the institutional market, for an OID typically will not help lower interest rates as much in a retail offering.

▮ Zero Coupon Bonds

Zero coupon bonds are fixed rate debt instruments on which no interest payments are made until the final maturity of the bonds. The interest that normally would be paid on a conventional bond continues to accrue interest at the stated rate on the bond. The interest is compounded periodically as though it had been paid out like a conventional bond and reinvested at the same interest rate. At maturity, the entire amount of principal and accrued interest is paid. The face amount on these bonds reflects the total amount that will be due at maturity. As a result, these bonds are issued at a very large discount, which represents the present value of the stream of interest payments that will not be received until maturity. As time passes, the amount of interest that is earned is added to the original price of the bonds to determine the accreted value of the bonds. The *accreted value* is the value that is used as the principal amount in the event the bonds are called or sold to someone else.

Zero coupon bonds are sometimes referred to as *zeroes* and are also sometimes referred to as *capital appreciation bonds (CABs)*. The value of zero coupon bonds tends to be more than twice as volatile relative to changes in interest rates as the value of conventional coupon bonds. This volatility is due to the fact that the reinvestment of interest is locked into the same interest rate as the principal on the bonds. With current coupon bonds, the bondholder is locked into the return received on the principal amount of the bonds, but is able to reinvest any interest payment in the current market when it is received. Zeroes take away the ability to reinvest interest payments in the current market and this accounts for their greater price volatility—the longer the term to maturity, the greater the volatility.

The interest rates on zero coupon bonds tend to be higher than those on current coupon bonds issued in the same market, although there are times when there will be no premium over conventional bonds. This premium might be as much as 100 basis points (1.0 percent) in some markets, and may disappear entirely in markets where the zero coupon bonds are in high demand. However, this cost to the borrower frequently can be more than offset by allowing more principal to be paid in early years, resulting in more serial bonds. The interest savings to the borrower derived by issuing more serial bonds frequently exceeds any higher interest cost of zeroes. Zero coupon bonds tend to be most attractive to the market during periods of falling interest rates and when the yield curve is steeper. As a result, they are not always an attractive alternative for a borrower, although they should be considered during the development of any capital plan.

Because the attraction of zeroes for the bondholder is the ability to lock in the reinvestment rate of all semiannual interest payments for the life of the bonds, many issues of zeroes are noncallable. The borrower does not maintain the right to call the bonds prior to maturity solely at its option. While this makes an issue of zeroes more attractive to the market, it could prove to be disadvantageous to the borrower if rates drop during the life of the bonds or there is a desire to refund the bonds for some other reason. It should be possible to include optional call provisions in a zero coupon bond issue if there is sufficient demand for the bonds.

▮ Book Entry

Until a few years ago, bonds were issued in certificate form and delivered to the buyer or the buyer's custodian. Now, most bond issues are done in *book entry* form, where a single bond is delivered to a depository company that keeps track of the beneficial holders of the bonds (i.e., the purchasers) and issues receipts to them to confirm their holdings. Book entry streamlines the process of transferring bonds between beneficial holders when they are sold in the secondary market because no bonds actually are transferred, only the beneficial interest in the bonds. As a result, there is no need for the trustee to issue new certificates because the depository continues to be the actual bondholder.

Some individuals still like to hold a bond certificate rather than a receipt and may avoid book entry offerings, but as more and more issues are done this way, fewer and fewer bonds actually are held by the public. Because it is simpler and less expensive for the borrower, book entry is the trend of the future. Individuals can still purchase the bonds, but they cannot physically hold a bond certificate. Virtually all derivative bond issues use the book entry procedure.

5 The Process of Issuing Tax-Exempt Debt: An Overview

Once a healthcare institution and its financial advisor have developed a capital plan and have determined the amount of tax-exempt financing they will need, the process of issuing that debt begins. Details of each major step in the process will be covered in significant detail in later chapters.

The capital plan should have determined the amount of debt to be incurred, and the nature of the bonds to be issued, i.e., long-term versus short-term, fixed rate versus variable rate, conventional versus derivatives, etc. In addition, the capital plan should recommend whether the bonds will be offered through a competitive sale method or a negotiated sale method (this topic is discussed in Chapter 8), and whether the offering should be public or private in the event the negotiated sale method will be used.

∎ Public Offering versus Private Placement

A key decision to be made when putting together a bond issue is whether to sell the bonds through a public offering or a private placement. In a *public offering,* the minimum denomination of a tax-exempt fixed rate healthcare bond is typically $5,000, and the bonds are offered to both the *retail market* (consisting of individuals) and the *institutional market* (consisting of large, "sophisticated" investors such as banks, insurance companies, bond mutual funds, and sometimes very wealthy individuals). A *private placement,* or *institutional offering,* is implemented when bonds are offered to a limited number of sophisticated potential buyers, as defined in the securities laws, and the minimum denomination frequently is $100,000 or more. Bonds are not offered to the retail market, which consists of the general public.

The lowest interest rates usually are obtained in a public offering because more buyers are competing for the bonds. However, in a public offering, securities law requires more extensive disclosure about the borrower than is required in a private placement. Another potential drawback to a public offering is that there usually will end up being many bondholders, so the likelihood of obtaining bondholder consent for a future amendment to the bond documents is greatly reduced. A private placement often allows a closer working relationship between the borrower and the lenders, and the lenders frequently have some input as to the final structure of the deal. With a limited number of lenders, a healthcare institution may have a greater ability to amend its documents in the future if the need arises.

❚ Selecting the Working Group

The first step in actually implementing the financing is selecting the remainder of the financing team. It is preferable for the financial advisor to be selected prior to the development of the capital plan, and to be instrumental in the development of that plan. If a financial advisor was not used to develop the capital plan, then this should be the first member of the financing team to be selected, since one of the key roles of the financial advisor is the coordination of the financing team. The financial advisor should review the capital plan and then assist in the process of selecting the remaining members of the working group that will best be able to execute the capital plan. Some conduit issuers of tax-exempt debt require input as to the selection of certain members of the financing team, so this should be a consideration in the selection of an issuer if more than one entity is able to serve as issuer. Once the financial advisor and issuer have been retained, the remaining members of the team can be selected. The members of the financing team and their respective roles are discussed in Chapter 6.

∎ Working Group Meetings

Once the financing team has been assembled, an *organizational meeting* is scheduled to bring each member of the team up to speed on the financing plan. During that meeting, the hospital administrators and financial advisor should explain the nature of the project, the types of bonds they expect to be issued, and the time frame under which they expect all the necessary requirements to be fulfilled for the issuance of the bonds. By the end of the organizational meeting each member of the financing team should have a good understanding of their marching orders.

During this meeting, the borrower and its financial advisor should be prepared to provide the group with information on any relevant topics, including the following:

The Borrower

- What is the identity of the borrower?
- What is the legal organizational structure of the borrower and its related affiliates?
- Will a master trust indenture be used?
- Will there be an obligated group or a single borrower?

The Issuer

- Who will issue the bonds?
- What is the process required by the issuer (e.g., number of meetings, timing requirements, uncommon policies, etc.)?

The Project

- Will the project consist of new money (i.e., financing a project that has not been financed in the past), refunding, reimbursement, or a combination of these?

- What is the description and cost of any new money project, or any project from which the proceeds of any debt to be refunded were used (e.g., construction, renovation, equipment, etc.)?

- What will be the total amount financed?

- Is any portion of the project not eligible for tax-exempt financing?

- Is a certificate of need required?

- What is the description of all approvals required and the process for obtaining them?

Structure of the Financing

- Will it be fixed rate or variable rate?

- Will the bond offering be competitive or negotiated?

- What is the anticipated security for the bonds?

- Will there be credit enhancement?

- Will the issue be rated?

- Will a debt service reserve fund be included?

- What will be the term (final maturity) of the bonds?

- What will be the amortization of the bonds?

- What types of bonds will be offered (conventional, derivatives, etc.)?

- Is the financing *interest rate sensitive,* i.e., if interest rates go up by 100 or 200 basis points, is the borrower prepared to proceed with the financing?

During the organizational meeting, a preliminary distribution list should be passed around the table and additional information and corrections for a master distribution list obtained from all parties. The distribution list will contain address, telephone, and fax information on each person who is to receive any documents, and should be prepared and distributed to the working group by the financial advisor or underwriter shortly after this meeting. A schedule for the financing should be agreed upon at the organizational meeting, providing for two or three drafting sessions, due diligence meetings, meetings with rating agencies and/or bond insurers, specific meeting dates of the conduit issuer, a mailing date for the preliminary official statement, the pricing date, closing dates, and any other items that are necessary for the issuance of the bonds.

Prior to the first drafting session for the documents, bond counsel prepares and distributes a first draft of the necessary bond documents. This usually includes a bond trust indenture and a loan agreement (or their equivalents) as a minimum. Prior to any drafting session, each member of the team should have reviewed the documents distributed by various counsel so that comments on the documents can be given at the meeting. Prior to the second drafting session, underwriter's counsel should have prepared a first draft of the preliminary official statement.

■ The Official Statement

An *official statement* (generally referred to as an *OS*) is the offering document of which the purpose is to disclose all relevant information about the bonds and the borrower to prospective purchasers of the bonds in a publicly sold tax-exempt bond issue. A *preliminary official statement* (generally referred to as a *POS*) is prepared prior to the sale of the bonds and should contain all the final information except for those details that will not be known until the bonds have been sold—such as the final interest rates, the final size of the issue, and the amounts of bonds that will mature each year. The POS is sometimes referred to as a "red herring" because it displays a cover statement printed in red ink along the left margin and top warning that the document is not a final OS.

Both the OS and the POS contain complete disclosure of relevant information on the bonds, the borrower, any credit enhancement, the issuer, potential risks to bondholders, and any other information that the working group feels is relevant to the potential purchaser of the bonds. A legal opinion from one or more of the counsel in the working group is required before the bonds are issued, to the effect that all relevant information has been included in the OS and that none of the information is misleading. The bonds are sold based on the information in the POS, and the final OS must be delivered to each purchaser prior to, or at the time the bonds are delivered.

Traditionally, a borrower and its financial advisor determined the type of bond to be issued in the early stages of the financing process, and the characteristics of that bond are then described in the POS to be distributed to the market. However, the advent of derivative products has changed the way bonds are described in the POS in many issues. Because different derivative products offer different benefits to potential bondholders, certain derivative financings will be more attractive to the market than others, given market conditions on any day. Because of the uncertainty as to which structure will be most attractive on a given day, it has become customary to offer more than one derivative structure when bonds go to market. As a result, many POSs now use more of a smorgasbord approach in describing the bonds that are to be issued. In this approach, brief descriptions of each of several different derivative type financings that are to be offered to the market are included in the POS. In many cases, a half dozen or more different types of bonds are described.

On the date of pricing, the market will determine which of these different derivative financing structures are most desirable by offering lower interest rates on those bonds that are most attractive to them. The borrower, financial advisor, and underwriter then determine which mix of different bonds to sell. The final OS will then describe only those bonds that actually are issued. The POS describes all the different structures that are offered, while the final OS describes only those bonds that are actually sold. This strategy allows the borrower to make sure a product that is attractive to the market is offered on the day its bonds are sold. The old approach, where the exact structure of the bonds is determined early in the process, limits the borrower in such a way that it might not be able to offer the types of bonds that are most attractive to the market on the day its bonds are sold.

▮ The Trust Indenture

A *trust indenture, bond resolution,* or some similar document is the document used to instruct the trustee on the terms, conditions, and procedures to be followed on a bond financing. It describes the security for the bonds and most of the covenants that the trustee is expected to monitor. There may be other documents that contain additional legal covenants—or actually grant any security interest to the trustee—but the trust indenture essentially is an instruction manual for the trustee on how to oversee the bond issue. A standard trust indenture is designed to govern an issue of bonds and sometimes additional issues of bonds that share in all the rights granted to bondholders under the indenture. A *master trust indenture* is a document that contains covenants and security like a trust indenture, but is designed to govern multiple obligations or bond issues.

Any obligation issued pursuant to a master trust indenture shares a parity (equal) interest in whatever security and covenants are contained in the master trust indenture. This becomes particularly helpful when a healthcare organization wishes to incur debt from several different sources. For example, it may issue bonds through a tax-exempt issuer, then wish to obtain a bank loan at a later date, and might also wish to participate in some other financing program from another issuer. Each of these lenders can receive a parity security interest each time debt is issued by securing their notes with an obligation issued under the borrower's master trust indenture, without modifying the underlying documents that grant the security to the master trust indenture.

A master trust indenture often includes an obligated group structure to combine the credit of several entities. The *obligated group* structure works like a set of cross-guarantees so that each member of the group is obligated to pay on any debt issued by any member of the group if that debt is secured by a master note. This has become desirable for many healthcare organizations since the trend began in the early 1980s to reorganize into multi-corporate organizations. Some healthcare organizations found that they had reorganized to the point that the credit quality of the remaining healthcare corporation itself was no longer sufficient to obtain attractive financing. The use of an obligated group allows a multi-corporate organizational structure while preserving the ability to present a unified credit to the financial markets.

▌ Obtaining Necessary Approvals

Unless a healthcare institution is owned by a governmental body, it will require the use of a conduit issuer to make its bonds tax-exempt. Each issuing body has its own system and approval process. It is important for the borrower to investigate this process early on, so the schedule for the financing can be worked around the schedule of the issuing body.

In addition to the issuer, approvals may be necessary from local planning and zoning departments. Some states also require a certificate of need for certain projects, which can require a lengthy process to obtain. Bond counsel typically will require all necessary approvals to be in place by the time the bonds are issued, or at least to have evidence that the necessary approvals will be forthcoming.

▮ Obtaining Bond Ratings or Credit Enhancement

During the development of the capital plan, the decision should be made as to whether the upcoming bond issue will be rated based on the credit of the borrower, or if credit enhancement will be sought. Many of the derivative product bonds that are offered to finance healthcare institutions require a AA/Aa rating or better to sell the bonds. Since there are very few healthcare organizations rated AA/Aa or better, this means that most institutions will need to obtain either bond insurance, a letter of credit, or some other form of credit enhancement if they are to make use of derivative products. Conventional bonds, on the other hand, can be issued either with or without credit enhancement. Many institutions decide to "dual track" their bond issues by proceeding to obtain ratings and credit enhancement at the same time. This option allows the borrower to wait until the last minute to make the decision as to which alternative is most economical.

The first step in obtaining bond ratings or credit enhancement is to prepare a package of information and pertinent materials to send to the rating agencies, bond insurers, and/or letter-of-credit providers. If a rating is being sought, meetings with the various rating agencies should be scheduled, either at their offices or at the facility of the borrower. Presentations to the rating agencies typically involve a more formal presentation than what is required by bond insurers or letter-of-credit providers. The materials should be sent to the agencies at least one week prior to any meeting, and final approval is not likely to be received until one or two weeks after the meetings. Ratings are discussed in Chapter 9, and credit enhancement in Chapter 10.

▮ Selling the Bonds in a Negotiated Offering

When the working team has determined that the financing documents are in final form, all necessary approvals have been received, ratings and/or credit enhancement are in place, and the POS is in final form, the borrower is ready to enter the market to sell bonds. The POS typically will contain financial information on the borrower. This information can become stale if an extended period of time goes by before the bonds are sold. Usually the market requires financial information current to within 90 days from the time bonds are sold, and within 120 days from the time the bond issue closes. There may be some flexibility on this timing, but it makes sense to include the most current financial information available in the POS so as to build some leeway into the time frame within which the bonds must be sold.

In a negotiated offering, the POS typically will be distributed to prospective bondholders roughly one week before the bonds are expected to be offered for sale. There are certain situations where the underwriter will be comfortable offering bonds for sale when the POS has been in the hands of prospective bondholders for as little as a day, and sometimes the underwriter wants the bondholders to review the information for two or more weeks. The actual timing is determined by several factors, such as expectations for market movements in the near future, the complexity of the issue, and the need to tell a story about either the bonds or the underlying credit. Bonds that have some unusual characteristics or are issued by a credit that requires a special sales effort are referred to as "story bonds" by the underwriters. Conventional bonds issued by a strong credit that is well known to the market will require a relatively short period of time for the POS to be in the hands of bondholders before they can be sold effectively. Conversely, a bond issue for a difficult credit that is new to the market (i.e., story bonds) may require the underwriter to provide additional information besides what is contained in the POS to prospective bondholders before they are willing to purchase the bonds, thereby requiring the POS to be distributed earlier.

Once the POS has been distributed and held by prospective bondholders for the desired amount of time, and the market appears to be in a favorable condition for the sale of bonds, the bonds will be priced.

Pricing bonds is the process of negotiating interest rates at which the borrower is willing to sell and the underwriter is willing to buy. It generally is advisable to schedule a preliminary pricing call on the afternoon prior to the day the bonds actually are priced. This call should include the borrower, the borrower's financial advisor, and the underwriters. The purposes of this call are for the underwriters and the financial advisor to discuss the current market conditions and the conditions expected for the following day, to agree upon a scale of interest rates for the bonds, and to develop a marketing strategy for the bonds.

The *scale* of interest rates is a listing of the interest rates (coupon rates) and prices for each maturity of the bonds. The price and the coupon rate determine the yield at which the bonds in each maturity will be issued. The shorter the maturity, the lower the yield in most market situations. The scale typically will contain interest rates for maturities in each year from one to 10 (sometimes out to year 15), and then one or two term bonds in the later maturities.

The bonds may be offered with, or without, original issue discount, and any other aspects of marketing strategy should be discussed during this telephone call. In most cases, the parties participating in that call will agree upon a scale of interest rates so the underwriter can offer the bonds for sale first thing the following morning without the need to contact the borrower and its financial advisor. In the event there is any change in the market and the underwriter determines there needs to be some revision in the scale of interest rates, another call would be placed the morning of pricing. Most underwriters will not offer to underwrite (purchase) the bonds unless they have obtained verbal orders from their customers for almost all the bonds at the designated scale of interest rates. Figure 2-2 shows an example of an interest rate scale for a long-term, tax-exempt healthcare bond issue.

On the day of pricing, the underwriter will broadcast the proposed scale of interest rates to the market on the various wire services. The scale is set at levels that are expected to result in offers to purchase the amount of bonds that are offered. If interest rates are set too high, the bonds are likely to be *oversubscribed*. This means the underwriter receives orders for more bonds than they have to sell in a given maturity. Conversely, if interest rates on the scale are set too low, sufficient orders for the bonds will not be received.

The inverse relationship of price to yield can cause some confusion when the pricing of bonds is discussed with underwriters. The underwriters usually are the initial purchasers of the bonds. Their interests are opposed to the borrower in that they will always prefer a higher yield on the bonds while the borrower will always prefer a lower yield. When underwriters refer to bonds as being "cheap," they mean that the yield is relatively high for the current market and the price is, therefore, relatively low. Conversely, when they refer to the bonds as "rich," they mean that the yields are relatively low for the current market, and the price is relatively high. Therefore, when the bond market is *up,* it means that prices on outstanding bonds have risen and interest rates have lowered. When the market is *down,* prices on outstanding bonds have declined and interest rates (yields) have risen. Since they are selling the bonds, borrowers prefer the market to be up and their bonds to be sold rich.

When the scale is broadcast over the wire services, an *order period* is established within which time all orders must be received by the lead underwriter. Usually, it will run from the morning of the pricing until early afternoon. If enough orders for the bonds have not been received by the end of the order period, the borrower either must raise the yields on the bonds and again attempt to sell them, or pull the issue from the market. When an issue has entered the market and the market has not been receptive due to the interest scale being too "aggressive" (low), it usually takes a fairly good bump in yield to get the market to seriously reconsider purchasing the bonds. In other words, it usually is not sufficient to raise the yields on the scale by only five basis points (.05 percent) or so. In many cases, it will take increasing the rates anywhere from 10 to 25 basis points for the market to regain interest in the issue. Because of this, it generally is advisable to enter the market with an interest rate scale at which the underwriter and financial advisor are fairly comfortable that sufficient orders will be received to sell the bonds. If the bond issue is oversubscribed, it is fairly easy to reduce the interest scale and then verify which orders will hold at the new scale. In other words, it generally is more effective to set the interest scale a little too high and then reduce it than it is to set the interest rate scale too low and then have to increase it. For example, if a particular maturity of a bond issue is offered to the market at 7.00 percent, and sufficient orders to sell the bonds are not received, it might be necessary to increase the yield on that bond to 7.10 percent or even 7.25 percent in order to sell it. Conversely, if the market is at 7.05 percent, the bonds could be offered at 7.10 percent or 7.15 percent and then reduced to 7.05 percent if the bonds are oversubscribed. Obviously, the ideal situation is to offer the bonds at 7.05 percent in the first place.

Some underwriters offer to have representatives from the borrowing institution come to their offices during the pricing session. This practice is of questionable value to a borrower because it may tend to reduce the objectivity of the borrower if a situation arises where it is necessary to push the underwriter to perform. It can be extremely difficult for the borrower's financial advisor to persuade the borrower to take a strong position against the underwriter relative to the pricing of the bonds when the representatives of the borrower are being wined and dined by the underwriters on their own turf. On the other hand, there can be some situations where it is beneficial to have representatives from the borrower at the underwriter's office, especially in cases where prospective bondholders are expected to ask a significant number of questions during the pricing. It can be quite expeditious to have representatives of the borrower on hand to respond immediately to such questions. Borrowers should evaluate the potential benefits and pitfalls of visiting the offices of their senior underwriters during the pricing of their bonds.

During the initial pricing call, a follow-up pricing call should be scheduled for shortly after the end of the order period. On this call, the underwriter will explain to the borrower and its financial advisor the results of the sales effort during the order period. The ideal situation is for the underwriter to have orders for roughly 75 to 90 percent of the bonds. This means the interest rate scale was not so high that the bonds were oversubscribed, but high enough so the majority of the bonds were sold. If a sufficient number of the bonds have been sold, the underwriter should agree to underwrite the remaining portion of the bond issue at the interest scale that was proposed. If sufficient orders were not obtained, the underwriter still might offer to underwrite all the bonds, but at a slightly higher interest scale than was initially proposed. The borrower's financial advisor should have conducted research throughout the day to develop an educated opinion as to whether or not a change in the interest scale is appropriate. The only options open to the borrower at this point are either to agree to sell the bonds at the underwriter's offer, or to pull the issue from the market and try to sell the bonds on another day.

Pulling a bond issue from the market is not done very often. When it is done, the bonds usually are not put back into the market the next day, but in a week or two following the initial sales attempt. This is to avoid the situation where prospective bondholders lose interest in the issue because they rejected it only a day earlier. During a delay of a week or two, there is a fair likelihood that the market will change, in which case the borrower may lose a significant amount in terms of interest cost if interest rates rise, and actually may save money if interest rates fall. The amount of interest expense either saved or lost during this period may well exceed the disputed amount that prevented the borrower from agreeing to the initial sale in the first place. In a successful pricing, the borrower will have determined that interest rates are at an acceptable level, and the bonds will be priced in such a fashion that the underwriter will agree to underwrite the bonds at the end of the order period.

Bond issues are usually priced on either Tuesday, Wednesday, or Thursday of any given week. The rationale for this is that Monday is used to ascertain whether or not there has been a shift in the market over the weekend. If there is a need to price the bonds on a Monday, the order period would normally not begin until afternoon for this reason as well. In situations where pricings begin in the afternoon, the order period often will flow over to the next morning.

Once the terms of the pricing have been agreed upon, a verbal award is made, and a purchase contract is prepared. The *purchase contract* is the binding written contract that details the terms and conditions under which the borrower agrees to sell, and the underwriter, or other purchaser, agrees to purchase the bonds. The purchase contract normally is executed a day or two after the verbal award is made, due to the number of specific details that have to be finalized. Bond issues rarely are priced on Fridays because underwriters are hesitant to hold a bond issue over a weekend on a verbal award alone.

∎ Closing the Bond Issue

Once the purchase contract has been signed, and all approvals obtained by the borrower and issuer, the lawyers finalize all the documents for *closing* when, under normal circumstances, the money from the proceeds of the bond issue is received by the borrower's trustee and the bonds are released for distribution. At closing, the legal counsel responsible for the disclosure will be asked to give an opinion that everything in the final OS is true and correct, and no relevant information that should have been included was omitted. Frequently, different legal counsel representing different parties will opine to the sections of the official statement that are relevant to their respective clients. Before the bond issue closes, all sections of the official statement will be covered by one or more legal opinions confirming the adequacy of disclosure.

The actual closing of a bond issue usually is a two-day process, and sometimes longer than that. The day prior to the actual closing is usually referred to as the *pre-closing*, and most documents are finalized and executed on that day. In a well-executed closing, all the documents will be signed and executed on the day of the pre-closing, except perhaps for the cross-receipts, which evidence receipt of the actual funds and the bonds. In this situation, the underwriter will initiate wire transfers for the bond proceeds first thing in the morning on the day of the closing. When everyone assembles for the closing, all that is necessary is for the trustee to verify that the funds have arrived. At that point, the bond issue is closed and the bonds are released to the underwriters. In many situations, however, many of the documents are not finalized until the day of closing. This can cause some excitement, especially in situations where the bonds are going to be issued in book-entry fashion. This is because the depository companies that hold the bonds have cut-off times by which the issue must close, or else they will not accept bonds until the next day. Currently, the cut-off time used by most of these institutions is 1 p.m. Eastern time (although they have been known to accept bonds as late as 1:15 p.m.)

These are brief descriptions of the steps typically involved in issuing tax-exempt bonds for a healthcare organization. Many aspects of this process are discussed in greater detail in later chapters. The first of these is a closer look at the members of the financing team and their specific roles.

6 The Financing Team for a Healthcare Financing

The process of implementing a healthcare bond transaction involves a group of specialized professionals brought together to form the *financing team,* which is also referred to as the *working group.* The working group on a typical bond issue usually is formed at the time the borrower decides to begin the process of issuing the debt, although some members of the group may be brought in earlier. For example, the borrower's management typically works with the organization's financial advisor or an investment banking firm to develop a preliminary structure that is consistent with the organization's capital plan, and an initial schedule for the financing. Preliminary discussions with bond counsel also may be held to determine any tax consequences of the proposed financing structure if it will be tax-exempt. The full group should be assembled by the time the deal is structured and it is time for documents to be drafted.

The working group members serve at the pleasure of the borrower, and it may serve the borrower well to remind these various parties of this from time to time. For most of the roles of the team members, there are other firms throughout the United States that are capable of providing the needed services. The borrower and its financial advisor should remain in control of the working group at all times, and demand excellence from each member. Too many healthcare organizations tend to limit their financing teams to those participants who have been used in the past, regardless of their performance. Healthcare finance is big business today, and there is no reason that a healthcare organization should settle for mediocre service from any members of its financing team.

As a rule, it is advisable for a borrower to avoid locking into contracts with the various members of the working group. A borrower should always be free to replace any member of the team who is not providing satisfactory service at any time it chooses to do so. Some professional firms regularly use written contracts, but few will refuse to work without one. If a contract is used, the borrower should make sure that it is free to terminate the engagement, *with no penalty,* any time. For firms working on a contingency basis (meaning that they do not get paid unless the financing closes), no fees are owed if services are terminated. It is then up to the borrower to decide whether the services that have been provided by any terminated parties warrant any compensation. Depending on the structure of the financing, some or all of the following parties may be needed in the working group.

▮ Financial Advisor

The financial advisor may be retained either by the issuer (if a separate issuer is used) or directly by the borrower. In either case, the purpose of a financial advisor is to provide state-of-the-art expertise with regard to the capital planning and acquisition process in the borrower's particular industry. As a result, it is important to select a financial advisor that has a great deal of experience with, and knowledge about, all the potential financing strategies and vehicles that may be appropriate. However, the borrower ultimately is responsible for all final decisions made regarding the creation and implementation of the capital plan.

The role of the financial advisor is to help the borrower make the most educated decisions possible. With the municipal finance industry constantly changing it is a full-time job to keep abreast of the changes and new developments that become available to borrowers, just as it is a full-time job for the borrower's chief financial officer to manage the financial aspects of the organization. No single person can do both jobs well at the same time. The financial advisor is the borrower's link to the world of public finance and is the financing team member on whom the borrower should rely the most to implement successful financings. A less than excellent financial advisor can inadvertently mask many issues that should be brought to the borrower's attention, resulting in less desirable financing. Unfortunately, it is highly probable that the borrower will never realize the potential that is lost when a less qualified financial advisor is used.

There is some debate over whether a healthcare organization is better served by an independent financial advisor or by a firm that also underwrites or trades bonds. The argument for seeking advice from underwriting (investment banking) firms is that they may be more aware of the market since their business is selling bonds. Arguments for independent financial advisors are that the better ones use the same market information sources that the underwriters use when they price bonds, and independent advisors have no vested interest in any particular financing plan. The most experienced independent financial advisors should be well versed in the various structures used by many different investment banking firms, as opposed to most investment bankers who gain experience only in the types of financings offered by their particular firms.

A potential conflict of interest arises when an investment banker or a firm that prepares feasibility studies is used as a financial advisor because that firm might benefit from one financing option more than another. The primary role of the underwriter is to sell bonds, and it is easier to sell bonds with tighter covenants and higher interest rates. However, the borrower is better off with more flexible covenants and lower interest rates. Even if an underwriter does not participate in the sale of the bonds in question when serving as financial advisor, a potential conflict still exists because underwriting firms depend on other underwriters for inclusion in various syndicates and selling groups for other bond issues. No underwriting firm generates enough business by serving only as senior manager to survive on that income alone without participating in the syndications and selling groups put together by other underwriters. In other words, an underwriter serving as financial advisor may be unwilling to take a strong position on the pricing of the bonds or the use of additional co-managing underwriters if the action carries the potential to alienate other underwriters.

Similarly, a firm that performs feasibility studies and serves as financial advisor may be more inclined than an independent financial advisor to recommend the use of a feasibility study. Feasibility studies typically are not required by the market or rating agencies unless the historical debt service coverage of projected debt is less than 1.5 times; the project is a start-up venture; or repayment of the bonds will depend upon the revenue stream generated by the new project. Even when a financial advisor claims to be independent, the borrower should always satisfy itself that no potential conflicts threaten to influence the financial advisor's recommendations.

The problem with many independent financial advisors is that they lack the experience and specialization to provide the services needed for a healthcare organization to make the most educated decisions regarding its capital planning and issuance of debt. As a result, some independent advisors are too reliant upon the investment bankers for expertise in structuring and implementing bond issues. This situation is less likely to result in the best financing possible for the borrower, due to the inability of the financial advisor to effectively serve as an advocate for the borrower. A good independent financial advisor should be able to help the borrower develop a financing plan that is designed to fit the needs of the borrower rather than those of the underwriter. When an underwriter is brought in, the financing plan should be in place already so that the underwriter can focus on implementing the plan and selling the bonds.

∎ Duties of the Financial Advisor

Capital Planning

The financial advisor should expect to begin an engagement with a healthcare organization by gaining an understanding of its long-term business strategy for at least the next five years. The financial implications of this strategy should then be examined to determine the projected long-term capital needs of the organization.

Next, the financial advisor should study the projected financial position of the organization and advise on its rating potential. During this process, advice can be given on the establishment of any financial goals that will help the organization reach its full rating potential. The next step is to explore alternative plans for obtaining the needed capital while evaluating the impact of these alternatives on the projected rating potential of the organization. This process will include the analysis of any potential refundings and will continue until one or two alternatives are developed that maximize the potential benefits for the organization.

The product of these efforts will be one or more long-term capital financing plans. The recommended plan should be reviewed with management, modified if necessary, and then presented to the finance committee and board of the borrower. The financial advisor should take part in these presentations and answer questions as to why the recommended plan makes the most sense. If the plan is not accepted, it must be modified and resubmitted until management and the board agree on a final capital plan.

Another task for the financial advisor is to evaluate the organization's existing bond documents to determine whether they provide the needed financing flexibility going forward, and whether any particular covenant or provision should be amended or eliminated. The evaluation should determine whether there are worthwhile advantages in adopting new financing documents or a new financing structure, if any refundings are appropriate, and whether there is an ability to make amendments to the existing documents.

Selection of the Financing Team

Once it is determined what kinds of financing needs the healthcare organization anticipates for the next five years (and beyond), the financial advisor should then work with the organization in the process of interviewing and selecting financing team participants that can best meet the financing objectives. Since every firm has different strengths and weaknesses, it is best to select financing team participants only after the organization has determined precisely what skills are needed based on the capital plan and immediate financing strategy. To help in the selection process, the financial advisor should draw up requests for proposals (RFPs), join in conducting interviews, negotiate fees, and assist in making the final selections of the financing team members.

One of the most useful tasks the financial advisor can perform in this process is to evaluate the feasibility and applicability of the many financing schemes with which the healthcare organization will be presented. When in competition, investment bankers are motivated to present all their latest financing techniques, whether or not they can be applied to this particular financing. The financial advisor can sort out which ideas are applicable and which are not, so the healthcare organization does not end up selecting a firm for the wrong reasons.

Coordination of the Financing Process

Once the financing team is selected, it is the financial advisor's job to represent the healthcare organization's interests throughout the process of putting together financings. This includes the following:

- establishing and revising a time and responsibility schedule for each financing
- working with the investment bankers (if a competitive sale is not being utilized) to come up with the optimal financing structure
- attending all meetings of the working group, and any necessary meetings of the borrower's board or finance committee, or any necessary meetings of the issuer
- explaining and evaluating the consequences of all proposed terms and financial covenants
- negotiating on behalf of the borrower when a particular proposal is not in its best interest, or is not the best that can be obtained
- assisting in the preparation of the POS and final OS
- preparing an outline and assisting in preparation for presentations to the rating agencies and bond insurers
- advising on market conditions
- advising on the timing of the bond issue
- assisting in the selection of a financial printer and trustee(s) (if any)
- eliciting and critiquing the marketing strategy of the investment banker (if a negotiated sale is being utilized)
- advising the borrower on the advisability of including co-managers to assist in the marketing of the bonds
- working with the borrower and the lead investment banker in the selection of other securities dealers to be included in any

syndicate or selling group

- providing expert and unbiased advice on the pricing of the bonds
- assisting in establishing investment strategies for the project fund and any escrows or debt service reserve funds
- advising on and bidding out the investment of bond proceeds, and
- assisting with last minute details to ensure a timely closing

Pricing the Bonds

As bond issues approach the marketing period, the financial advisor should review the underwriters' proposed marketing plan and strategy, and make sure that it is consistent with the requirements of the financing—not just what is convenient to the underwriters or what makes the deal most profitable to them. The financial advisor should participate in a series of "pricing calls" between the investment banker (underwriter) and representatives of the borrower. The role of the financial advisor at this point is to critique all marketing and bond pricing proposals.

In terms of dollars and cents, this is the function where a really good financial advisor can have the most impact and generate the greatest savings for the borrower, other than in the development of the overall structure of the issue. Experience confirms that it practically is impossible for anyone who is not in the tax-exempt market on a continuing basis to know with confidence whether an underwriter is proposing the most favorable terms on a tax-exempt financing. A financial advisor that is involved in the pricing of tax-exempt issues for healthcare organizations on a frequent basis may be better able to know, at any one time, the proper market interest rate levels and competitive underwriting spreads. The financial advisor's job is to make sure the underwriters "sharpen their pencils" and offer the borrower the best terms available.

Investment Advice

Bond issues tend to generate significant amounts of money that need to be invested in various trustee-held funds such as the project fund, debt service reserve fund, or any refunding escrows. Borrowers often receive significant amounts of money as reimbursement for projects on which they had spent their own funds prior to the financing. These funds also need to be invested. The borrower's financial advisor may or may not be qualified to assist in this area, but assistance is definitely recommended. The underwriters working on the financing will be more than willing to assist the borrower with these investments, because there is a significant amount of money to be made if a qualified financial advisor is not on hand to make sure the prices and yields for the securities are as competitive as possible. Ideally, all such investments will be bid out by the financial advisor to ensure the most competitive yields for the borrower.

The investments predominantly used by healthcare organizations are highly rated fixed income securities rather than equities (stocks), which usually are deemed too risky to be "permitted investments" for bond proceeds. Some healthcare organizations do invest in equities with their own funds with the goal of increasing the overall return on their reserves, but usually on a limited basis due to the greater risk of these types of investments. Chapter 14 deals with fixed income investing for healthcare organizations.

After the Financing

One of the most important functions of the financial advisor is to continue to advise after the financing is completed. After one series of bonds is issued, the healthcare organization's financing needs do not stop. The borrower should continue to work with the financial advisor on a continuing basis, between financings, to make sure that the organization is operating in conformity with its long-term strategic financing plan and that the plan continues to meet the foreseeable needs of the organization. If adverse circumstances or new capital needs arise, the financial advisor should work with the organization to develop a modified plan, and to recommend changes in strategy or operating procedures that will assure the ability to finance under the changed circumstances.

■ The Issuer of the Bonds

In the case of a tax-exempt bond issue, the issuer of the bonds usually will be a city, county, or authority, although some hospitals are set up as *hospital districts* that can issue their own tax-exempt bonds. Some issuers take an active role and are represented at the working group meetings, whereas others have very little contact with the other members of the working group. It is advisable to learn the preferred procedures of the issuer, thereby encouraging its cooperation, because most healthcare organizations have a limited number of alternative tax-exempt issuers available to them. No separate issuer should be needed for a taxable financing, although one may be desirable in some situations where taxable debt is being issued along with a tax-exempt issue, or if there is a potential for greater market acceptance with a better-known conduit issuer.

Some bond insurers are only able to issue insurance to cover the obligations of municipal entities. As a result, a hospital that desires to use one of these companies to enhance taxable debt might need to issue that debt through a conduit issuer so there would be a municipal entity involved. In most cases, however, it should be possible to develop a structure in which no conduit issuer is needed for a taxable financing.

■ Investment Bankers (Underwriters)

The primary role of the underwriter/investment banker is to sell bonds. The terms "underwriter" and "investment banker" tend to be used interchangeably when referring to a firm because these services are two different functions that typically are provided by different departments from within the same firm. The *investment bankers* are the people at the firm who coordinate the development of the bond issues for their firms and have the most direct contact with the borrowers. They frequently assist in structuring the financings, and sometimes serve as financial advisor to the borrower if a separate financial advisor has not been retained. The investment bankers attend all drafting sessions and are key players in the working group if the negotiated sale process is used. Their primary function is to generate bonds in a form that the underwriters in their firm like to sell.

The *underwriters* are the people at the firm who establish the pricing for the bonds and conduct the sales efforts. When an investment banking firm serves as an underwriter, it purchases all the bonds, whether or not it has orders to resell all of them. This is what is meant by *underwriting* the bonds and is the approach used for most fixed rate, public bond offerings for healthcare organizations. When bonds are underwritten, the borrower enters into a purchase contract for the bonds with the underwriting firm. The underwriter purchases the bonds and resells them to the ultimate bondholders. The borrower usually has little contact with the actual people referred to as underwriters until the bonds are ready to be priced, at which time the investment bankers typically take a back seat while the underwriters run the sales effort. In practice, it is common to refer to all people from these firms interchangeably as either investment bankers or underwriters.

If more than one underwriter (firm) is used by a borrower, one firm is usually designated as the *senior manager* and runs the deal from the underwriters' perspective while the other firms become *co-managers*. Co-managers usually have little, if any, input other than on the pricing of the bonds. Their role is to assist in the distribution of the bonds and in the underwriting of any unsold bonds. The senior manager is listed first on the cover of the OS, followed below by any co-managers. In the unusual situation where there are more than one senior manager, only one is responsible for "running the books," meaning that firm is responsible for coordinating all the orders for bonds. The senior manager that is running the books is customarily listed to the left on the first line of managers listed on the cover of the OS.

The senior manager typically is involved in the development and structuring of the issue if the decision has been made to use a negotiated offering as opposed to a competitive sale of the bonds. In a competitive sale, the underwriter is not involved until the bonds are sold. More healthcare organizations are keeping the option of a competitive sale open, and not hiring an underwriter until the bonds are offered or until the decision is finally made to use a negotiated offering. Virtually all healthcare organization revenue bond issues ultimately have been negotiated, although there have been a few successful competitive offerings. More discussion of this option follows in Chapter 8.

When a bond issue is being sold as a *private placement,* the investment banking firm serves as a *placement agent* rather than an underwriter. This means the placement agent finds purchasers for the bonds and never underwrites them. Private placements usually are used for financings that are somewhat out of the ordinary and are only offered to a limited number of institutional investors. When the bonds are sold, the borrower typically enters into the purchase contract with the ultimate bondholders rather than with the placement agent.

Most VRDB issues are sold as private placements, and the investment banking firm that serves as placement agent typically also serves as *remarketing agent.* The role of the remarketing agent is two-fold. First, the remarketing agent usually is responsible for setting the periodic interest rate on the VRDBs. To do this, the remarketing agent determines the lowest rate at which it believes all the bonds could be sold in the market on the day the interest rate is reset. That interest rate becomes the rate on the bonds for the next interest period. In the event bondholders believe the interest rate is too low, they are free to put the bonds and receive full par value once the appropriate notice period has ended. In the event bonds are put, the remarketing agent is called upon to attempt to find new buyers for those bonds, thereby remarketing them. In the event no new buyers can be found, the borrower will be forced to draw upon its liquidity facility to make payment to the existing bondholders on the put date. The remarketing agent will continue to search for new purchasers for the bonds until they have been successfully remarketed.

Occasionally, the pricing function on a VRDB issue is separated from the remarketing function. In these situations, the interest rates are reset by a *pricing agent,* and the remarketing agent is only responsible for remarketing the bonds. Problems can occur with this system if the pricing agent is overly optimistic and the remarketing agent is made to pay the consequences by having to remarket the bonds on a frequent basis. Conversely, there is a conflict of interest when the remarketing agent also serves as pricing agent. The remarketing function is made extremely easy if the interest rates on the bonds are set slightly higher than what the market demands. The remarketing agent can collect its fee without having to remarket any bonds.

∎ Bond Counsel

Tax-exempt debt requires a legal opinion from nationally recognized bond counsel to the effect that the interest on the bonds is exempt from federal, and in many cases, state income taxes if it is to be broadly accepted in the market place. The term "nationally recognized" means that the bond counsel firm is listed in a directory entitled *The Bond Buyer's Municipal Market Place.* Currently, this directory is published semiannually by Thomson Financial Publishing, Inc., of Skokie, Ill. It is readily recognized by its bright red cover, and is referred to in the municipal finance industry as the "Red Book." The contents of the Red Book have been expanded in recent years from its tradition of listing investment banking firms and municipal bond attorneys, to the inclusion of financial and investment advisors, credit enhancers, corporate trust departments, rating agencies, derivative specialists, arbitrage rebate specialists, various government officials, associations, and other information that is relevant to the municipal finance industry. Any legal firm that is selected as bond counsel should be listed in the Red Book if the borrower is to obtain the broadest market acceptance for its bonds.

Bond counsel primarily represents the interests of the bondholders. The role of bond counsel is to draft bond documents that reflect the structure of the deal and to deliver an unqualified legal opinion that the bonds are validly issued and binding, tax-exempt (if applicable), and in compliance with all laws governing the issuance of debt. Bond counsel as a discrete role normally is not needed for taxable bonds, although some counsel must be responsible for drafting the documents.

It is beneficial for a borrower and its financial advisor to develop a close working relationship with the bond counsel that is expected to be used in a tax-exempt bond issue. Advice from bond counsel can be sought as to tax law implications resulting from structures proposed by the financial advisor, as well as the circumstances of the borrower. Early determination and resolution of tax issues will prevent false starts in putting together the bond issue and will save a significant amount of time for the working group.

Bond counsel firms tend to interpret various aspects of tax law differently. This means that some firms may not be willing to give an opinion on bonds that utilize a certain structure, while other nationally renowned bond firms will be willing to do so. The borrower's financial advisor should be experienced enough with different bond counsel firms to advise on whether the positions of a particular firm are generally consistent with those of most other firms. In the event a particular bond counsel firm will not allow a financing technique that has been utilized by other borrowers around the country, the borrower may deem it advisable to investigate the use of a different firm as bond counsel.

■ Other Legal Counsel

The **underwriters' counsel** represents the underwriters during the development of the purchase contract for the bonds, and is primarily responsible for the adequacy of disclosure in the offering document (the official statement in a tax-exempt bond issue). The underwriters' counsel is also responsible for surveying the various state "blue sky" laws that govern the sale of securities and for instructing the underwriters on compliance with those laws as well as federal securities laws. In a competitive sale of bonds these functions are performed by counsel referred to as **disclosure counsel**, because the underwriter is not involved with the development of the financing.

In some cases, bond counsel serves as underwriters' counsel as well. This practice may reduce the overall cost for these services, but the situation should be evaluated carefully to expose any potential conflict in the event there is a problem with the bond issue in the future.

The **issuer's counsel** represents the interests of the issuer in a tax-exempt bond issue, and provides written legal opinions relating to the powers of the issuer to issue the bonds and to the disclosure about the issuer in the offering document. Issuer's counsel typically does not play an active role in structuring the financing unless there are specific issues that deal with the powers or policies of the issuer.

The **borrower's counsel** represents the legal interests of the healthcare organization (borrower) and provides opinions concerning the organization's corporate powers and the disclosure on the healthcare organization contained in the offering document. It is not necessary, in most financings, for the healthcare organization's counsel to have expertise in the area of bonds, although it can be helpful.

■ Bond Trustee and Master Trustee

The **bond trustee** for the bond issue receives the bond proceeds at closing, disburses funds as directed by the bond indenture, collects debt service payments from the borrower, makes the principal and interest payments to the bondholders, and implements all the directions found in the trust indenture. Basically, the trustee is responsible for overseeing the bond issue and monitoring the borrower's compliance with legal covenants throughout the life of the debt. The trustee usually is brought into the working group after several drafts of the documents have been revised by the group.

When a master trust indenture is used, a **master trustee** is also required. The typical structure is for a master trust indenture to govern over various bond indentures and other documents related to debt issued pursuant to the master trust indenture. The master trustee carries out the directions found in the master trust indenture. There usually is little work for the master trustee to perform unless there is a default on one of the underlying debt instruments, at which time the role of the master trustee kicks in to look out for the interests of all underlying debt holders.

In some cases, borrowers have used the same firm to serve as bond trustee and master trustee. This practice is becoming less common because there may be a conflict of interest in such situations. The argument can be made that no conflict exists as long as the same firm is master trustee and trustee on *all* underlying debt issues. However, in the event one firm is master trustee and trustee on some but not all underlying debt issues, then that firm may have a vested interest in how the various underlying lenders are treated in the event of a default. The concern is that the bond issues for which that firm is trustee will receive more favorable treatment than the other debt issues. Some trustees try to avoid this conflict by agreeing to resign if there ever is a default under the master trust indenture. This solution makes little sense for two reasons. First, there is likely to be significant difficulty in finding a replacement for the master trustee if there is a default—due to the potential for large amounts of work as well as increased liability. Second, the original master trustee would have collected a fee during the years there was no default and little work, only to be excused from the increased workload due to the default. For these reasons, it is advisable to retain separate firms to serve as bond trustee and master trustee.

■ Other Professionals

A **feasibility consultant** may be required if the proceeds of the financing are to be used for a project expected to generate significant additional revenue that is needed for the debt service on the bonds, and if the historical income available for debt service is not sufficient to demonstrate coverage of at least 150 percent of the projected maximum annual debt service. Even if a feasibility study is not required, the healthcare organization board may want a limited version of a study for its own use in evaluating the advisability of going forward with the project. Limited feasibility studies for the borrower's own use generally cost significantly less than full-blown feasibility studies that are sometimes published in the official statements of tax-exempt bond issues.

Financial auditors may be brought into the working group meetings periodically to discuss the financial information to be included in the offering document. Usually, three to five years of audits are prepared in comparison format for a public offering, along with comparative "stub" financial statements for the current interim period and the same period for the prior year. These stub statements typically are not audited. Accountants usually are required to provide "comfort letters" at the time the bonds are sold and again when the issue closes. *Comfort letters* declare, in effect, that the auditors are not aware of any material negative financial developments that have occurred since the release of the most recent audited financial statements. The borrower's auditors frequently are also retained to serve as **verification agent** on any refunding issues, although not all accounting firms offer this service. The role of the verification agent is to verify the calculations of the underwriter concerning the funding of the refunding escrow. Any miscalculation in setting up the escrow could result in a shortfall on the refunded bond issue. The services of the verification agent provide comfort to the bondholders that the escrow is funded in the appropriate manner.

Representatives of a **letter of credit provider** or a **bond insurer** will join the working group if the financing is to be credit-enhanced. Frequently, they will also involve their own counsel.

These are the primary parties who work with the healthcare organization to implement a tax-exempt financing, and some of them are not needed for a taxable financing. Special circumstances may require the involvement of other professionals. Any healthcare organization should expect its financial advisor to coordinate the working group to make efficient use of time and to minimize costs. One of the key areas where this can be helpful is in the negotiation of fees for each member of the working group.

7 Negotiating the Fees of the Working Group Members

Issuing debt tends to be an expensive proposition for a healthcare organization. Some methods of incurring debt cost less initially, but may cost more in terms of interest expense in the long run. Conversely, issuing tax-exempt debt tends to be quite expensive in terms of cost of issuance, but the reduction in interest expense usually benefits the healthcare organization far beyond the initial cost.

The initial cost of incurring debt is probably lowest with a direct loan from a bank or other financial institution. Some healthcare organizations may be able to utilize boilerplate (standard) documentation provided by their banks, with a quick review of the documentation by their own counsel. If the borrower wishes to enter the public markets, thereby reducing its interest cost and perhaps reducing its covenants, then the cost of issuance will increase. Publicly offered debt requires disclosure of all pertinent information for prospective purchasers. Preparing this disclosure entails retaining experienced counsel.

The largest single fee for professional services that a healthcare organization is likely to incur in the issuance of a bond issue is that of the underwriter, followed by the financial advisor, and various legal counsel. The fee for the financial advisor typically should be negotiated first, as the financial advisor usually is the first member of the team brought onboard by the borrower. The financial advisor should then be able to assist the borrower in negotiating the fees for the remainder of the working group.

■ Financial Advisor Fees

There are several methods of setting financial advisor fees. The most common is a small percentage of the total financing. For example, financial advisory fees on a bond issue typically range from roughly $1 to $2 per bond. One dollar per bond ($1/bond) is one-tenth of one percent (.001) of the issue size. When fees are quoted in dollars per bond, it is assumed that the face value of a bond is $1,000—although bonds are rarely issued in this denomination. A fee of $1/bond would most likely be agreed to for a very large issue, while a fee of $2/bond would be more appropriate for a smaller issue. The borrower should clarify which expenses of the financial advisor, if any, will be included in this fee, and whether any expenses will be passed through to the borrower.

While there may be an incentive for a financial advisor to recommend a larger financing if the fee is based on the size of that financing, the borrower ultimately determines the size of any bond issue. If the financial advisor is serving the borrower well, an educated decision should be made as to the size of any bond issue, eliminating the ability of the financial advisor to artificially increase the size of the financing, and thus its fee.

One argument for the appropriateness of structuring the fee for the financial advisor based on the size of the issue is that the fee increases as the size of the issue increases. Financial advisors tend to be named in lawsuits if there is a default on the bonds, along with the borrower and other members of the financing team. Consequently, the risk to a financial advisor increases as the size of the bond issue increases. While it is possible that a $100 million bond issue does not take any more work on the part of the financial advisor than a $30 million bond issue, the exposure to financial risk is proportionately greater.

A second fee structure used by some financial advisors is an hourly fee basis. The problem with this approach is that it encourages low productivity and excessive time in structuring and implementing the issue. A healthcare organization hires a financial advisor for the expertise that can be provided, which should result in a financing that fits the needs of the borrower better and hopefully reduces its overall cost. This benefit is derived from the expertise of the financial advisor, as opposed to the number of hours spent on the issue. For example, some financial advisors are experts at generating reams of reports that are of questionable value to the borrower. These reports take a significant amount of time but may not generate the value the healthcare organization should demand.

A third method for healthcare organizations that regularly make use of a financial advisor is a monthly retainer. Under this method, the financial advisor is paid a certain amount whether or not a financing is implemented. The argument for this approach is that the financial advisor has no potential interest as to the size of any bond issue. The retainer approach typically is only appropriate for organizations that expect to enter the financial markets at least every year or two.

A fourth method for establishing a fee with the financial advisor is for the healthcare organization and the advisor to discuss the anticipated scope of the project as well as the anticipated issue size, and then agree upon a fixed fee for the project. This eliminates any potential conflict of the financial advisor recommending a higher than needed issue size. In the event the scope of the project changes, and the size of the issue increases or the work required by the financial advisor increases, it should be understood that the financial advisor is free to request a re-evaluation of the fee. Most financial advisory firms will be willing to work on whichever fee structure is most amenable to the borrower.

Healthcare organizations should evaluate the different alternatives and work with their financial advisers to develop a fee structure that is fair and workable for both parties. A good, experienced financial advisor may be able to save a healthcare organization hundreds of thousands or even millions of dollars in a short period of time, while a financial advisor with less experience and creativity may spend tens or hundreds of hours on a financing with little benefit ensuing to the borrower.

However the fee structure is established with the financial advisor, it is advisable to allow the fee to accrue throughout the process of issuing debt. This avoids the problem of creating a conflict of interest for the financial advisor if the fee is entirely contingent upon the completion of the financing. It may not be in the best interest of the borrower for the financial advisor to have incentive to complete a financing in order to get paid. Establishing clear points in the financing schedule at which portions of the fee are earned can alleviate this potential conflict of interest. For example, 20 percent of the expected total fee may be considered earned after the organizational meeting. An additional 50 percent could accrue when the second draft of bond documents is distributed, and the balance due if the financing closes.

▌ Fees for Investment Banking and Underwriting Services

The underwriter's fee usually is referred to as the underwriter's "discount" or "spread." Like financial advisor fees, the underwriter's fee typically is structured in terms of dollars per bond, although it is significantly larger. Underwriting spreads for healthcare bond issues typically range from less than $5/bond for very large issues to $20/bond, or more, for non-rated bond issues that will be sold on a retail basis. Placement fees for VRDB issues should be in the range of $2/bond to $5/bond.

The underwriter's fee is referred to as a *discount* because the underwriter subtracts the amount of its fee when paying the borrower the net proceeds of the bond issue—in essence, discounting the payment for the bonds. When the underwriter is serving as a placement agent, as opposed to an underwriter, a placement fee is paid rather than an underwriter's discount. The placement fee may be paid either to the placement agent at closing or deducted by the placement agent as a discount from the bond proceeds.

Depending on the nature of a financing, the investment banking firm may be asked to serve as an underwriter, placement agent, remarketing agent, pricing agent, or any combination. The fee structures for each of these different roles differ, as do the strategies that are most appropriate for their negotiation. In general, when bonds are being offered in a negotiated sale, the earlier that certain portions of the underwriter's spread are agreed upon, the more negotiating leverage the healthcare organization has. In some cases, however, certain parts of the spread are best left undetermined until the bonds are priced, or the results may be less favorable to the borrower.

There are four components to an underwriter's spread on a fixed rate bond issue. The *takedown* is the largest component and is the commission paid to the people who actually sell the bonds, although other participants from the firm may also share in this component. Under normal circumstances, there may be a direct correlation between the size of the takedown and the amount of effort a bond salesman will put into selling a healthcare organization's bonds. The second component is the *management fee*. This portion usually compensates the individual investment bankers who structure the issue and work with the healthcare organization on a day-to-day basis. The third component is the *underwriter's risk*, which is compensation for buying bonds for which there are no existing orders at the time the deal is verbally awarded. The last component is *expenses*, which consist of reimbursement of direct out-of-pocket expenses incurred during the development and implementation of the financing.

The most effective strategy for negotiating the spread depends upon whether the healthcare organization is issuing fixed rate or variable rate debt. On a fixed rate financing, it is advisable to negotiate the management fee when the underwriters are first retained. This way, the borrower has the most leverage. The longer this negotiation is delayed, the more the leverage shifts to the benefit of the underwriters.

At the same time that the management fee is negotiated, a cap on expenses should be negotiated, including the fee for the underwriter's counsel. Because expenses can accumulate rapidly unless the underwriter has some incentive to contain them, a cap will encourage the underwriter to watch travel and other expenses, and to negotiate a competitive underwriter's counsel fee. The fee for underwriter's counsel usually is the largest expense incurred by the underwriter.

The underwriter's risk component and takedown often should be left open until the bonds are in the market. If the bonds end up being *oversubscribed* (more orders for bonds than there are bonds available) then there should be no underwriting risk and no fee for this component. In other situations, however, it may be desirable to ask the investment banker to underwrite a large amount of unsold bonds to get the deal done. In that case, a fair underwriter's risk component would be appropriate.

Setting the takedown too early in a fixed rate financing can have a negative impact on the overall cost to a healthcare organization. If the takedown is too low, then the salesmen might concentrate first on selling other bonds with higher takedowns. In a volatile market, this could cost the healthcare organization 10 to 15 basis points (.10 to .15%) on its bonds, which could result in millions of dollars of increased interest expense over the life of a large issue. Similarly, in a stable market it may be appropriate to negotiate a lower takedown if there is little risk that it will affect the yield on the bonds. The appropriate takedown can be determined only on the day of pricing and generally should be left open until then, when the healthcare organization's financial advisor can advise the borrower on making that determination. Another factor to consider is whether the bonds are being sold in the retail market or the institutional market. The sale of bonds in the retail market typically requires a higher takedown because individuals tend to place smaller orders than institutions, resulting in more work for the salesmen.

While the above strategy generally has been the most advisable approach for negotiating an underwriter's spread (discount) on a fixed rate bond issue, there are times when an alternative approach may be more beneficial to the borrower. During the 1980s, most of the investment bankers that did the work of putting a bond issue together and worked day-to-day with the borrower were paid entirely out of the management fee of the underwriter's spread. Since the early 1990s, investment banking firms have been so eager to be named as senior managers on bond financings, they have been compensating these people out of the overall spread on the bonds and not just the management fee. This means that some firms are willing to serve as the senior manager on a financing with little or no management fee component to the spread. Likewise, some firms have been willing to reduce the average takedown they pay their salesmen in an attempt to attract more bond issues. The net effect to the borrower has been a significant reduction in total underwriting fees being paid on a bond issue, especially when a competitive process is used in the selection of the underwriter.

Total underwriting fees proposed when healthcare organizations solicit proposals from underwriters have become very aggressive. The borrower's financial advisor should be experienced enough to advise the borrower on the advisability of accepting a bid for an overall underwriter's spread rather than leaving negotiations for the takedown and underwriter's risk components until the bonds are being priced. If the financial advisor is knowledgeable about the investment banking firms who are proposing, and is also able to access current market information at the time of pricing to make sure the bonds are being priced aggressively, then this alternative approach may result in a lower total under-writer's fee for the bond issue.

On a VRDB issue, the initial interest rate is only set for a week or for some other short period of time. The ultimate success of the issue will depend on the periodic repricing rather than on the initial interest rate. Therefore, it is advisable to negotiate the entire spread as early as possible, preferably before the underwriter is hired. As mentioned ear-lier, the longer the negotiation is put off, the more the leverage shifts to the favor of the underwriter. With a VRDB issue, the borrower has little to lose, even if the placement agent does a lackluster job on the initial pricing of the bonds.

While the trend has been for underwriting fees to decline, there has been another trend that healthcare organizations should be aware of. As investment banking firms have been receiving less compensation for their services in structuring and selling bond issues, there has been an increased effort to provide other services beyond the normal scope of those typically provided by underwriters to generate additional fees. Ex-amples of these services might be the sale of securities to the borrower for the investment of the proceeds of project funds, debt service reserve funds, or escrows. While the underwriter will purchase these securities and resell them to the borrower at "market," there can be significant variation as to what "market" actually is. Failure to seek competitive bids on these investments can cost a borrower a significant sum.

Similarly, many underwriters are pushing the use of various deriva-tive products, which provide alternatives for generating fees on the part of the underwriters by selling the borrower swaps or other financial in-struments that are integral components of the derivative structures. The borrower's financial advisor must be keenly aware of the various areas where underwriting firms attempt to make up revenues that may have been foregone in their underwriting spreads, to be able to protect the borrower from hidden costs that are avoidable. The best way to avoid these hidden costs is to competitively bid all these various services out to several different firms so the true market value may be determined. Failure of a borrower to utilize a financial advisor who is free of any conflicts in this area may result in significant added cost, which may remain totally unrecognized by the borrower.

Remarketing Agent Fees

The fees for remarketing agent services on VRDB issues tend to be fairly standardized. They typically are a flat rate that ranges from .10% to .125% per annum on the amount of the bonds outstanding for the combined services of pricing and remarketing the bonds. In some cases, the remarketing agent gets paid a fee only for the actual remarketing, with a cap at the levels mentioned. Although this fee structure is not common, it is preferable to the borrower since the remarketing agent only gets paid if bonds are actually put. It may be in the best interest of the borrower for the bonds to be put periodically, because this means the interest is being set at aggressive levels that are not palatable to all bondholders. If a VRDB issue is never put, an argument can be made that the remarketing agent is setting the interest rates too high so the existing bondholders are never dissatisfied. This situation allows the remarketing agent to collect its fee while doing very little work.

Remarketing agreements typically serve as the documentation that establishes the relationship between the borrower and the remarketing agent. If a remarketing agent wishes to relinquish the position for some reason, the remarketing agreement should provide that the remarketing agent must give the borrower at least 30 days' notice, and that a replacement remarketing agent must be appointed before the existing agent is no longer responsible for setting interest rates and remarketing bonds.

Conversely, if a remarketing agent is not doing a good job, and the borrower wishes to find a replacement, the borrower should only have to give that remarketing agent about three days' notice before the replacement takes effect. While this approach may appear to be inequitable at first glance, it makes sense. The remarketing agent is in a position to do significant harm to the borrower, thereby necessitating the short notice period for removal. The borrower is in no position to cause harm to the remarketing agent, and thus the longer termination notice requirement.

Borrowers who utilize VRDBs are well advised to develop some method of verifying that the remarketing agent is setting the interest rates aggressively on the bonds. One of the few ways of doing this is by obtaining the VariFact™ report, which is published by Ponder & Co., in Bedford, Tex., on a weekly basis. The VariFact report is a weekly compilation of the interest rates from a database of more than 100 VRDB issues. The average of these rates is published in *The Bond Buyer* each week. Subscribers to this service are able to obtain a report that compares the interest rates on their bond issues with the average for the entire database. A distribution analysis of all the various data is also included, which allows borrowers to see exactly how the pricing of their bonds compared to those of the various issuers of VRDBs that report to this database. This database was created in 1986 after a large number of healthcare organizations issued VRDBs in anticipation of the Tax Reform Act of 1986. Prior to the development of the VariFact database, organizations that issued VRDBs had no way to determine whether or not their remarketing agents were doing a good job in establishing the interest rates on the bonds.

■ Fees for Legal Counsel

Fee negotiations for legal counsel retained directly by the borrower usually are done on a competitive basis where the borrower sends out requests for proposals (RFPs) and then selects legal counsel based on the responses to the proposals received. Typically, the borrower uses its regular legal counsel to represent its interests during the process of issuing debt. As a result, sending out RFPs for this service does not make much sense if there is only one firm that the organization wishes to use. It does make sense, however, to establish a fee up front for the entire service, or to establish an hourly rate with a cap. As long as the fee, or the cap, is acceptable to the borrower, there should be no need to look further for its counsel.

While an RFP process may result in a bond counsel at the lowest possible fee, the borrower may not be well served. Depending on the planned financing structure that has been developed by the borrower and its financial advisor, some bond counsel firms may be more experienced than others with the given financing structure. Similarly, if an underwriter has been retained, that underwriter will have specific structures it has utilized in the past for the bonds it has sold. Some bond counsel will have had experience with these structures and some may not. Therefore, it may be advisable to limit the field of potential bond counsel to those that the financial advisor and underwriter are confident can efficiently handle the proposed bond structure. Once the field has been narrowed in this way, the RFP approach can be a highly efficient way to negotiate legal fees. As with the borrower's counsel, the fee structure may be based on issue size, a flat fee, or an hourly basis with a cap. The cap is a good idea because bond issues tend to end up being more complicated than initially anticipated, and this results in bond counsel usually spending more hours than they anticipate in documenting the bond issue.

Legal counsel fees are usually quoted "plus expenses." As legal fees have been declining over the years, expenses have increased in some cases. It is not unusual to see photocopying expenses billed at 25¢ to 30¢ per page. Therefore, a borrower should negotiate a cap on expenses as well as on the rate charged for copied pages as the number of pages copied for a bond issue can be quite substantial.

▮ Other Members of the Working Group

As with the strategies for negotiating fees with the professionals described above, a borrower is well advised to take one of two different approaches with the rest of the professionals in the financing team. Where the borrower has a specific firm or individual that it wishes to use for a specific role, it is advisable to negotiate a fee up-front. If an acceptable fee cannot be negotiated, then the position should be subject to an open competitive bidding process through the use of an RFP. When the borrower does not have a specific firm that it wishes to use for a specific role, the RFP process should be used wherever possible. This will result in the lowest fees for the borrower. Again, the borrower will have to rely on its financial advisor to limit prospective bidders to those that are capable of providing the required services in the most efficient and professional manner possible. The goal in the selection of each member of the working group should be to obtain the highest caliber of service at a fair fee.

8 Negotiated Sale versus Competitive Sale of Bonds

The healthcare industry customarily has used the negotiated sale process when bonds are issued. Municipalities, counties, school districts, and many other issuers of tax-exempt debt typically use the competitive bid process instead. Competitive bids can often result in a lower cost to the borrower because the bonds are sold to the underwriter offering the highest price (lowest interest rate) for the bonds. Another benefit of competitive bidding is that it is an objective process, and it generally eliminates the political problems of selecting an underwriter.

▮ Negotiated Sale of Bonds

The primary differences between a competitive sale and a negotiated sale of bonds are the timing and degree of involvement of the underwriter. In a *negotiated sale,* the underwriter is selected early in the process and becomes a member of the working group that structures and documents the bond issue. When the time comes to sell the bonds, the underwriter, the borrower, and the borrower's financial advisor agree upon a scale of interest rates for the various maturities of the bonds. The underwriter then proceeds to "enter the market" for an agreed-upon period of time to obtain orders for the bonds at the designated interest rates. Once enough bonds are pre-sold, the underwriter offers to purchase them.

When the borrower and its financial advisor agree with the underwriter on the final scale of interest rates, a purchase contract is executed and a closing date is set. If no agreement can be reached with the underwriter as to the appropriate scale for the bonds, the borrower has only two alternatives: accept the underwriter's offer or pull the issue from the market and try again another day. The alternative of pulling the deal from the market is rarely used, and most borrowers end up accepting the underwriter's offer even if they do not believe it is as good as it should be. In theory, a perfectly executed negotiated offering should result in interest rates and an underwriter's discount as low as that which could be derived from a competitive sale. However, that assumes that the hospital and its financial advisor are able to get the underwriter to accept terms that are as aggressive as those that would be offered by any other underwriter in the country.

■ Competitive Sale of Bonds

A *competitive sale* differs from a negotiated sale in that no underwriter is involved until the bonds are ready to be sold. The working group for a competitive sale consists of the same members as for a negotiated sale, with the exception of the underwriter. The borrower's financial advisor structures the financing to fit the needs of the borrower and orchestrates the sale process. Disclosure counsel (called "underwriter's counsel" in a negotiated financing) prepares the POS and the OS, and gives the necessary opinions as to the adequacy of disclosure to the winning underwriters. Bond counsel and the other members of the team play the same roles that they do in a negotiated financing.

When it is determined that it is time to go to market in a competitive sale, the sale is advertised in appropriate trade publications and a notice of sale and bid form are circulated to a group of underwriters. The notice of sale solicits bids on the issue and establishes bidding requirements. Seven to 10 days usually are allowed before the bids are due. Each underwriter, or group of underwriters, wishing to bid on the bonds submits its bid within the prescribed time, detailing the coupon rates and yields for the various maturities and any premium or discount on the bonds. The borrower accepts the bid that offers the lowest interest cost (which is the same as offering the highest price for the bonds), or the bid that best satisfies other criteria specified in the notice of sale. The bond issue then proceeds to closing. The borrower should always reserve the right to reject all bids.

Under the right circumstances, a competitive sale can offer substantial cost savings to the borrower because no single underwriter has the exclusive right to purchase the bonds. All the underwriters submitting bids compete to offer the lowest interest cost because that is the only way they will get the bonds. This assures the borrower that it will receive the lowest interest rates and underwriter's discount that were available for that particular type of financing that day—since all interested underwriters had the chance to buy the bonds. In a negotiated sale, only one firm is allowed to make an offer. This is why a competitive sale can frequently cost a borrower less than a negotiated sale.

The competitive sale approach has not been used to a great extent by the healthcare industry, largely due to the misconception that healthcare credits are not readily accepted by the market and require a special sales effort. This may have been true years ago, before many healthcare organizations had entered the tax-exempt market, but this argument is no longer valid since the market has readily consumed billions of dollars in tax-exempt healthcare revenue bonds. Local municipalities and school districts have made use of the competitive sale method for years, and there is no reason that healthcare organizations cannot enjoy the savings offered by this approach as well.

Determining When a Competitive Sale May Be Appropriate

While it is true that a competitive sale can offer a more economical financing for the borrower under most circumstances, and may eliminate some of the political problems associated with the selection of an underwriter, there are some situations where a competitive sale may not be appropriate. There are at least four conditions that optimize the likelihood of success of a debt issuance under the competitive sale method, and any borrower should reevaluate the advisability of using this approach if any one of them is not in place at the time the bonds are sold:

1. a normal, or "vanilla," structure to the deal;

2. sufficient creditworthiness of the borrower;

3. a relatively active secondary trading market for the type of security being offered; and

4. stability of market rates.

If the structure of the financing is unusual or the healthcare organization is not perceived as a particularly strong credit, underwriters will assume that a more strenuous marketing effort will be required to sell the bonds, and they will compensate for this in their bids by increasing the yield on the bonds, increasing the discount, or both. The result is a higher financing cost for the healthcare organization. This should not present a problem for a borrower if the issue is fairly standard and is insured, but a healthcare organization that does not have a rating of A1/A+ or higher may want to evaluate whether there would be a problem with a competitive sale without enhancing the rating with bond insurance.

An active secondary market for a particular type of security facilitates the sale of an initial issue of debt because bondholders take comfort in knowing that they can dispose of their bonds before maturity if necessary. In other words, the bonds have a degree of liquidity. The secondary market for healthcare bonds has reached the degree of activity where, in most cases, there should be no concern about the ability of bondholders to sell their bonds in the secondary market. The concern should be greater if there are any unusual aspects of the structure of the bond issue to which the market is unaccustomed.

If the market is unstable when bids are delivered, with fluctuations in interest rates occurring relatively quickly, increased yields and discounts are likely to be built into underwriters' bids to protect the underwriters from such fluctuations. Again, the result is increased cost to the issuer. If a healthcare organization decides to use the competitive bid approach, it should make sure that the bids are solicited during a period of stable markets.

When all these preconditions are in place, the competitive sale of an issue can often result in a lower cost to a healthcare organization than a negotiated sale. If, however, any one of these conditions is not met, or there are other extenuating circumstances, a negotiated sale may be preferable. In any case, it makes sense for the borrower to include this process as one option to review with its financial advisor, rather than dismissing it out-of-hand as has been done frequently in the past.

▌ Competitive Negotiation of Bonds

An additional alternative for hospitals to consider is a hybrid between a negotiated sale and a competitive sale—a process sometimes referred to as a competitive negotiation. In a *competitive negotiation,* the financial advisor puts the financing together with the borrower, as in a competitive sale, but the underwriter is brought into the working team late in the process in time to give some final input as to the structure of the financing and to perform a pre-sales effort on the bonds. In this situation, the hospital is in a very strong negotiating position with respect to the underwriter and can negotiate significantly lower fees than on a normal negotiated offering because the underwriter is not being asked to spend the time and effort on the front end of the financing. This approach eliminates many of the shortcomings and uncertainty of a competitive sale, while maintaining some of the savings.

▌ Considerations Related to Selecting the Best Approach

Each of the three approaches to selling bonds described above is more appropriate than the others under certain circumstances. The mistake that many hospitals make is that they do not consider all three alternatives with their financial advisors before they retain an underwriter. Once an underwriter is retained, the options of a competitive sale and a competitive negotiation are eliminated. None of these alternatives will give optimum results to a borrower every time bonds are issued, and all three alternatives deserve consideration by any healthcare organization that is in the process of planning a financing and developing a capital plan. As healthcare financial officers seek new ways to reduce costs, more and more institutions are likely to use more creative and lower-cost financing methods, including competitive negotiations and competitive sales.

When a healthcare organization determines that it wishes to use either the competitive sale or a competitive negotiation, the role of the financial advisor takes on additional importance. The financial advisor is responsible for assisting in putting together the financing team and coordinating the entire process without the assistance of an underwriter. Because of this, most borrowers should not begin the process of a competitive sale or a competitive negotiation without a competent financial advisor on board.

The Competitive Sale of Derivative Bonds

While the argument can be made that the competitive sale approach should offer a healthcare organization a lower cost financing as long as the bond issue is fairly standard, the introduction of derivative products to the market has raised a question as to the desirability of the competitive bid process. Properly structured derivative bonds should allow a healthcare organization to access the tax-exempt bond markets at interest rate levels that are 10 to 20 basis points below the rates for conventional bonds. It is fair to question whether a competitive sale approach on conventional bonds could match this level of savings. The ideal approach might be to use a competitive bid process for derivative products. This has proved to be difficult, however, because each underwriting firm has its own derivative products, which have not yet become standardized, and because each firm has its own documentation for its own particular products.

One of the difficulties in attempting to implement a competitive sale of derivative products is the fact that a description of the bonds to be issued must be included in the POS. Because each firm's derivative products are different, this means that there would need to be a description of each product in the POS. Until recently, this would have proved to be unwieldy, but a new approach in describing bonds in an OS may make a competitive sale of derivative products a viable option. This approach involves briefer descriptions of each product in the POS, with complete descriptions of the actual products that are issued in the final OS. This should allow interested bidders to supply the disclosure counsel with language about their specific derivative products that they would like to be included in a competitive sale. These products could then be described in the POS and the competitive bid process implemented. This could mean the POS might include anywhere from 10 to 30 or more different potential derivative products, but the final OS would only include descriptions of the derivative products that are actually sold once an award has been given to a specific firm for the bonds. The competitive bid of derivative products is a fairly new concept, but it is a viable option that a healthcare organization should review with its financial advisor. The benefits and pitfalls of derivative products are described in Chapter 13.

Selling Advance Refunding Bonds

If the financing being considered is exclusively an advance refunding of another bond issue, then a negotiated sale may be more appropriate than a competitive sale. This is because of the added complexity of having to calculate escrow requirements at the same time the bond issue is sized. If the proposed financing includes some new money project as well as an advance refunding, this problem is much less of a concern because usually there is some play in the amount that can be financed for the new money project. This allows the escrow to be sized at the same time as the bond issue, because the bond issue size does not have to be exact.

Large Issues

If the size of the issue is extremely large, it may be desirable to allow an underwriter to do a significant amount of pre-selling of the issue to enhance the likelihood that it will be sold in a timely manner. Also, there may be heightened desirability to include derivative products in a very large issue to tap different buyers at specific points in time. Because of these points, a negotiated sale may make more sense than a competitive sale if the bond issue is extremely large.

Timing

If the timing of the issue is extremely important, a competitive sale adds the potential uncertainty of market turmoil at an inappropriate time, thereby causing the issuer to delay the financing. While the financial markets may appear to be stable for a period of time, they can become unstable very quickly for a variety of reasons. New economic data are being released to the markets fairly consistently, and any negative news can cause a significant change in the market—or at least expectations for the future of the market. A negotiated sale allows sufficient pre-selling so the impact of market instability is not as great as if a competitive sale is used.

Control of Which Underwriters Participate

Another potential drawback to the competitive sale approach is that it eliminates the ability of the issuer to dictate which firms, or which types of firms, get the bonds. Many borrowers desire to have local firms receive a significant amount of bonds so local individuals will have the opportunity to purchase them. In other cases, issuers have determined that it is desirable to include minority-owned firms in their bond issues. Neither of these considerations can be given much weight with a competitive sale. Typically, whichever firm offers the lowest interest rates will get the bonds, regardless of whether they offer local distribution or minority participation. However, it might be possible to include other criteria in the documentation requesting bids indicating that such factors as local distribution or minority participation will be given some weight in the final decision.

■ Conclusion

Perhaps the best plan of action for large and frequent issuers of debt is that they review each of the three marketing alternatives each time they consider going to market, and use whichever is most appropriate at the time. This should result in a mix of all three alternatives, depending on the particular conditions that exist each time the borrower goes to market.

9 Bond Ratings

Bond ratings are designations of creditworthiness assigned to bond issues by certain rating agencies. Bonds with higher ratings are supposed to have a greater likelihood of having principal and interest repaid on schedule than bonds with lower ratings. Bonds issued on behalf of healthcare organizations may be rated by a recognized rating agency, or not rated at all. Bond issues that are not rated require prospective purchasers to do their own credit evaluations to determine the likelihood of repayment and the associated risk. While purchasers of healthcare bonds should not rely exclusively on the ratings bestowed by the rating agencies, bonds that are rated save purchasers a significant amount of effort in evaluating the underlying credit and likelihood of repayment of the bonds.

Just because a bond issue is non-rated, does not mean that the underlying credit is not strong or that there is significantly more risk to the repayment of those bonds than there is to an issue that is rated. It only means that the issuer of the bonds did not apply for, and pay for, a rating on that particular issue. In reality, the vast majority of healthcare issues that are able to obtain investment grade ratings do so, and most bond issues that are brought to market without at least one rating probably were not able to obtain an investment grade rating from a recognized rating agency.

When a rating is issued on a series of bonds, that rating applies only to that particular security and not the underlying borrower. While it is technically incorrect to refer to the credit rating of the organization, it is common to categorize organizations by the highest rating that they have been able to obtain on an outstanding debt issue that is not credit enhanced by another institution. When a corporation is referred to as "an A credit," this means that this particular corporation either has an A-rated bond issue outstanding, or it is the speaker's belief that the corporation could obtain an A rating if it issued a reasonable amount of bonds under its own credit at that time. Any organization may have different debt issues outstanding that hold different ratings either due to subordination to other debt, or based on a different level of security. An organization whose most senior debt is rated A may have debt outstanding that is rated BBB+/Baa if it is subordinated to the senior A-rated debt. Therefore, it would not be uncommon for that organization to be referred to as "an A credit."

There currently are three rating agencies that primarily are used to rate municipal healthcare bonds: Moody's Investors Service (Moody's), Standard and Poor's Ratings Group (S&P), and Fitch Investors Service, Inc. (Fitch). These are not the only firms that rate debt, but they account for virtually all the outstanding ratings on healthcare bond issues. Other rating agencies may be more popular for rating debt of institutions in other industries. Some bond investors value the ratings from one agency or another more highly than the others. As a result, a decision needs to be made as to the most effective rating, or ratings, to be used on an issue. Most rated healthcare bond issues are rated by two rating agencies, although many issues only carry one rating. Different underwriting firms have different preferences as to whether one or two ratings is desirable, and which rating agencies are preferable. This depends upon their customer base, as some customers have preferences for one rating agency over another, and some investors insist that all issues they purchase have two ratings.

■ Categories of Ratings

S&P and Fitch use uppercase letters to denote their long-term rating categories, with the rating of AAA (referred to as "triple A") being the highest, followed by AA ("double A"), A, BBB ("triple B"), BB ("double B"), B, and so on. Plus or minus signs after the letters indicate relatively stronger or weaker standing within the letter categories. Moody's uses a similar structure with an initial upper-case letter followed by one or two lowercase *a's*. The highest Moody's rating is Aaa ("triple A") followed by Aa, A, Baa ("B double A"), Ba ("B A"), B, and so on. Moody's indicates a stronger rating on municipal long-term ratings within a letter category by adding a numeral "1" as a modifier, but does not use a modifier to indicate weaker than average credits within a letter category. Thus a rating of Ba1 is higher than a rating of Ba. Figure 9-1 depicts the scale of long-term bond ratings used for tax-

---

Figure 9–1   A Comparison of Long-Term Bond Ratings for Tax-Exempt Healthcare Bonds

Moody's [1]	Standard & Poor's [2] and Fitch	Comparable Description [3]
Aaa	AAA	Highest quality
Aa	AA	Very high quality
A	A	High quality
Baa	BBB	Adequate or medium grade
Ba	BB	Speculative in some ways
B	B	Lacking some desirable characteristics
Caa	CCC	Demonstrates some vulnerable characteristics
Ca	CC	Very speculative
C	C	Lowest-rated class of bonds
	D	Bonds in default

(1) Those issues that are relatively stronger within a rating category may have a "1" added to the end of the rating.

(2) Those issues that are relatively stonger within a rating category may have a "+" added to the end of the rating.

Those issues that are relatively weaker within a rating category may have a "–" added to the end of the rating.

(3) See Appendix A for more complete information on the ratings provided by these three companies.

---

exempt healthcare debt by each of the three agencies primarily involved in the rating of healthcare bond issues. Other rating categories may be used for other types of healthcare debt, or for debt obligations in other industries.

When a bond issue is rated by more than one agency, the ratings typically are separated by a slash when presented together, and designated like A1/A+ or BBB+/Baa1. There is no established protocol for which rating goes first. When two agencies give ratings on the same bond issue that indicate different opinions as to the credit quality, it is called a "split rating." Examples of split ratings would be A/A1 and AD/Baa. When S&P or Fitch assign a rating with a "D" modifier, such as AD, Moody's offers no comparable rating. The result must be a split rating. The borrower in this example can only hope that Moody's chooses to assign an A rating rather than a Baa rating. Since each rating is assigned based on the credit criteria of each particular agency, it is possible for ratings to be widely split, such as A+/Baa, although it is unusual for ratings from different agencies to be split by more than one or two comparable degrees.

Ratings can be divided into two different broad groups: investment grade and speculative grade. *Investment grade* ratings compose the higher group, which includes long-term ratings of BBB-/Baa and higher. There are no healthcare organizations rated AAA, unless their bonds are credit-enhanced. *Speculative grade* ratings include all ratings of Ba1/BB+ and lower. The rating categories described above reflect long-term ratings for tax-exempt bonds. Different designations are used for short-term ratings and ratings for other types of obligations.

Bonds issued with speculative grade ratings, or no rating at all, are sometimes referred to as "junk bonds." This term is a misnomer in that it implies that there is little likelihood that the bondholder will receive payment of principal and interest on its investment. Certain situations can prevent an organization from obtaining a rating on its debt, thereby falling into the category of junk bonds, while the actual credit quality and likelihood of repayment on the bonds can be fairly high. As a result, any bonds that are not rated, or contain speculative grade ratings should undergo careful scrutiny before they are purchased so that the investor determines a level of comfort with the overall credit quality of the borrower before funds are committed.

In some cases, ratings from each of the agencies may be designated as "conditional." This means the rating is based upon the successful completion of a project or the occurrence of some specific event sometime in the future. Once the project is completed or the other necessary event has occurred, the conditional aspect of the rating is removed. There are other modifications that the agencies use to indicate certain characteristics of the debt to which a rating applies, such as when interest is not being paid on the bonds. Appendix A contains more detailed descriptions of each of the ratings supplied by the various rating agencies and the various modifiers that they each use. Please refer to Appendix A for selected information provided by each of the three rating agencies that are most frequently used to rate healthcare bond issues.

▌ The Relationship of Ratings to Interest Rates

Many institutional investors are precluded from purchasing bonds that do not hold an investment grade rating, so there are fewer potential buyers of speculative grade bonds. There tends to be a strong correlation between the rating of a bond issue and the relative interest that is paid on those bonds. For example, bonds that are rated A are considered to be of stronger credit quality and have a higher likelihood that principal and interest will be paid in a timely manner than bonds rated A− or lower. Since investing in A-rated healthcare bonds is perceived to entail less risk, investors will most likely be willing to purchase them at a lower interest rate than other healthcare bonds that are rated A− or less. The net result is the higher the rating on the bonds, the lower the overall interest cost to the borrower.

The spread between the interest rates that the market will demand for healthcare bonds with different ratings varies depending upon market conditions. For example, in a market where there is a shortage of bonds and many interested investors, it is likely that the spread between yields on bonds of different credit qualities will narrow. Yields on bonds rated A− will not be much higher than yields on bonds rated A. Conversely, in markets where many bonds are available, or fewer than normal investors are ready to purchase them, the spread between comparable bonds of different credit quality will likely widen. Issuers of bonds rated A− will have to pay a higher interest rate to induce potential investors to purchase those bonds rather than bonds that are rated A. As a result, it is extremely important for a healthcare organization to obtain the highest rating possible on its debt.

■ The Rating Process

Once a borrower has begun the process of developing a bond issue that will be rated, a decision needs to be made as to whether the issue should be rated on the borrower's own credit, whether the borrower should "enhance" its own credit with that of a bank or insurer, or whether the borrower should proceed on a "dual track" and keep both options open until the bonds are ready to be priced. If a rating is to be obtained on the healthcare organization's own credit, the rating agencies should be called to schedule a rating presentation to be held either at their offices or at the healthcare organization.

About two weeks prior to the meeting, the healthcare organization should send a package of information to the agencies. This package should include the following:

- audited financial statements for the past three to five years
- internal year-to-date financial statements compared to the prior year and to the budget
- management letters from the auditors for the past three fiscal years and management's responses
- historical utilization data for the past three fiscal years and for the year-to-date period for the current and immediately prior years
- projected payer mix, utilization and financial statements for the next three to five years, including relevant underlying assumptions
- description of current managed-care contracts and plans for dealing with managed care in the future
- description of any integration underway or planned
- information on competition (locations, size, and market share)

- most recent Joint Commission on Accreditation of Healthcare Organizations (JCAHO) letter and comments

- listing of the top-10 admitting physicians, their specialties, ages, percentages of total admissions, and any group practice affiliations

- per-case costs and rates for the 10 most active diagnosis related group (DRG) categories

- historical rate increases

- list of insurance claims paid during the past three years

- resumés on key management personnel

- demographic information on the service area

- preliminary sources and uses of funds statement and a debt service schedule

- drafts of the POS, the feasibility study, if any, and the relevant bond documents

- any other information that will help the agencies evaluate the credit of the borrower

The rating agencies will request any additional information needed at the time of the meeting.

It is very important that the rating presentation be carefully orchestrated, and that it communicate an accurate impression of the borrower. The presenters should take the process seriously because a bad impression could cost the borrower in its final rating, which could translate into a significantly higher interest cost. The rating presentation should include participation by the president of the healthcare organization, the chief financial officer, a board representative, chief of the medical staff, and any other key personnel that are necessary to communicate the strengths of the healthcare organization effectively. The overall goal of the presentation should be to convince the representatives of the rating agencies that:

1. the borrower understands its industry and the external factors that will affect its success in the future;

2. the borrower is preparing for the future with confidence and proactivity; and

3. the borrower is vital to the community and will pay off the debt issue as it comes due with little difficulty.

The following areas should be covered, as a minimum, in a good rating presentation:

- history of the organization
- organizational structure
- management experience and background
- nursing and labor relations
- service area
- market share and competition
- strategy for the next three to five years in terms of integration and coping with changes in the industry
- efforts in dealing with managed-care contract payers
- description of the board of directors
- board's role regarding the management and medical staff
- composition, credentials, and other information on medical staff members
- involvement and support of medical staff
- financial goals and policies
- budgeting and financial management
- control procedures and information systems
- overview of operating results
- discussion of insurance coverage
- discussion of the project
- the feasibility study, if any
- the upcoming bond issue and any unusual provisions in the bond documents

- strategic capital planning

- future capital needs and anticipated future financings

- any other areas that point out strengths of the organization

The healthcare organization's financial advisor and investment banker should assist in preparing for the rating agency presentations due to their frequent contact with the agencies. A well-organized presentation should result in the highest possible rating for the organization. If the bond issue is credit-enhanced, a presentation to the rating agencies should not be necessary, but presentations to the prospective credit-enhancing organizations may be requested.

In the event a healthcare organization receives a rating on a debt issue that it believes is not correct, each rating agency has an appeal process. In most cases, the agencies will not want to begin an appeal process unless the borrower can present some new information to support the claim that the initial rating was not correct. Borrowers should not hesitate to use the appeal process when they feel that a higher rating should have been assigned. If split ratings were assigned to an issue, it may be worthwhile to appeal the lower rating.

The rating agencies have recently begun to charge the same fees for credit-enhanced ratings that they charge for ratings on bond issues based on the credit of the borrower alone. Their primary argument is that they need to invest the same amount of time and effort in evaluating the underlying credit on a credit-enhanced bond issue in determining whether the credit enhancer's rating will remain the same after incurring the added potential liability of the bond issue.

The market has begun to take greater interest in the credit of the underlying borrower in credit-enhanced bond issues. The reason for this increased scrutiny is that a AAA/Aaa insured bond issue with an underlying credit of BBB/Baa may be more likely to be called prior to maturity due to a default on the bonds than an insured bond issue whose underlying credit is rated A. As a result, sometimes it is easier to sell insured bond issues with underlying credits in the A category than to sell bond issues with underlying credits in the BBB/Baa category. The rating agencies will release underlying ratings on the borrowers on credit-enhanced bond issues, if requested, and any borrower with an underlying rating of A or better probably is well advised to request that the underlying rating be released.

If a healthcare organization does not have an outstanding rating on any debt, the rating agencies are willing to perform a more cursory review and tell the prospective borrower what the likely rating would be on a proposed financing. This can be useful in developing the capital plan and evaluating the debt capacity of an organization.

Appendix A contains a significant amount of information provided by Fitch, Moody's, and S&P. This information is included to serve as a resource for healthcare organizations that anticipate working with these rating agencies in the future.

10 Credit Enhancement

The term "credit" generally deals with an entity's ability to repay its debt obligations and other liabilities in a timely manner. In some situations it is desirable, or necessary, to obtain *credit enhancement* on a bond issue—which means to increase the credit standing (or credit rating) of the bond issue above what it would otherwise be. When a bond issue is credit-enhanced, the credit risk becomes that of the credit facility provider rather than that of the underlying borrower. This means that the bond issue will be given a rating based on the credit strength of the credit facility provider rather than on the credit strength of the healthcare institution incurring the debt.

Credit facilities on healthcare bond issues almost always are provided by one of two sources: letters of credit from banks, or insurance from municipal bond insurers. Other forms of credit enhancement may be available from time to time, such as FHA insurance. A guaranty of the debt of an institution by a related entity with a higher credit rating, such as a parent corporation, also could be considered credit enhancement.

When a bond issue is credit-enhanced, bondholders must be protected from any event of bankruptcy on the part of the underlying borrower if the debt is to receive the higher credit rating. One of the key elements of current bankruptcy law is that it attempts to protect creditors from favoritism on the part of the debtor when bankruptcy is looming. If an entity goes bankrupt, some of the payments that it made for a certain period of time immediately prior to the filing of bankruptcy may be "disgorged" from the recipients of those payments. *Disgorgement* means that the bankruptcy court would attempt to reverse the payments and get the money back from the intended recipients. The intent of these laws is to make it so that a bankrupt entity cannot favor certain creditors over others when it becomes evident that bankruptcy is inevitable. The period of time prior to a bankruptcy during which disgorgement is allowed by law is referred to as the *preference period*. The most common preference period is 90 days, but some states require longer periods. Payments made to any creditor by the debtor during this period may be deemed by the bankruptcy court to be *preference payments,* and may be subject to disgorgement. Any bond issue that is substituting the credit of one institution for that of the underlying borrower must make provisions to insulate bondholders from any bond payments made by the borrower during the relevant preference period. This effort of protecting the bondholders is referred to as *preference proofing* the bonds, and it is necessary whenever bonds are credit enhanced.

▌ Bank Facilities

The most common form of credit facility provided by banks is a letter of credit. A *letter of credit (L/C or LOC)* is a document that requires the issuing bank to make payment, according to its terms, no matter what happens to the underlying borrower. In other words, the bank is obligated to pay even if the borrower goes bankrupt. With a *line of credit,* the bank is obligated to pay unless the borrower is bankrupt or in default of the line of credit agreement in some other way. A L/C provides both credit and liquidity to a bond issue, meaning that the bond trustee can draw funds under the L/C regardless of the financial condition of the borrower. A line of credit provides liquidity but does not change the credit, meaning that a bond trustee can draw funds under the line of credit only if the borrower is not in default of the line of credit agreement. When a line of credit is used, the rating of the bank is not transferred to the bonds.

The tightest possible line of credit would be one in which the bank is obligated to make payment under any situation other than if the underlying borrower is bankrupt. Beyond this, lines of credit can be structured so that there can be any number of different "outs" for the bank in which it will not have to make payment if the line is drawn upon. For this reason, when a bond issue uses a line of credit to provide liquidity, the underlying long-term credit rating on the bond issue is that of the borrower, not the bank. With a L/C backing a bond issue, the rating on the bonds reflects either the rating of the bank, or the rating of the underlying borrower, whichever is higher. There is little point in paying for a L/C if the rating of the borrower is higher than that of the bank, so it would be unusual to structure a bond issue with a L/C unless the intent was to obtain the rating of the bank on the bonds.

Letters of credit are used primarily to secure VRDB issues because the market requires a long-term credit rating of AA/Aa or better on the bonds for maximum buyer acceptance, which results in the lowest interest rates. Some VRDBs are issued with lower ratings, but their marketability may be limited. A L/C also provides the liquidity that a VRDB issue requires for the purchase of any bonds in the event they are put and not remarketed.

Some fixed rate bond issues are secured with L/Cs, although there are drawbacks to this structure if the maturity of the bonds exceeds the expiration date of the L/C. The primary drawback is that L/Cs are available only for periods of up to about 10 years, with maturities of three to five years being more common. This means that a long-term fixed rate issue will need to contain a special call provision, to be exercised if the bank does not renew its L/C. This special call provision may add to the interest rate on the bonds due to its conflict with the standard call protection of 10 years that is customary in the market.

Another drawback to securing a long-term (30-year) fixed rate bond issue with a L/C is that the borrower is limited to two ways of pricing the bonds, neither of which is ideal. The first way is to price the bonds for the full 30 years. In this case, the healthcare institution will pay a 30-year interest rate, but if the L/C is not renewed or replaced with a L/C of equal or higher rating, the bonds will be subject to a mandatory tender. The bonds will have to be resold at the then current market rate for the remaining maturity, with whatever rating the bonds hold at that time. The result could be that the borrower pays the higher 30-year interest rate but does not get the benefit of the fixed rate for 30 years.

The second way to price fixed rate bonds backed by a L/C is to set a mandatory tender at the expiration of the L/C. In this case, the healthcare institution pays a lower interest rate but automatically ends up with a variable rate financing because it is obligated to reprice the bonds every time the L/C is renewed, even if the same bank is willing to continue renewing its L/C. The net result of these two alternatives is that a borrower can price bonds either at a 30-year rate and risk having to reprice if the L/C is not renewed, or price at a shorter-term rate but be certain that the bonds will have to be repriced, thereby foregoing a fixed interest rate for the life of the bonds.

When a L/C is used to secure a bond issue, the bank typically will require a term loan agreement to provide for repayment to the bank in the event a draw is made on the L/C and the borrower is unable to repay the funds immediately. The L/C will be drawn upon if it expires and is not replaced before the bonds are paid off. The bank then is faced with a draw for the full amount of the L/C at the end of its term, which must be amortized by the borrower according to the provisions of the term loan. Most banks limit their total commitments to a borrower to 10 years, which includes the L/C and the term loan. Because of this, a five-year L/C usually will have a five-year (or less) term loan, and a seven-year L/C usually will have a three-year (or less) term loan. The bank will want to satisfy itself that the borrower can realistically pay off the entire obligation over the life of the term loan. The stronger the healthcare institution's credit, the more comfortable a bank should feel with a shorter term loan and, therefore, the longer the L/C can be. Some banks try to limit their total commitments to five to seven years, and a few will go beyond 10 years for a strong credit.

In a VRDB issue, if bonds are put and not remarketed for a predetermined period of time, the term loan goes into effect and the borrower typically loses the ability to resell the bonds in the public market. In other words, when the borrower is forced to begin amortizing the debt under the term loan, the L/C terminates. A potentially better way to structure the L/C is to have it run for the full term of the commitment, but reduce in later years as the bank's exposure would if there were a term loan. This would require the borrower to pay down the debt as if it were paying down the term loan, but the bonds would remain outstanding at a lower interest rate. Suppose a bank is willing to issue a five-year L/C, with a five-year term loan, for a total commitment of 10 years. The bank also might be willing to offer a 10-year L/C that reduces over the last five years just as the term loan would. The healthcare institution is better off during the last five years because the bonds remain in the market at the tax-exempt rate, rather than going to the bank at prime or higher. The bank is better off because it never needs to fund a term loan as long as there is market demand for the bonds.

One situation where this structure may be disadvantageous to the bank is if it plans to sell off part of its exposure under the L/C to a foreign bank. Many foreign banks will not accept L/Cs for longer than five years, so they would not be interested in taking part in a 10-year L/C. If a bank balks at this structure, it may be because it is planning on selling off part of the exposure. Selling off exposure under a L/C can lead to other problems if the bank also gives away its right to amend the documents without approval from the other participants. The borrower may find its bank less able to accommodate amendments to the agreement.

When a bond issue is backed by a bank facility, in the form of either a L/C or a line of credit, documentation is needed to formalize the agreement for the borrower to repay the bank if there is a draw that is not immediately repaid by the mechanics of the bond issue. In other words, if the bank facility is drawn upon and bonds are not remarketed immediately to repay the bank, the underlying borrower is obligated to repay the bank. These documents generally take the form of either loan agreements, or bank bond purchase agreements. Whichever document is used, it generally is desirable to structure it in such a manner that the underlying bonds are not extinguished at the time the bank facility is drawn upon. If a bond is *extinguished,* it is deemed to have been paid off and cannot be resold again. Since most bank facilities are used to back bond issues that are intended to stay in the public market, it would be unfortunate if the bond issue is terminated (extinguished) whenever there is a draw on the bank.

Borrowers should make sure the underlying repayment document to the bank is structured in such a fashion that the ability to resell the bonds is always maintained, without it being deemed a reissuance by the bond counsel. A *reissuance* implies that the old bonds were extinguished and new bonds are being issued when they are sold. This is an unfortunate situation for the borrower because there are certain provisions in the tax law that must be complied with each time bonds are issued. If, on the other hand, the documentation can be structured in such a way that the outstanding bonds are temporarily warehoused by drawing on the bank facility, instead of being extinguished, and those same bonds are then sold to new holders when they are found, then the borrower is spared the inconvenience, expense, and effort of having to comply with tax law for the issuance of new bonds. The borrower also avoids the risk that tax law has changed since the initial issuance of the bonds, perhaps prohibiting a feature of the old bonds.

Direct Pay versus Standby Letters of Credit

There are two basic types of L/Cs. The first is a *standby L/C* where the instrument is drawn upon only in the event there is a default on the part of the borrower. In other words, a standby L/C is drawn upon only when an unexpected event occurs. The other form of L/C commonly used in healthcare financings is referred to as a direct pay L/C. A *direct pay L/C* is used in bond structures where routine payments to the bondholders are made by the bank under draws on the L/C, and the bank is reimbursed by the borrower.

Direct pay L/Cs accomplish preference proofing because the payments to the bondholders come from the bank rather than from the underlying borrower. When payment is due on the bonds, the trustee draws on the L/C to make those payments and the underlying borrower repays the bank on the same day that the L/C is drawn upon. Because the bondholders never receive any payments directly from the borrower, they are not subject to disgorgement of any payments made by the borrower in the event the borrower goes bankrupt. The bank providing the L/C takes that risk. If the institution providing the L/C goes bankrupt, then the bondholders may be subject to disgorgement of any payments received during the bank's preference period, but that is the credit risk the bondholders took when the bonds were purchased.

Bond issues using standby L/Cs must preference proof the bonds in another fashion. When a bond issue is structured making use of a standby L/C, payments to the bondholders typically are made by the underlying borrower. The L/C will only be drawn upon if the borrower fails to make payments on time. If the borrower were to file for bankruptcy, the payments that it made during the preference period could be subject to disgorgement.

To avoid this, most bond issues of this type "age" any payments made by the borrower before they are passed on to the bondholders. The payments are held by the trustee for the applicable preference period. Once the preference period has passed and there has been no filing for bankruptcy, the funds are deemed to be "aged" and thereby preference proof. They can then be used by the trustee to make payments to the bondholders without fear that the payments might be disgorged at a later date. Because preference proof funds must be available to pay bondholders when bond payments are due, this structure requires the borrower to make its debt service payments to the trustee earlier, so the funds have time to age before being paid to the bondholders. This structure is more cumbersome than using a direct pay L/C, but it provides the bondholders with the same result of bond payments that are preference proof to any bankruptcy on the part of the underlying borrower.

Negotiating Bank Facilities

Fees on L/Cs and lines of credit typically are charged as a percentage of the total exposure on a per annum basis. For example, if the fees on a $10 million L/C were 1.0 percent per annum, the annual fee would be $100,000. In actuality, the fee most likely would be more than $100,000 due to a method of calculating interest and fees that the majority of banks use—unless the borrower is able to negotiate otherwise. Most banks calculate their interest rates and their fees on a formula that charges the borrower for every single day of the year, but calculates the daily charge as though there were only 360 days in a year. This is referred to as the "365/360 day" (pronounced "365 over 360 day") method or "actual over 360 day" method of calculating interest. As a result, the annual fee in our example would be $101,388.89. This is calculated by taking the 1.0 percent of $10 million, dividing it by 360 days to obtain the per diem fee, and then multiplying the daily fee by the actual 365 or 366 days in the year. In this fashion, bank fees frequently are higher than what the borrower might assume given a fee quote.

Banks often collect their fees on a quarterly basis (or more frequently), and at the beginning of the quarter. Again, unless it is negotiated otherwise, the borrower does not get the benefit of any reductions in the amount of exposure to the bank during that quarter, or other fee period, because the fee is paid at the beginning of the period when the exposure is the greatest. Banks often are willing to negotiate a feature whereby a credit will be given on the borrower's next fee payment in the event a reduction was made in the exposure to the bank during the preceding fee payment period. A more simple approach is for the fee to be paid in arrears, based on the average amount of exposure outstanding throughout the fee period.

During the 1980s, fees for bank facilities were very aggressive. It was not unusual to see fees on L/Cs from AA/Aa and AAA/Aaa rated banks as low as one-eighth of one percent per annum (.00125), or even lower. Fees for L/Cs have increased dramatically, and it is advisable for a borrower to seek competitive quotes from several banks before selecting one. The willingness of a bank to offer aggressive fees depends on the overall nature of its portfolio and the desire to add more business in this industry or product. As a result, a bank that was very aggressive in its fees several years ago may no longer be as aggressive today.

The primary reason that the fees on bank facilities have increased so dramatically is that banks are now required to fund reserves for most of these facilities. The amount of reserve that is required for each facility depends on how committed the bank is to funding that facility. For example, the reserve requirement for a L/C is greater than the reserve requirement for a line of credit, because the bank has a higher level of obligation to make payment on the L/C than with the line of credit. Likewise, a line of credit that is committed to for more than one year requires a certain reserve, but a line of credit that is committed to for less than one year, currently does not require any reserve. Because of this, fees on L/Cs generally are higher than fees for lines of credit, and lines of credit for more than one year cost more than lines of credit that have commitments of less than one year. Healthcare institutions are likely to find that the most economical bank facility they can obtain, to provide liquidity for a VRDB issue, is a line of credit with a commitment on the part of the bank for less than one year.

The primary disadvantage of a line of credit that is committed to for less than one year is that it requires frequent renewals. If a healthcare institution is able to obtain a five-year L/C, that institution will not have to worry about renewing that facility for at least four years. In the event the facility is not renewed by the bank, the healthcare institution has a full year to seek an alternative facility, or to refund the bonds. With a one-year line of credit, the healthcare institution will want to seek renewal at least every six months, so it will have a six-month period to find an alternate liquidity facility if the bank declines to renew the line.

Some banks are willing to offer facilities with an "evergreen" feature, where they automatically renew periodically unless they give the borrower notice. For example, if a bank is willing to provide a 364-day line of credit, it might be willing to include a feature where the facility automatically renews itself each week, unless the bank gives notice to the borrower that it declines to renew the line. This is a good alternative for the borrower because it may avoid the necessity of going through a formal renewal procedure every six months. The borrower knows the facility will always have just a few days short of a year remaining in the event the bank should decline to renew it. Given the desirability of shortening the exposure to the bank with the goal of reducing fees, an evergreen feature can be a very desirable feature for a borrower.

However the commitment from a bank is structured, the borrower should make sure that there is a provision for the bank facility to be terminated at the discretion of the borrower. This could be desirable if the bonds are paid off, converted to fixed rate, or a more attractive facility becomes available from another institution. Because the bank will have incurred some up-front expenses in structuring the credit facility, it is not unusual to provide for a termination fee if the facility is terminated within the first year. After that time, the borrower should have the ability to terminate the agreement without any penalty whatsoever. Most banks will charge initial fees to cover their up-front expenses in any case. Many bank agreements do not automatically contain termination provisions, in which case the borrower is obligated to make all the fee payments required under the facility, or negotiate a termination fee with the bank. Including these termination provisions in the initial negotiations can save the borrower a great deal of inconvenience and expense.

The borrower should also be able to terminate the bank facility without penalty if the rating of the bank drops below a specified level, usually AA/Aa. As discussed in the section on VRDBs, the market typically requires a AA/Aa rating on VRDB issues for broadest market acceptance. If the bank's rating on its own senior debt drops below this level, the rating on the bond issue is likely to drop as well, thereby reducing its marketability. If this happens, the borrower should be free to obtain a more marketable credit facility.

Bank facility agreements typically include a provision whereby the bank is allowed to increase its fee in the event certain additional reserve requirements or other governmental regulations that add to its cost for providing the facility are implemented. The borrower should maintain the ability to terminate the bank facility without penalty in the event the bank chooses to exercise its right to increase the fee under its existing commitment.

■ Bond Insurance

Municipal bond insurance is a form of credit enhancement that can be used to increase the rating on a healthcare institution's bonds to AAA/Aaa. Most bond insurers will not accept an issue for insurance unless they believe that it would be rated at least BBB-/Baa (the minimum rating for investment grade bonds) if it were rated on its own. Although most insured bonds receive ratings of AAA/Aaa, they tend to sell in the market more like bonds rated AA/Aa. This is because the market recognizes that a credit that is rated less than AAA/Aaa is the primary source of repayment on the bonds. In some markets, insured bonds sell at yields higher than AA/Aa bonds, and in other markets insured bonds sell at yields lower than AA/Aa bonds.

As more and more bond issues are insured, portfolio managers are attempting to select which of them will outperform the general market for insured bonds. To this end, they are looking "through" the insurance and evaluating the underlying borrower on many bond issues. If an underlying borrower goes into default, the bond insurer has the option of accelerating the bonds and prepaying them. In periods of lower interest rates than when the bonds were issued, it might be desirable for the bond insurer to exercise this option. The early redemption of an insured bond issue reduces the average life of those bonds and may be disadvantageous to the investment strategies of many portfolio managers.

There are six municipal bond insurance companies that currently account for virtually all the bond insurance in municipal healthcare finance. The three oldest firms—AMBAC Indemnity Corporation (AMBAC), Financial Guarantee Insurance Company (FGIC), and Municipal Bond Investors Assurance Corporation (MBIA)—are the three largest players in this market. AMBAC began issuing municipal bond insurance policies in 1971, followed by MBIA in 1974. Bonds insured by these three firms have traded at fairly comparable levels, offering the lowest yields available on insured bonds. The other three firms active in insuring healthcare bonds are Capital Guaranty Insurance Company (Capital Guaranty), Connie Lee Insurance Company (Connie Lee), and Financial Security Assurance Inc. (FSA). Bonds insured by these three firms typically have sold at slightly higher yields than bonds insured by the first three firms mentioned, but market conditions and perceptions change, so any borrower should investigate the differential in market acceptance and interest rates associated with the various bond insurers before committing to one. Information provided by these firms relating to their histories, policies, approval processes, and other topics is included in Appendix B.

Bond insurance is effective for the life of the bonds, so there is no danger of an insurer failing to renew its commitment. As a result, no special call provisions are needed on a long-term fixed rate issue as there are when a L/C is used. Bond insurance serves as a credit facility, with the bonds receiving the rating of the credit enhancer, but it does not serve as a liquidity facility. In other words, insurance provides for the payment of principal and interest when it becomes due, but not for puts on VRDBs or other instances that require liquidity. Bond insurance may be combined with a liquidity facility from a bank to enhance a VRDB issue as an alternative to a L/C.

The decision as to whether or not to use bond insurance usually is an economic one. An evaluation is made of the likely rating of the borrower without insurance, and then what the likely interest rate differential would be if the borrower issued bonds under its own rating compared to the insured rating. If the savings in interest expense are greater than the cost of the insurance premium, then it may make sense to use the insurance. Since the entire premium for bond insurance typically is paid when the bonds are issued, the likelihood of calling the bonds prior to maturity also must be taken into consideration in the decision process. Calling the bonds early will have the effect of increasing the overall yield on the bonds. This is because the insurance premium must be amortized over a shorter period.

There are other reasons why a healthcare institution may choose to use insurance. For example, bond documents frequently contain language providing that so long as the bonds are insured, amendments to the documents can be made with the consent of the bond insurer, and no consent is required on the part of the bondholders. If a healthcare institution feels that it may be necessary to amend its documents in the future, it may feel it will be easier to do so if it only has to obtain the consent of the bond insurer as opposed to many individual bondholders.

Bond Insurance Fees

Municipal bond insurance fees typically are charged as a percentage of the total principal and interest (total debt service) that will be paid on the bond issue. This formula makes it fairly difficult to compare bond insurance fees with L/C fees from a bank that will be paid annually. With the explosion of VRDB issues in the 1980s, some bond insurance companies established annual fees to provide credit enhancement on these issues so they could compete more effectively with bank facilities. While annual fees may be an option from some insurance companies on VRDB issues, the vast majority of bond issues that are insured are charged an up-front premium based on the total amount of debt service.

The amount of the premium charged on a bond issue will vary depending upon the creditworthiness of the underlying borrower, just as do the fees for bank facilities. As a result, it generally makes sense for the borrower to solicit competitive bids on fees for bond insurance so the borrower can determine which insurer is willing to be most aggressive on its fee at that time. The borrower then can have its financial advisor run an analysis on the fees proposed and the trading differential of each firm's name in the market to determine the best offer.

One disadvantage of the up-front premium paid to bond insurers is that it assumes the bond issue will remain outstanding for its entire life. Since most bond issues do not remain outstanding for their entire lives, bond insurance usually ends up being more expensive for the borrower than is anticipated at the time bonds are issued. Most bond insurance companies are willing to offer a lower premium for a bond issue that is refunding bonds that were insured by that same bond insurer. This certainly makes sense because the bond insurer has been paid for its exposure for the entire life on the bonds that are being refunded, and the exposure to the bond insurer will be virtually eliminated once the bonds are advance refunded. If the bonds are *advance refunded*, the bond insurance policy will only be drawn upon in the event there is a problem with the escrow of government securities that defeased the bond issue.

If the bonds are *current refunded,* the bonds are paid off, and the exposure to the bond insurer disappears on those bonds altogether. In either case, the bond insurer is let off the hook. (See Chapter 12 for further discussion of advance and current refundings.)

The lower fee that bond insurers typically offer on a refunding issue reflects a credit for the elimination of that bond insurer's exposure on the refunded bonds. In most cases, however, the credit that is reflected in the lower premium does not come very close to the premium that was paid to the insurer but not yet earned. The net result of this practice is that most bond insurers give enough credit on their premium for a refunding bond issue so it makes it very difficult for another bond insurer to outbid them. The amount of that credit generally does not come close to the value of the excess premium that was paid to that bond insurer for the exposure that ultimately resulted from the original bond issue.

Appendix B contains information provided by several of the municipal bond insurance companies. The information includes descriptions of the process of obtaining bond insurance, the philosophies of some of the companies, and the materials that should be provided to the bond insurers when a borrower seeks credit enhancement.

11 Key Covenants Found in Healthcare Bond Issues

Covenants are legal obligations of the borrower that are found in bond documents and other debt instruments, and are designed to protect the lender's ability to receive timely payment of principal and interest. A borrower violating a covenant is in default of the agreement containing the covenant. A default can result in different consequences depending on the terms spelled out in the document, the most severe of which may be an *acceleration* of the debt, requiring immediate repayment of the remaining outstanding principal.

As a rule, the stronger the credit, the fewer covenants the market requires. For example, a healthcare organization rated AA/Aa can issue debt with few covenants, while an organization rated BBB/Baa is likely to be required to comply with significantly more. Bond insurers and banks typically require a more restrictive set of covenants than the rating agencies. In addition, tax-exempt bond issues contain certain tax-related covenants that are not necessary for taxable issues. It is important for a healthcare organization to explore what covenants the market truly requires, as opposed to those suggested by members of the working group based on what they have used in the past. A good financial advisor or underwriter should be able to provide examples of current covenants that are satisfactory to the rating agencies, credit enhancers, and the market in general. Bond financings for healthcare organizations typically contain similar covenants, or at least covenants that address similar areas of importance to lenders.

■ Alternative Security for a Bond Issue

Prior to the early 1980s, it was common for healthcare organizations to secure their bond issues with mortgages on their primary healthcare facilities. In addition to a mortgage, they usually were required to pledge their revenues or gross receivables as additional security. A pledge on gross revenues and a pledge on gross receivables are considered equivalent by the market. Bond counsel differ as to which form of security is more appropriate or enforceable. Both attempt to achieve the same purpose of attaching any revenues of an organization after a default on the bonds.

Mortgages currently are rarely required by the market for healthcare financings with debt rated in the A category or better. A typical healthcare bond issue without a mortgage will still be secured by a pledge of revenues where all revenues of the organization would be available first to pay down bonds in the event of a default. In this case, there would also be a *negative pledge* on the borrower's healthcare facilities to prevent the borrower from giving a lien on the real estate to any other creditor. The strongest credits—A1/A+ or better—can get rated and sell bonds with just a negative pledge on both revenues and real estate. Many healthcare organizations believe that a negative pledge leaves them with more flexibility than a mortgage or pledge of revenues. This additional flexibility is questionable because these assets cannot be pledged to any other creditors. The true appeal may be that the healthcare organization appears to be a stronger credit when bonds are sold with only a negative pledge. Weaker credits (BBB/Baa and below) may be required to secure their financings with mortgages if they are to obtain the best possible interest rates.

■ Debt Service Coverage

Debt service coverage is a concept that is used in many of the covenants and tests found in healthcare bond documents. It measures the number of times that annual debt service on the bonds (principal and interest payments that are due that year) could be covered from the revenues that are available to pay debt service. The formula typically is stated as income available for debt service divided by annual debt service. Income available for debt service includes net income (profit) plus depreciation and interest expense. Income available for debt service is intended to include all the cash flow that the borrower generates and is available to pay debt service after the normal operations of the borrower are covered. Debt service coverage can be calculated for any period of time, but most tests evaluate either coverage for the most recent fiscal year for which an audit is available, or the income available for debt service relative to the maximum annual debt service in any future year—given the current debt outstanding and any proposed debt.

▮ Rate Covenant

A *rate covenant* requires a healthcare organization to charge sufficient fees to produce enough revenue to cover the debt service on its bonds by a certain amount, in addition to the revenue needed to operate the healthcare facilities. This coverage requirement is frequently set at 125 percent of annual debt service, but has been reduced on many financings to 110 percent. In the event that a borrower does not meet the required coverage, it may be required to retain a qualified consultant to review the situation and make recommendations to the healthcare organization that are intended to allow it to reach the required coverage in the following fiscal year. The borrower can avoid a default on its bond issue if it retains the consultant within a specified period of time and follows the consultant's recommendations. In the event that the coverage is not increased to the required level, the borrower usually is required to retain a consultant every two years. There should be a provision that allows the required debt service coverage to drop to 100 percent if a consultant's report is delivered to the trustee stating that government regulation has prevented the healthcare organization from obtaining the required coverage, and that the organization has operated so as to maximize its revenues.

▮ Liquidity and Excess Margin Tests

While not common in healthcare financings, some tax-exempt conduit issuers require covenants that obligate the healthcare organization to maintain a certain level of liquidity and/or earn at least a certain excess margin. The argument of these issuers is that the rate covenant does not warn the issuers and bondholders soon enough in many cases, with the result that the required consultant is not hired in time to be effective. The *excess margin test,* which requires a certain level of profitability or else a consultant must be retained, is intended to be triggered earlier than the normal rate covenant. The *liquidity covenant,* which requires that the borrower maintain a certain level of liquid assets such as cash or marketable securities, is intended to make sure that the resources are available to allow the borrower to continue operations for a longer period of time in the event of a problem, so the recommendations of the consultant will have time to take effect.

▮ Additional Debt Provisions

Additional debt provisions restrict the ability of the healthcare organization to incur additional indebtedness in the future. There normally are different covenants for long-term and short-term debt.

The ability to incur long-term indebtedness usually is restricted by several alternative sets of tests. There typically is one alternative that looks at historical debt service coverage of the projected maximum annual debt service of all long-term debt, assuming issuance of the proposed debt. If a healthcare organization can meet this test, then it can proceed to issue debt. As an alternative, the healthcare organization is allowed to retain a consultant to project expected coverage of maximum annual debt service for the two years following the completion of the project being financed. Until a few years ago, the coverage for these alternative tests typically was set at 125 percent. It is now common to see these tests at 110 percent for healthcare organizations rated in the A category or better. There usually is a provision similar to the one found in the rate covenant that reduces these coverage ratios to 100 percent in the event that a consultant's report can be obtained showing that government regulation prevented the healthcare organization from meeting the test. There is often a third alternative test that allows the organization to incur additional long-term debt if the total amount of long-term debt to be outstanding is not more than two times the amount of the fund balance of the healthcare organization.

Additional Debt Basket

In addition to the tests for additional debt described above, bond covenants should also allow the healthcare organization to issue a restricted amount of additional long-term or short-term indebtedness without meeting any tests. A common limitation is an amount not to exceed 25 percent of the prior year's total operating revenue. This provision is commonly referred to as a "basket" for additional debt.

Guarantees

Bond documents typically contain special provisions for the way certain forms of debt are to be treated for purposes of the debt service coverage tests. When a healthcare organization guarantees another party's debt—for purposes of calculating debt service coverage—the guaranty frequently is treated as though 20 percent of the amount of actual debt is incurred by the guarantor. The result is that the guarantor need only include 20 percent of the actual debt service requirement when calculating its debt service coverage. Some documents use a graduated approach where the amount of the guaranty treated as debt by the guarantor is dependent upon the debt service coverage of the actual debt by the party benefiting from the guaranty. In this case, the guarantor usually would be required to treat 100 percent of the guaranty as debt if the debt service coverage by the guaranteed party is below 125 percent, but it would not have to treat any of the guaranty as debt if the coverage by the guaranteed party is more than 200 percent. The amount of the guaranty that must be treated as debt of the guarantor decreases as the debt service coverage by the guaranteed party increases. Whichever method is used, in the event that the guarantor actually has to make a payment under the guaranty, 100 percent of the guaranty amount is treated as debt for a period of one year, and then the lower percentage goes back into effect.

Balloon Debt and Variable Rate Debt

Bond documents also should contain special provisions for the calculation of debt service coverage that allow for balloon indebtedness to be treated as though it is amortized over 20 to 30 years at an appropriate long-term rate. Balloon indebtedness usually is defined as debt in which 20 to 25 percent or more of the original principal amount is due in any one year. Similar provisions are made for variable rate debt, in that the borrower is allowed to assume a fixed rate for debt service calculations and a 20- or 30-year amortization if there is a put feature associated with the debt.

Other Debt Provisions

Subordinated debt, debt to complete the project being financed *(completion indebtedness)*, and debt incurred for the purchase of certain assets and secured solely by those assets without recourse *("non-recourse debt")* frequently are allowed without limit. Long-term indebtedness is also allowed for the purpose of refunding existing indebtedness, so long as the maximum annual debt service amount is not increased by more than 15 percent. In some cases, there are no restrictions on refunding debt.

In all additional debt sections, there should be a provision that allows debt incurred under one of the provisions just listed to be reclassified under another provision if the test for that provision can be met. An example of when this can be useful is when the healthcare organization wants to incur several smaller debt obligations under the basket, and then demonstrate compliance with the coverage tests only once for all to reclassify it all as debt incurred under one of the other tests. This frees up the basket to be used for the same purpose over again and avoids the necessity of proving debt service coverage for every small piece of additional debt.

■ Transfers of Assets

Covenants restricting transfers of the borrower's assets are intended to protect the bondholders' interest in the healthcare organization remaining a viable, revenue-producing healthcare facility. These covenants usually allow transfers of obsolete assets, sale of assets on an arm's-length (fair market value) basis, and transfers of assets that total a maximum of five to 10 percent of the total book value of assets in any year.

Frequently, an additional provision allows transfers of a greater amount of assets if it can be demonstrated that the borrower could have passed the additional debt coverage tests for the incurrence of $1 of additional debt, assuming the assets had been transferred prior to such calculation. In other words, more assets can be given away if the revenue producing capability of the healthcare organization is not reduced below a specified amount. In addition, current tax law restricts the transfer of property financed with tax-exempt debt.

■ Consolidation or Merger

These covenants typically allow a consolidation or merger if it can be demonstrated that the consolidated entity could pass the coverage tests for the incurrence of $1 of additional debt after the merger. Again, this test allows a merger if the revenue producing capability of the new entity is not below a certain amount. Evidence is also required that such a merger will not create a default under the terms of the bonds and will not adversely affect the tax exemption on any outstanding tax-exempt bonds.

■ Corporate Existence and Maintenance of Properties

The borrower is required to maintain its legal existence and to maintain its property in good working order. These covenants generally contain a series of common sense requirements such as complying with laws, paying taxes and assessments, making timely payments on debt, maintaining licenses, and maintaining tax-exempt status (if applicable).

■ Insurance

The borrower typically is required to maintain insurance in the form and amount customary for similar corporations and activities. There typically is a requirement for a review by an insurance consultant at least once every two or three years for commercial insurance, and more frequently for self-insurance.

■ Use of Insurance or Condemnation Proceeds

Covenants covering the use of insurance or condemnation proceeds require that if the proceeds of insurance or condemnation exceed a certain specified amount, then the healthcare organization will either repair or replace the facility that was affected, or use the proceeds to repay the debt that was issued to finance the facility. There may be exceptions to these requirements if certain coverage ratios can be demonstrated.

■ Limitation on Liens

Limitation on liens covenants limit the ability of any other lender to obtain a security interest that is prior (senior) to the interest of the bondholders in any of the borrower's property. It is customary to have certain exceptions to these restrictions that allow a limited amount of senior indebtedness, and for the exclusion of property not necessary for the operation of the healthcare organization.

■ Joining or Leaving the Obligated Group

In the event the financing contains an obligated group structure, there will be restrictions limiting the ability of entities either to join, or to be removed from the obligated group. These tests usually conform to the coverage tests for mergers and additional debt.

■ Default

In the event that any of the covenants contained in the documentation of a bond issue are breached, the borrower is potentially in default. The documentation of the bond issue will outline what has to take place for a borrower to be in default, and may contain certain grace periods during which the borrower may correct the problem and escape an actual default. In the event there is a default, the trustee of the bond issue generally has several possible remedies. The most severe remedy is to *accelerate* the bonds. This means that the trustee will declare all the principal and accrued interest due and payable as of a certain date, regardless of the maturity on each bond. In the event the bonds are accelerated, the borrower will be forced to attempt to repay the bond issue in full. In reality, the bondholder most likely will not be able to pay off all the bonds, otherwise, there would not have been a default in the first place. A trustee is most likely to declare a default and accelerate the bonds if it is determined that it will be beneficial to the bondholders to do so in terms of realizing on any security for the bond issue. If a trustee failed to accelerate the bonds and realize on any collateral, other creditors might get paid off first.

Some covenants do not require an acceleration of the bonds. For example, the remedy under a default of the rate covenant generally requires that a consultant be hired to evaluate the operations of the healthcare facility. As long as the recommendations of the consultant are implemented, the borrower is deemed to no longer be in default, for a certain time, even if the rate covenant still cannot be met.

▌ Funds Created in Bond Indentures

The trust indenture of a tax-exempt bond issue typically establishes certain "funds" for the purpose of holding moneys from specific sources and for specific purposes. Tax law requires that earnings on the moneys held in most of these funds that is in excess of the yield on the bonds must be rebated to the United States government. An exception to this rebate requirement is for a bona-fide debt service fund, which is the fund into which the borrower makes periodic payments of principal and interest. Under certain circumstances, the project fund may be exempt from rebate also, but if a project fund is not likely to earn a sufficient yield to require a rebate, it might be advisable to specifically include it in the rebate calculation to offset any excess earnings in other funds.

When any moneys held in any fund by a trustee are invested at yields that exceed the allowable yield on the bonds, this creates positive arbitrage. If the funds are invested at yields below what is allowed by tax law, this creates negative arbitrage. The actual amount earned in excess of the allowable yield is referred to as the *positive arbitrage,* and the actual amount earned below the allowable bond yield is referred to as the *negative arbitrage.*

Debt Service Fund

A *debt service fund* is created to receive payments from the borrowing organization and hold them until they are needed to make payments on the bonds. Sometimes this fund is called the *bond fund,* and sometimes it is divided into separate principal and interest subaccounts. Long-term, fixed rate, tax-exempt bond issues usually require semiannual interest payments, and annual principal payments. Deposits into the debt service fund typically are made monthly, quarterly, or sometimes only a few days before they are needed to make payment on the bonds.

In most situations, earnings on the debt service fund are exempt from rebate, unless the borrower chooses to include them in the rebate calculations. To be exempt, this fund must be deemed to be a "bona-fide debt service fund," and must be cleared out almost entirely at least once every 13 months. Certain other technical conditions must be complied with as well.

Project Fund

The *project fund* is a fund that is established under the trust indenture for the purpose of depositing the bulk of the proceeds of a "new money" bond issue that will be used to fund the project. If the project consists solely of construction, this fund is sometimes named the *construction fund.* The moneys in the project or construction fund are invested until their expected use. This can range from a very short period of time in situations where an organization will reimburse itself for its own resources that were spent on various projects, to very long periods of time for construction projects where draws will be made over a period of several years. As previously mentioned, in certain situations this fund can be exempt from the rebate requirement of the tax law, but it may or may not be desirable to make it exempt.

Debt Service Reserve Fund

A *debt service reserve fund (DSRF)* provides payment of principal and interest to bondholders for a period of time in the event the borrower fails to make its payments to the trustee. The purpose of such a fund is to provide a troubled healthcare organization with some time to correct its problems and resume making payments on the bonds before there is a payment default on the bonds.

Prior to the enactment of the Tax Reform Act of 1986, virtually all healthcare tax-exempt bond issues contained DSRFs equal to the maximum annual debt service on the issue, or sometimes set at amounts of 10 to 15 percent of the issue size. The Tax Reform Act of 1986 requires that the DSRF in a tax-exempt bond issue be limited in size to the *lesser* of (a) 10 percent of the bond issue; (b) the maximum annual debt service on the bond issue; or (c) 125 percent of the average annual debt service of the bond issue.

The tax law also made DSRFs subject to the rebate regulations. This made DSRFs less desirable from the healthcare organization's point of view, and many healthcare bond issues since 1986 have been sold without them. Prior to 1986, borrowers could keep any earnings of the DSRF. This provided incentive to include them in all tax-exempt financings. The 1986 tax law eliminated the upside potential of earning income on the DSRF in excess of the bond yield, but kept the potential downside risk of not being able to earn the bond yield on the fund, which would result in a cost of having the fund. With no recognized upside potential, borrowers began to push the market to accept bonds without DSRFs.

Healthcare organizations rated A or better probably can maintain their ratings on non-insured bond issues without including a DSRF. Most underwriters will tell them that a DSRF is not necessary for the successful marketing of their bonds. By not including a DSRF, the borrower can reduce the total size of the bond issue, thereby reducing issuance costs and reducing the amount of overall debt on its balance sheet. These are good reasons why there may be situations in which a healthcare organization may choose not to include a DSRF in its bond issue. In many cases, however, it is desirable to include a DSRF in a tax-exempt bond issue. There are at least two benefits that are foregone when no DSRF is provided for, and these are frequently overlooked by borrowers. The first is loss of all the insured bond funds as potential buyers. The second is the loss of the ability to make up negative arbitrage on construction funds, escrows, and even debt service funds in some cases.

Elimination of Insured Funds as Potential Purchasers—There are many bond funds that insure their portfolios. They are referred to as *insured bond funds.* They either purchase bonds that already are insured, or purchase uninsured bonds and then acquire bond insurance on those bonds even though the remainder of that bond issue continues to be uninsured. As a result, an uninsured bond issue may well end up having some of its bonds insured by some of the purchasers. For an insured fund to do so, the bonds must be *insurance qualified.* This means that the borrower could have obtained insurance on the entire issue if it had wanted to, and the requirements of the bond insurance companies have been met, even though the issue was not insured.

Currently, all the municipal bond insurers require either a funded DSRF, a surety bond, a letter of credit or, for stronger credits, a liquidity covenant with a requirement to fund a DSRF if the covenant is breached. The insured bond funds represent a significant portion of the institutional market that purchases most healthcare bonds. All these potential buyers will be eliminated if no provision is made for a DSRF, as outlined above. Fewer potential purchasers may lead to higher interest rates. The broader the appeal of a bond issue to different segments of the market, the lower the interest rate is likely to be.

Ability to Make Up Negative Arbitrage Created by Construction Funds, Debt Service Funds, and Escrows—Another good reason to include a DSRF is it may be used to recapture some negative arbitrage that is created in other funds. Since the debt service fund holds payments from the borrower until they are needed for principal or interest payments on the bonds, this fund will contain moneys that must be invested for less than a year. Some of the money in the debt service fund may be invested for less than 30 days. As a result, it is unlikely this money will be able to earn a sufficient yield to meet the allowable yield on the bond issue, thereby creating negative arbitrage. Likewise, most project funds are expected to be spent within three years. Again, the short periods of time for which these funds can be invested are likely to create negative arbitrage. Since the project fund is funded with bond proceeds, and since it frequently is the case that these funds cannot be invested at the allowable yield, there is a real cost to these funds until they are spent unless there is some mechanism to make up the negative arbitrage.

Perhaps the most significant situation where negative arbitrage is likely to be created is in an advance refunding escrow. Frequently, these funds cannot be invested at the allowable yield, due to market conditions. The size of the escrow and the length of time that it is invested below the allowable yield determine the magnitude of the negative arbitrage.

A DSRF can be invested for longer periods of time than these other funds, thereby frequently allowing it to earn positive arbitrage. In calculating the allowable yield on the bond issue, all the negative arbitrage created in the various funds is included in the calculation, thereby increasing the allowable yield above the interest being paid on the bonds. If there is no DSRF, there is no way to make up this negative arbitrage. If there is a DSRF, then the allowable yield is increased by all the negative arbitrage in these various other funds, and the borrower has the opportunity to invest the DSRF in as high a yield as it can possibly obtain until all the negative arbitrage is made up. Once the interest earnings on the DSRF have recouped all the negative arbitrage, the borrower will be required to rebate any excess earnings beyond the bond yield.

It must be pointed out that a fully funded DSRF may, itself, generate some negative arbitrage initially. An appropriate strategy, in this case, would be to invest the DSRF in relatively short-term securities until rates increase enough to gain back some of the lost income by investing in longer maturities. The question to the borrower is whether interest rates are expected to be significantly higher between the date of issuance and the final maturity of the bonds. A derivative investment alternative discussed in Chapter 13, called a debt service reserve fund put agreement, frequently can allow an organization to lock into a sufficient yield at any point in time (markets permitting) to cover all the allowable yield on its bonds. This product can allow the organization to assure itself that all the available negative arbitrage can be recouped, and alleviates the uncertainty of being able to reinvest the proceeds of the DSRF in the future at rates sufficient to obtain the allowable yield. It is a useful tool for outstanding bond issues as well as new issues.

A borrower that does not actually fund a DSRF with bond proceeds may be throwing away hundreds of thousands of dollars in lost investment income. In any case, the DSRF should not cost the borrower anything in terms of negative arbitrage, but it has the potential to make up all, or a significant portion of, the negative arbitrage created by other funds. It makes sense to fully fund the DSRF with bond proceeds in financings where there is significant negative arbitrage in a construction fund or escrow, and to consider providing for the bond insurance DSRF requirements in other cases.

Cost of Issuance Fund

The *cost of issuance fund* is created for holding bond proceeds (and sometimes funds of the borrower as well) that will be used to pay the costs of issuing the bonds. Current tax law limits the amount of tax-exempt bond proceeds to be used for the cost of issuance, excluding any fee for credit enhancement, to 2 percent of the total size of the bond issue. In the event the total cost of issuance exceeds the 2 percent limit, the borrower may be required to add moneys of its own to this fund so sufficient moneys will be available to pay all the anticipated costs of issuance.

Renewal, Replacement, and Depreciation Fund

The concept of a *renewal, replacement, and depreciation (RR&D) fund* recognizes that principal payments on a bond issue with a level debt service structure are relatively small in the earlier years of the issue and relatively large in the later years. Medicare used to reimburse healthcare organizations for depreciation on a level basis, over the life of the assets. As a result, there was a concern that a healthcare organization might receive depreciation reimbursements from Medicare but not be obligated to reduce the principal of bonds used to finance those assets in a like amount for several years. The RR&D fund was set up to hold excess depreciation funds until later years in the bond issue when principal requirements would exceed depreciation reimbursement. The RR&D fund is not required by the market anymore, but it is found in the documents of bonds issued in the 1970s and 1980s.

12 Refundings

A series of bonds issued for the purpose of providing for the repayment of another series of bonds, or other debt, is referred to as a *refunding*. Refundings usually are implemented either to take advantage of lower interest rates or to gain the benefit of a new set of documents and eliminate restrictions in the old documents.

If the proceeds of a tax-exempt bond issue are used to pay off an outstanding tax-exempt bond issue within 90 days from the date of the issuance of the new bonds, it is deemed to be a *current refunding*. If the proceeds of tax-exempt refunding bonds are deposited into an escrow to provide for the repayment of the old bonds as they come due until they can be called or they mature, and the final payment date is later than 90 days past the date of issuance of the refunding bonds, it is deemed to be an *advance refunding*. Advance refundings are necessary when the debt being refunded cannot be redeemed within the 90-day period immediately following the date the refunding bonds are issued. For example, most long-term tax-exempt bond issues cannot be called and redeemed at the option of the borrower for roughly 10 years from the date they are issued. Bonds that cannot be redeemed (paid off) within 90 days must be advance refunded, and redeemed from the proceeds of the refunding escrow when they mature, or can be called.

The Tax Reform Act of 1986 limits most tax-exempt bonds issued after 1985 to one advance refunding during their lives. Tax-exempt bonds issued for healthcare organizations prior to January 1, 1986, are allowed to be advance refunded twice, and are allowed one additional advance refunding if they already had been advance refunded two or more times prior to January 1, 1986. The effect of these rules is that every outstanding healthcare tax-exempt bond issue is allowed at least one more advance refunding as of the time the new tax law went into effect, and those issues that were issued prior to the effective date and have not yet been advance refunded are allowed two advance refundings. Under present tax law, there is no specific limit on the number of current refundings tax-exempt bond issues may enjoy. Taxable refundings (using taxable or tax-exempt bond proceeds to refund taxable debt) are not restricted in number by tax law, and are limited only by the specific provisions contained in the documents of the debt being refunded.

When a bond issue is paid off and the bonds are redeemed, the documents pertaining to the old debt are no longer effective, and the borrower is no longer constrained by the covenants contained in those documents. If the old debt cannot be paid off immediately, and the documents governing the old bonds allow it, the proceeds of the refunding bonds can be deposited into an escrow to pay off the bonds, either at an early call date or at their maturity. The money in the escrow usually is required to be invested in U.S. Treasury obligations, and the original security for the bonds is released. Once the escrow has been established and the old bonds are secured by a portfolio of U.S. Treasury obligations, the indenture that governed the old bonds is deemed to be *defeased,* after which the borrower is no longer obligated to comply with any of its provisions; nor is the borrower required to show the old debt on its balance sheet. For all practical purposes to the borrower, the debt has been paid off. To the bondholders of that debt, those bonds will remain outstanding until they are paid off by the escrow. If the borrower has the old bonds re-rated, they will be rated AAA/Aaa because they are now secured by obligations of the U.S. Government and no longer are dependent upon payments from the borrower for their repayment.

Refunding escrows must be set up to provide funds to make the required payments on the bonds when they are due. They may be made up of investments that are purchased in the open market (thereby creating *open market escrows)* or made up of special U.S. Treasury obligations referred to as *State and Local Government Series (SLGS),* which the Treasury will issue on a customized basis for the funding of tax-exempt refunding escrows. SLGS (pronounced "slugs") can be tailored to meet the specific needs of an escrow, with specific maturity dates to correspond with the due dates of the refunded bonds. They are issued at any interest rate that is needed as long as it is below the maximum rate offered for the SLGS of any given maturity. The maximum SLGS rates are always slightly below the rates at which U.S. Treasury securities of comparable maturities were sold at the most recent Treasury auction. The ability to subscribe for customized SLGS often allows tax-exempt bond refunding escrows to be 100 percent *efficient,* meaning that the maximum allowable yield is earned on the escrow. SLGS must be subscribed for prior to the time they are issued, and there are some other restrictions that must be complied with when they are used.

Treasury securities purchased on the open market mature on the dates specified on each security at the time it is issued, and it is not likely that those dates will coincide exactly with the due dates of all the refunded bonds. As a result, it is likely that securities in an open market escrow will come due a number of days before they are needed, due to the requirement for funds to be available when they are needed to make payments on the bonds. This often creates some inefficiencies in the escrows because the money sits uninvested for a period of time. However, there are some techniques for reducing or eliminating these inefficiencies that can be applicable in many cases, and open market securities usually can be purchased at higher interest rates than SLGS. Because of the added restrictions that must be followed when using SLGS to set up a refunding escrow, it may be preferable to use open market securities if the escrow can be made efficient. This might allow more flexibility in the future if laws change and there is an ability to restructure the escrow. The strategy for setting up the escrow is one that warrants careful evaluation by a borrower and its financial advisor because choosing the wrong strategy could be expensive for the borrower.

Open market escrows can be made more efficient if the payment dates on the bonds coincide with payment dates on the open market securities that are funding the escrow. To this end, it may make sense to consider making the payment dates on tax-exempt bonds on the fifteenth of the month rather than the first of the month. This is because most Treasury obligations make payments on the fifteenth of the month. If the payment dates on the bonds are also on the fifteenth, then any open market advance refunding escrow will be more efficient.

▮ High-to-Low Refundings

A *high-to-low refunding* is the term used for a refunding when the average interest rate on the new bonds is lower than the average interest rate on the old bonds. In a high-to-low advance refunding, it is preferable for the escrow to pay off the old bonds at the earliest call date, assuming there is not an excessive premium required to do so. This will allow the borrower to benefit the most from the lower average interest rate on the new bonds. As long as the old bonds remain outstanding, the borrower will have to provide for the higher interest rate to be paid on those bonds through the escrow.

To make matters worse, tax law limits the yield that can be earned on tax-exempt advance refunding escrow of tax-exempt bonds to the yield on the new refunding bonds. For example, if the tax-exempt bond issue being refunded is paying interest at 10.0 percent, and the tax-exempt refunding bond issue will pay interest at 7.0 percent, then the escrow will be allowed to earn only 7.0 percent. Because of this, for every dollar that is to be advance refunded, the borrower must fund the escrow at something more than $1 to make up for the shortfall in interest earnings due to the yield restriction. The borrower must incur a larger amount of debt in a high-to-low advance refunding than the amount of the outstanding indebtedness that is to be refunded. A one-time extraordinary loss is reflected on the income statement for the borrower in the year that the refunding bonds are issued. The greater the period of time that the escrow must remain outstanding, and the greater the difference between the old bond yield and the yield on the escrow, the larger this extraordinary loss will be.

To demonstrate this point with an oversimplified example, assume that a borrower has $70 of debt outstanding that is paying 10.0 percent per year, and that no principal amortizes for an infinite number of years. This means that the borrower is obligated to make an interest payment of $7 per year as long as the principal of $70 remains outstanding. If the borrower implements an advance refunding of this debt, and the interest rate on the refunding debt is 7.0 percent, then the borrower will need to fund the escrow with $100 in order for the escrow to provide interest of $7 per year. In this case, the borrower would show an extraordinary loss of $30 because the $70 of debt on its books has been replaced by $100 of debt. This example exaggerates the extraordinary loss because it does not take into account any payments of principal, but it demonstrates the concept of why a borrower must incur an extraordinary loss in a high-to-low advance refunding. The extraordinary loss is due to the need to fund the escrow with more principal than existed on the old debt because of the tax law requirement that the yield earned on a tax-exempt advance refunding escrow be limited to the yield on the new bonds.

The net present value savings to a borrower that takes advantage of a high-to-low refunding will equal roughly the present value of the difference in the interest rates between the old bond issue and the new bond issue, but only for the period of time from the call date on the old bond issue until the final maturity of the new bonds. There is no way for the borrower to enjoy any savings on the differential in interest rates for the period prior to when the old bonds are paid off, due to the yield restriction required by tax law. This assumes that the refunding bond issue is structured identically to the old bond issue in every way other than with different interest rates. Any additional deviations between the two bond issues will result in additional savings or added cost. Structuring the refunding bonds with an amortization that pays off the old debt over a longer period than the original amortization (i.e., a longer average maturity) will result in decreased gross savings, but the borrower will have the use of the bond proceeds for a longer time. Conversely, structuring the refunding bonds with an amortization that is shorter than that of the original bonds will increase the gross savings, but the borrower will have use of the bond proceeds for a shorter period of time.

Figures 12-1, 12-2, and 12-3 attempt to depict the concept that savings from a high-to-low advance refunding can only be derived for the period after the call date on the old bonds. Figure 12-1 depicts the debt service requirements of a bond issue with level debt service at an average coupon of 10.0 percent. Figure 12-2 depicts the debt service requirements of a refunding bond issue with level debt service at an average coupon of 7.0 percent. The dotted line at 10.0 percent, above the required debt service on the refunding issue represents the debt service requirements on the old debt. If the borrower could implement a current refunding and pay off the 10.0 percent bonds with the proceeds of the 7.0 percent bonds, then the savings would be represented by the area above the 7.0 percent debt service and below the 10.0 percent debt service of the old bond issue.

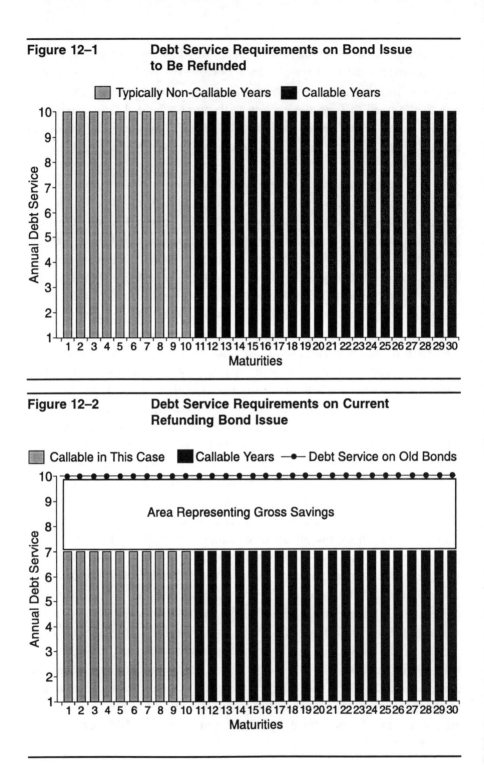

Figure 12–1 **Debt Service Requirements on Bond Issue to Be Refunded**

Typically Non-Callable Years Callable Years

Annual Debt Service

Maturities

Figure 12–2 **Debt Service Requirements on Current Refunding Bond Issue**

Callable in This Case Callable Years Debt Service on Old Bonds

Area Representing Gross Savings

Annual Debt Service

Maturities

Figure 12–3   Net Effect of High-to-Low Advance Refunding

Chart A

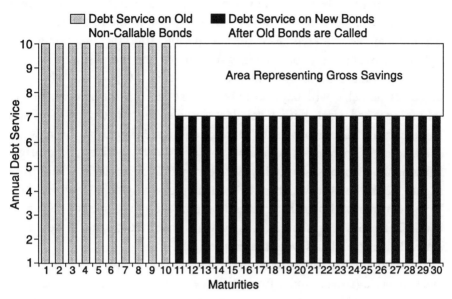

Chart B

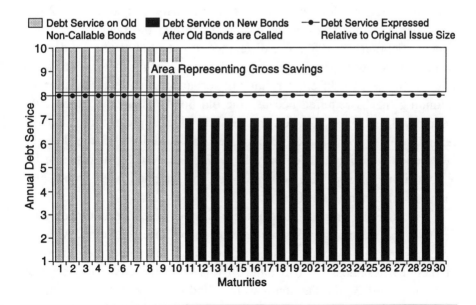

Figure 12-3 depicts the more typical situation where the borrower is not able to call the old bonds for 10 years and must provide for that debt service in an escrow. As depicted in Chart A of Figure 12-3, the escrow will provide for the payment on the old bonds at 10.0 percent until they can be called. The benefit of the new interest rate of 7.0 percent can be realized only for the period after the old bonds are called. However, the borrower will borrow an increased principal amount to fund the escrow, which can only earn 7.0 percent. While the borrower actually will pay the new interest rate of 7.0 percent on the refunding bond issue with level debt service, the amount of the issue has increased. The annual debt service requirement paid on the new issue size at 7.0 percent is equivalent to paying debt service on the original amount of bonds at roughly 8.0 percent. As depicted in Chart B of Figure 12-3, the borrower has realized savings equivalent to what could have been realized had there been a current refunding at about 8.0 percent. (The areas representing gross savings in Charts A and B would be equivalent if the charts were scaled precisely.)

Figure 12-4 shows a more precise numerical example of the difference in savings that results from an advance refunding of an issue with some non-callable bonds versus a current refunding of a bond issue in which all bonds are callable. In this example, bonds were first issued on February 1, 1983, at an average interest cost of 9.70 percent, in the amount of $20 million, and with a final maturity of February 1, 2013. The borrower in this example wanted to refund the bonds four years later on February 1, 1987. The difference in potential savings is demonstrated by comparing a column of statistics regarding the original bond issue with the two different refunding scenarios, one being an advance refunding that is required because the old bonds cannot be called until February 1, 1993, at 103 percent, and the other representing a current refunding under which the old bonds could be paid off on the date the new bonds were issued (February 1, 1987). The average interest rate for a bond issue on that date was 7.10 percent for bonds that would also mature on February 1, 2013.

Because the original bond issue could not be called until February 1, 1993, the refunding was structured as an advance refunding, with the proceeds of the new bonds placed in an escrow to pay off the old bonds at their earliest possible call date. In this case, the first call date was February 1, 1993, and the bonds were called at a 3 percent premium. To

Figure 12–4 **High-to-Low Advance Refunding versus Current Refunding**

	Old Bonds	New Bonds	
		Advance Refunding*	Current Refunding
Date of Issue:	2/1/83	2/1/87	2/1/87
Average Interest Rate:	9.70%	7.10%	7.10%
Maturity:	2/1/13	2/1/13	2/1/13
Principal Amount (2/1/83)	$20,000,000	—	—
Principal Amount (2/1/87)	$19,335,000	$22,700,000	$19,930,000
Annual Debt Service:	$2,064,750	$1,928,250	$1,692,790
Total Debt Service (2/1/87–2/1/13)	$53,683,550	$50,134,550	$44,012,600
Total Savings:	—	$3,549,000	$9,670,950
Gross Cost of Call Provisions:	—	$6,121,950	—

*First call date on old bonds is 2/1/93, at 103%

implement this advance refunding, a principal amount of $22,700,000 was required, which resulted in annual debt service of $1,928,250. This resulted in total debt service for this bond issue of $50,134,550 and gross savings of $3,549,000 compared to the original issue.

If the borrower had been able to implement a current refunding, whereby the old bond issue would be paid off on February 1, 1987, the principal amount of the new bond issue would have been $19,930,000, which equals the amount of outstanding bonds plus the cost of issuing the refunding bonds. The annual debt service on that bond issue would have been $1,692,790. This would have resulted in total debt service for that bond issue of $44,012,600, which would have resulted in gross savings compared to the original bond issue of $9,670,950.

The net effect of the requirement to leave the old bonds outstanding until the first call date (six years later) was that the borrower ended up paying a penalty of $6,121,950 over the life of the bonds. This reflects the cost of including the call restrictions at the time the original bonds were issued. Unfortunately, the borrower had no choice but to include the call restrictions at the time because the market would not have purchased the long-term bonds at any reasonable interest rate without call protection.

The purpose of this demonstration is to show that there is no way for a borrower to realize the savings of lower interest rates until the old bonds can be paid off. This is because the borrower still has the obligation to pay the higher interest rate on the old bonds as long as they are outstanding. A high-to-low advance refunding requires an increase in the bond issue size. The outstanding balance on the old bond issue as of February 1, 1987, was $19,335,000. The necessity of funding an escrow out to the first call date at the lower yield of the new bonds required that more bonds be issued to fund the escrow. In this case, the size of the advance refunding bond issue was $22,700,000, which reflected the cost of funding the escrow plus the cost of issuing the new bonds. The borrower would reflect an extraordinary loss due to this increase in debt outstanding, but would actually end up with gross savings of more than $3.5 million by implementing the advance refunding.

▌ Low-to-High Refundings

A *low-to-high refunding* means the average interest rate on the refunding bonds is higher than the average interest rate on the refunded bonds. When this is the situation, it usually is beneficial for the borrower to do an advance refunding and set up the escrow to pay off the old bonds as they come due until their final maturity. This gives the borrower the benefit of the lower interest rate on the old bonds for a longer period of time and results in a lower cost to the refunding.

Again, tax law requires that the yield on the escrow be limited to the yield on the refunding bonds. In this case, the yield on the refunding bonds is higher than the yield on the refunded bonds, so for each dollar of the old bonds that is to be refunded, the borrower needs to fund the escrow with something less than $1 due to the additional earnings that will be derived from the higher yield. For example, if the old bonds are paying interest at 8.0 percent, and the refunding issue will be paying interest on the bonds at 10.0 percent, then the yield on the escrow can be as high as 10.0 percent This will generate income in the escrow that is in excess of the 8.0 percent required to pay the bonds, so less money is needed to fund the escrow.

It is possible for a healthcare organization that is implementing a low-to-high refunding to eliminate any increased cash flow requirements due to the higher average interest rate through the appropriate structuring of the escrow. This is because the escrow can be invested at the higher rate of the new bonds, resulting in a smaller escrow required to pay off the old bonds. For example, (again ignoring the effect of principal on the calculation) if a borrower has a $100 bond outstanding that pays interest at the rate of 8.0 percent, then the borrower is obligated to pay $8 per year in interest. If that borrower refunds that bond at 10.0 percent, how much will need to be borrowed, and invested at 10.0 percent, to generate $8 per year? The answer is $80. In this situation, the borrower will be paying 10.0 percent rather than 8.0 percent, but will be paying that 10.0 percent on $80 rather than on $100, so the cash flow required for debt service on the refunding debt is the same as it was on the old bonds. This over-simplified example does not take into account the effect of the principal in the calculation, but it does demonstrate the effect that occurs in a low-to-high advance refunding. In most situations, the net result can be that the only cost involved in a low-to-high refunding is the actual cost of issuing the new bonds. If the escrow can be invested at the allowable yield out to the final maturity of the old bonds, the borrower should be able to negate the effect of the higher interest rate.

Figure 12-5 gives a more complete demonstration of the effects of a low-to-high advance refunding. In this case, bonds were issued on February 1, 1972, at an average yield of 5.90 percent, with a final maturity of February 1, 2002. The principal amount of bonds when they were issued was $20 million, and the borrower refunded these bonds on February 1, 1983, at current market interest rates. Even though the refunding bonds only had a remaining life of 19 years, the current interest environment at that time required an average yield on the refunding bonds of 9.95 percent. The principal amount of the new bonds to be issued was significantly lower than the remaining balance of $16,090,000 on the old issue because the escrow for the advance refund-

Figure 12–5   Low-to-High Advance Refunding

	Old Bonds	New Bonds	Difference
Date of Issue:	2/1/72	2/1/83	—
Average Interest Rate:	5.90%	9.95%	4.05%
Maturity:	2/1/02	2/1/02	—
Principal Amount 2/1/72:	$20,000,000	—	—
Principal Amount 2/1/83:	$16,090,000	$12,445,000	($3,645,000)
Annual Debt Service:	$1,431,655	$1,472,415	$40,760
Total Debt Service (2/1/83–2/1/02)	$27,201,450	$27,975,920	$774,470
Total Interest (2/1/83–2/1/02)	$11,111,450	$15,530,920	$4,419,470

ing was invested out to the maturity on the old bonds, and could earn the 9.95 percent average yield on the new bonds.

The issue size of the refunding issue was $12,545,000 (including cost of issuance), which was $3,645,000 less than the amount of outstanding bonds. This resulted in an extraordinary gain on the income statement of the borrower for that year, even though the organization would be paying higher interest rates for the life of the new bonds. The annual debt service on the old bonds was $1,431,655, and the annual debt service on the refunding bonds was $1,472,415. This reflects an increase of only $40,760 per year, which corresponds to the amortization of the issuance costs of the refunding bonds plus any inefficiencies in the escrow. Correspondingly, total debt service on the old bond issue, from February 1, 1983 to February 1, 2002, would have been $27,201,450, while the total debt service on the new bond issue will be $27,975,920 for an increase of only $774,470. This reflects the total cost of issuing the new debt and any inefficiencies in the escrow.

The total interest that would have been paid on the remaining original bonds was $11,111,450, while the total interest to be paid on the new bonds is $15,530,920 for an increase of $4,419,470. The outcome to the borrower was a significant increase in interest payments, coupled with a significant decrease in principal payments, for a net result that was equal to the cost of issuing the new bonds plus any inefficiencies in the refunding escrow. This demonstrates that a borrower frequently is able to go from a low interest rate on its tax-exempt bonds to a higher interest rate without bearing the full brunt of the higher interest costs, due to the ability to earn the higher yield in the refunding escrow.

▌ Historical Refunding Trends in the Healthcare Industry

During the 1970s, many healthcare organizations issued tax-exempt bonds with 30-year maturities and interest rates in the 7.0 percent range. Around 1980, the trend in the industry was to "restructure" healthcare organizations, and many organizations found their bond documents would not allow them to change their corporate structures in the ways they desired. Because of this, many of the outstanding tax-exempt bond issues were advance refunded in the early 1980s. Because interest rates were higher than they had been in the 1970s, these advance refundings were low-to-high advance refundings. The documents for the new bond issues often incorporated master trust indentures and the concept of an obligated group. This allowed the organizations to restructure as they wished, and gave them the flexibility for additional restructuring in the future.

In the early 1990s, interest rates dropped to the lowest they had been in 20 years. As a result, many of the bonds issued in the 1980s were advance refunded in high-to-low refundings for the purpose of reducing the interest rates. The healthcare organizations that implemented low-to-high advance refundings in the 1980s generated an extraordinary gain on their income statements in each of the years that a refunding was implemented. Those healthcare organizations that implemented high-to-low advance refundings in the 1990s showed extraordinary losses on their income statements in the years in which the refundings were implemented. The markets and the rating agencies tend to be very understanding about extraordinary gains and losses resulting from refundings. As a result, they generally have little effect on an organization's credit standing.

■ Crossover Refunding Bonds

Crossover refunding bonds are issued for the refunding of outstanding indebtedness, like all refunding bonds, but the proceeds are placed in an escrow to defease or pay off that indebtedness at a later date rather than immediately. In a normal advance refunding, the old bonds are defeased concurrent with the issuance of the refunding bonds. A crossover refunding does not defease the old debt until some date in the future. As a result, the borrower usually is required to show both the old debt and the new debt on its balance sheet until the old debt is either defeased or paid off. Although many uses for crossover bonds were eliminated under the Tax Reform Act of 1986, they are still used when it is desirable to issue bonds but not implement the actual refunding until some future date. The date on which the escrow is broken and the outstanding indebtedness is paid off or defeased is referred to as the *crossover date.*

One of the primary uses of crossover bonds in the early 1980s was to provide a fixed rate backup for a VRDB issue. A drawback of VRDB issues is that there could be certain situations in which it would be desirable for the borrower to convert the bonds to a fixed interest rate, or refund the bonds at a fixed interest rate, but it may be at a time when fixed interest rates are unattractively high. Crossover refunding bonds allowed the borrower to implement a fixed rate refunding of its variable rate issue at a time when fixed interest rates were favorable, but to invest the proceeds of the refunding issue at the fixed interest rate of the refunding issue, thereby incurring no additional interest expense. The earnings on the escrow covered the interest cost on the refunding bonds until they were used. The escrow typically would secure the crossover refunding issue until the crossover would take place.

For example, assume a borrower is paying roughly 3.0 percent on a VRDB issue. It would issue crossover refunding bonds at the fixed rate of 7.0 percent. The proceeds of that refunding issue would be deposited into an escrow and invested at 7.0 percent. A crossover date would be established at which time the securities in the escrow would mature and would be available to pay off the VRDBs. In the event the borrower chose to keep the VRDBs outstanding, the escrow could be reinvested, once again at 7.0 percent, and a new crossover date established. The borrower in this example could enjoy the low interest cost of the VRDB issue while being assured that the worse-case scenario would be to implement a crossover at 7.0 percent at some point in the future.

This use of crossover refundings eliminated the risk of higher interest rates in the future when a conversion to fixed rates might be desirable. However, the Tax Reform Act of 1986 severely restricted the ability for borrowers to utilize this structure by requiring that any advance refunding escrow must be used to call the refunded bonds at the earliest possible call date if the refunding was likely to result in a lower interest rate to the borrower. Because the interest rate on a VRDB issue could potentially exceed the fixed interest rate on the refunding bonds, it was determined that typical VRDBs need to be called at the earliest possible call date. Because most VRDB issues can be called on 30 days' notice, this eliminated the benefits of that strategy. Other uses for crossover refundings may offer a borrower some advantage from time to time, so it is beneficial to understand how they work.

■ Forward Purchase Contract Refundings

For borrowers unable to issue advance refunding bonds at a given point in time due to tax law restrictions, a technique using a forward purchase contract may provide a mechanism to lock in some of the savings that could have been derived from a refunding of outstanding high-coupon bonds that cannot be called for several months or years. This technique involves the use of a *forward purchase contract* between the borrower and a counterparty, which stipulates that the counterparty will purchase the borrower's tax-exempt bonds at a future date. The date of purchase frequently is the call date of the bonds that the borrower would like to refund. All terms of the future issue are specified in the contract, including the interest rate. The rate takes into account market conditions at the time the contract is signed, a premium reflecting the investment rate on funds to the date of the delivery of the bonds, and the reduced liquidity of the contract compared with the borrower's bonds in the cash market.

Various mechanisms are available to assure the borrower that the counterparty will deliver payment on the future date, and the contract also details the consequences if tax law changes or other developments prevent the bonds from being issued on that date. This structure may be an alternative for healthcare organizations that have exceeded the permitted number of advance refundings for a particular issue, or that wish to lock in their borrowing cost in advance of issuing bonds for a new money issue. Forward purchase contracts are covered in greater detail in Chapter 13, including an additional refunding technique to the one just described.

▌ Restructuring Advance Refunding Escrows

Restructuring a refunding escrow is the process of replacing existing escrow securities with more effective qualified investments that produce the same cash flows over time. The transaction is effected to reduce the investment cost of an inefficient escrow account employing open market securities. An *inefficient escrow* is one in which the investment yield is not equal to the allowable bond yield. Benefits vary, depending on the size and maturity of the escrow as well as the yield spread.

A critical determinant as to whether, and to what degree, an escrow may be restructured is the bond rate on the advance refunding issue and the extent to which a yield shortfall currently exists. An escrow yield verification will determine any potential savings from a restructuring. Bond counsel and the trustee should be consulted at the outset to ensure a legal and conforming transaction.

13 Derivatives

Prior to the enactment of the Tax Reform Act of 1986, a significant amount of creativity was demonstrated in healthcare institution financing. Exploring options beyond conventional ("vanilla") fixed rate financings, healthcare institutions issued VRDBs, tax-exempt commercial paper, pooled financings, and other creative vehicles to achieve their financing objectives. Financings subject to the new tax law tended to lack creativity for some time after it became effective on January 1, 1986.

The introduction of derivative products to the healthcare industry several years later breathed new life into the creative juices of the professionals who finance healthcare organizations. New financing structures were developed that provide benefits to borrowers and bondholders alike. The structures tend to be complex, but the benefits can be significant and genuine. Likewise, the potential risks that some of these instruments bear can be significant and genuine.

The term *derivative* implies that the benefits of an instrument are derived from another source. For example, the interest rate on a *derivative bond* might be derived from (or dependent upon) an interest index from another market, or the benefit of a fixed rate might be derived from an interest rate swap entered into at the time variable rate bonds are issued. The term is frequently used loosely to mean almost any unconventional or sophisticated financial product.

The demand for derivative products has exploded in recent years. These are complicated instruments, and the effects of various interest rate movements on the return that a holder of these securities will receive can be difficult to understand. Most underwriting firms will sell these securities only to "sophisticated" investors and not to "widows and orphans," as the general public is sometimes referred to. There has been some negative press about derivative products, but most of it has dealt with bondholders that may not have understood what they were buying. It is appropriate for borrowers to limit the sale of these securities to institutional investors, but a borrower should not necessarily be put off by negative press about derivatives, as the risks to the borrower tend to be identifiable, quantifiable, and less than the risks to the bondholder. An educated borrower can save significant sums by making appropriate use of derivative products, while saving significant additional sums by appropriately managing or avoiding the risks involved in their use.

Utilizing derivative bonds to obtain fixed rate financing at a lower interest cost is one of the primary uses of derivatives by the healthcare industry. Derivative products are engineered to provide specific benefits to potential purchasers of the securities. A purchaser of these securities should be willing to pay something—in terms of a lower interest rate—for these benefits. The benefit to the borrower in a fixed rate derivative financing is the lower interest rate that the purchaser is willing to accept.

There are two main types of derivative financings that result in fixed rate interest exposure to the borrower: those that use an interest rate swap as an integral part of the structure, and those that do not rely on an interest rate swap. Both are referred to as *synthetic* fixed rate financings because no fixed rate bonds are ever issued. The first general form of synthetic fixed rate financing is accomplished by issuing variable rate bonds with certain characteristics, and then entering into an interest rate swap to change the interest exposure of the borrower to a fixed rate. The other common form of fixed rate derivative financing is where the total financing is made up of two or more variable rate financings that result in a fixed interest exposure when added together.

The most common form of the latter type of derivative financing is where the issue is divided in half, with one half of the issue floating with the market, the other half floating inversely to the market, and both pieces moving in tandem so that the combination of their rates always equals the fixed rate. Each investment banking firm that uses derivatives comes up with its own names for them, and this form of derivative is quite common under many different names. The concept of splitting the issue into parts can be carried to the extreme where the cash flow of the payments made by the borrower on the bonds is sold off in many different parts that always add up to the fixed cash flow of the bond payments. These various tax-exempt payment streams frequently are designed to imitate characteristics of taxable securities with which the market is familiar. The ability of these securities to behave like taxable instruments, which are understood and accepted by the market, while providing tax-exempt income, makes them very attractive to some purchasers.

This chapter reviews several of the more prevalent derivative products being used by healthcare institutions, including some of the structures referred to above that result in synthetic fixed rate financings at lower interest rates than conventional fixed rate financings. Once these basic structures are understood, it should be easier to grasp new forms of derivative products as they are introduced to the healthcare industry.

The specific derivatives that will be covered are: interest rate swaps, embedded swap bonds, Dutch auction bonds, inverse floaters, forward purchase contracts, float contracts, and debt service reserve fund put agreements. *Interest rate swaps* are the basis of many of the derivative products in the market today. *Embedded swap bonds* usually result in lower interest rates for borrowers than conventional bonds. *Dutch auction bonds* are an alternative to VRDBs. *Inverse floaters* are floating rate bonds that can be used to generate fixed rate financings at lower interest rates than conventional bonds when combined with either floater bonds or interest rate swaps. *Forward purchase contracts* allow borrowers to lock into current fixed interest rates for bonds issued sometime in the future. *Float contracts* are a form of forward purchase contract where the borrower locks into a fixed yield for the investment of funds that periodically will be deposited into a debt service fund for payments on a bond issue, or any other fund (including a refunding escrow) where a determinable amount of money will become available for investment in the future. *Debt service reserve fund put agreements* allow borrowers to avoid market risk on the investment of a debt service reserve fund, at no cost to the borrower.

New derivative products constantly are being developed. This discussion is not intended to be exhaustive, but it will give a general understanding of current derivative products that should allow a quicker understanding of new derivatives as they become available.

■ Interest Rate Swaps

An *interest rate swap* is a contractual obligation between a party and a counterparty for the exchange of payments based on two different interest formulas as they relate to a single notional amount. Each party in the transaction refers to the other party as the *counterparty*. The *notional amount* is equivalent to the principal amount of a debt instrument, but it never becomes due and payable. Payments due under an interest rate swap are the result of the interest rate formulas, with no payment of the notional amount. The counterparties offering to enter into swap transactions with healthcare organizations tend to be large financial institutions such as banks, insurance companies, and investment banking firms. Most interest rate swaps are written with terms of 10 years or less, although a few counterparties will write swap contracts for as long as 30 years.

At least one party to an interest rate swap pays based on a variable interest rate. The other party usually pays a fixed interest rate. For example, a party might enter into an interest rate swap based on a notional amount of $30 million and agree to pay a fixed interest rate of 5.00 percent. This results in an annual payment obligation of $1.5 million. In return, the counterparty agrees to pay a variable interest rate on the $30 million notional amount equal to some variable index, such as a percentage of short-term Treasury obligations, LIBOR, or some tax-exempt index. Payment obligations are netted out on the payment dates, so the party with the fixed obligation would be required to make a payment to the variable counterparty if, and to the extent that, the variable rate averaged less than 5.00 percent. Conversely, the fixed party would receive a payment to the extent the variable rate averaged more than 5.00 percent during the period.

Swaps are most commonly used by healthcare institutions to offset interest rate exposure on a debt instrument. Swaps make it possible to change the interest exposure from fixed to variable, or vice versa. For example, note the effect of the swap transaction depicted in Figure 13-1.

Figure 13–1   SWAPS—Flow of Funds

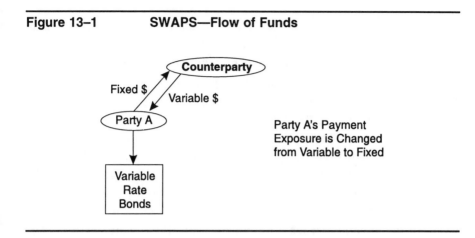

Party A's Payment
Exposure is Changed
from Variable to Fixed

In this example Party A, a healthcare provider, has variable rate bonds outstanding. Management of Party A determines that it would be beneficial to have a fixed interest exposure on the bonds, and enters into an interest rate swap with a counterparty. The notional amount of the swap equals the par amount of the variable rate bonds outstanding. The payment dates on the swap could be set up so they coincide with the interest payments due on the bonds. Under the terms of the swap, Party A receives a periodic variable payment from the counterparty equal to the interest exposure on Party A's variable rate bonds. Party A is required to make fixed payments to the counterparty based on a fixed interest rate as it is applied to the notional amount. Because Party A's interest exposure on the variable rate bonds is totally offset by the payments from the counterparty, the remaining obligation of Party A is the fixed payments to the counterparty. Party A's exposure has changed from variable to fixed, without refunding the variable rate bonds.

As previously mentioned, the payment obligations on an interest rate swap are netted out on each payment date. In the current example, Party A will only be required to make a payment to the counterparty whenever the variable rate under the swap (which generates payments to be *received* by Party A) averages less than the fixed rate (which generates payments to be *paid* by Party A) for that period. The amount of the payment will equal the amount of the fixed payment less the amount of the variable payment. Similarly, Party A will receive a payment from the counterparty whenever the variable rate exceeds the fixed rate for that period.

It is important to note that Party A continues to be obligated to make the payments required under the variable rate bond issue. The swap does not change those payment requirements. Instead, the swap offsets part, or all, of those required payments so that the net effect on total payments to be made by Party A is changed.

In the example, Party A has a variable rate bond issue outstanding that corresponds to the variable payments received from the counterparty. The payments due on the bonds are offset, or canceled out, by the payments received under the swap contract. The counterparty would be taking a risk if it does not have some payment obligation that corresponds to the payment stream that it will receive from Party A under the swap. In fact, counterparties usually hedge, or offset, their risk by entering into other interest rate swaps to balance out their exposure. An example of how this works is depicted in Figure 13-2.

Building on the previous example, the counterparty enters into a second swap with Party B. This swap with Party B cancels out the counterparty's exposure on the swap with Party A, and the counterparty makes a profit by earning a spread on each contract. For example, if the variable payment obligation of the counterparty is pegged to a particular index, then the variable payment that the counterparty will receive under the swap with Party B will be on the order of that same index plus 10 basis points (.10 percent). The 10 basis point spread is the profit that the counterparty makes. Likewise, if the counterparty is obligated to make a fixed payment of 5.00 percent under the swap with Party B,

Figure 13–2   **SWAPS—Flow of Funds**

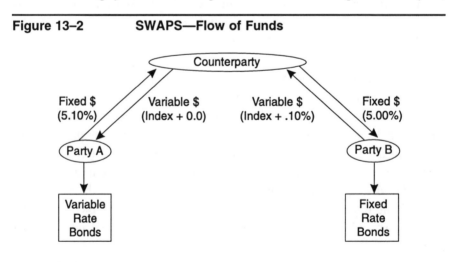

then the counterparty will be receiving a fixed payment of roughly 5.10 percent under the swap with Party A. If the counterparty has a perfectly balanced book of interest rate swaps, it can make significant profits with little, or no, risk. The counterparty acts as a middleman. Party A and Party B are not aware of each other. There are other ways that counterparties can also hedge their exposure on interest rate swaps, but this method is employed by every swap dealer because it happens automatically, to some extent, as each swap is booked.

Basis Rate Swaps

When a swap contract is written where both parties are obligated to pay variable rates, the contract is referred to as a *basis rate swap*. In this type of interest rate swap, the variable interest rate that each party pays will be calculated on a different basis. For example, one party might be obligated to pay on an interest formula based on LIBOR, while the other party makes payments based on U.S. Treasury obligations. The effect of a basis rate swap is that it allows a party that has a contractual obligation to make variable payments based on a particular index or formula to convert that payment obligation to some other basis. For example, a healthcare institution might have a VRDB issue outstanding with an obligation to make payments based on an index published by J. J. Kenny Co., Inc. In the event the borrower chooses to convert its payment obligation to a formula based on U.S. Treasury obligations, it could enter into a swap where it is obligated to make payments based on U.S. Treasuries while it receives payments based on the J. J. Kenny index, thereby offsetting its payment obligations under its bonds. Once again, the net effect of entering into this basis rate swap is to change the ultimate payment obligation of the borrower from one based on a tax-exempt index to one based on U.S. Treasury obligations.

Appropriate Uses of Interest Rate Swaps

As described above, one use for interest rate swaps is to change the payment exposure on existing debt from fixed to variable, or vice versa. An example of an appropriate use of this approach might be where a borrower wants to advance refund fixed rate tax-exempt bonds and end up with a variable rate exposure. When tax-exempt bonds are advance refunded, it is very difficult to do so with variable rate debt, due to tax laws. If a borrower desires to advance refund tax-exempt fixed rate bonds with variable rate bonds, it could issue fixed rate bonds to accomplish the refunding, and then enter into an interest rate swap with a similar notional amount at a later date to change its exposure to a variable rate. Tax counsel should be consulted to make sure that the swap is structured so that it is not included in the yield calculations of the refunding bonds.

Another example of an appropriate use of an interest rate swap might be in a large fixed rate issue of bonds, where a significant portion of the proceeds is going into a construction fund. Because the construction fund will be drawn down over two or three years, those funds will be invested in securities with relatively short maturities. It may not be possible to find short-term securities with yields as high as the long-term bonds, thereby creating an additional cost to the project. It might be possible to enter into an interest rate swap with a notional amount equal to the amount of the bond proceeds deposited into the construction fund, and reducing according to the expected draws on the construction fund. The swap would change the payment exposure for the construction fund from the long-term fixed interest rate to a short-term variable rate. In return, the borrower would receive a short-term fixed rate that would partially offset the interest exposure on the bonds. It may be possible for the borrower to purchase investments that will equal the new interest exposure, which is equal to the short-term variable rate paid by the borrower under the swap, plus the spread between the bond rate and the rate on the fixed payments that the borrower receives under the swap. This technique may work under some market conditions and not in others.

Another use for interest rate swaps is to create synthetic types of debt. The term *synthetic* applies to debt structures where variable rate bonds are issued but the net interest rate exposure to the borrower is a fixed rate, or fixed rate bonds are issued but the net interest rate exposure to the borrower is variable. In essence, interest rate swaps are entered into at the time the bonds are issued to change the nature of the interest exposure for the borrower. Synthetic bonds are used when they can provide the borrower with lower interest rates than conventional bonds. These bond issues can be structured so that the swap either is, or is not, taken into account when calculating the yield on the bonds for tax purposes. When the swap is an integral part of the bond issue, and included in yield calculations, the structure is called an *embedded swap bond*. This type of structure will be discussed in greater detail later in this chapter.

Caps, Floors, and Collars

Certain versions of interest rate swaps called "caps" and "floors" can be useful to healthcare borrowers. A *cap* is a contract where the counterparty will pay the difference whenever a variable rate goes above the cap rate. This may be appropriate in a situation where a healthcare institution has variable rate debt outstanding or about to be issued, and it does not want interest exposure above a certain level. For example, a borrower may desire to issue variable rate bonds, but not be willing to risk that variable rates could go above a certain level. If the current rate on variable rate bonds is at 4.0 percent, a borrower might find it desirable to purchase a cap at 6.0 percent so that the net interest exposure will not go above 6.0 percent for the life of the cap. The counterparty would pay the difference whenever interest rates exceed 6.0 percent.

In most cases, the borrower will have to purchase a cap based on some popular index that closely resembles the interest exposure on the borrower's debt, rather than on the actual exposure on the debt itself. In this situation, the counterparty would pay when the index exceeds 6.0 percent regardless of what the actual rate on the borrower's bonds is. This sort of transaction is most common so that the counterparty is shielded from the risk that a credit problem with the borrower could cause the interest rates on the bonds to exceed the cap even when the market remains stable. Some underwriters offer specific types of variable rate bonds for which they will be willing to issue a cap that exactly matches the borrower's interest exposure, thereby eliminating the risk that an interest rate index will not exactly match the actual interest exposure.

A *floor* is the converse of a cap. In a floor, the party (borrower) agrees to pay the difference when a variable rate goes below a certain level. It is not unusual for a borrower to buy a cap by selling a floor. The net result is a variable rate financing that will never go above the cap rate, or go below the floor rate. The combination of a cap and a floor is referred to as a *collar*, because interest exposure is prevented from going above the cap or below the floor. Figure 13-3 depicts the effects of a cap, a floor, and a collar.

Advantages of Interest Rate Swaps

The primary use of interest rate swaps is to change the interest exposure on a debt obligation from fixed to variable, or vice versa. This is beneficial because the nature of the borrower's payment exposure can be changed without refunding the bonds. Current tax law limits the number of advance refundings of tax-exempt financings, so interest rate swaps can provide some additional flexibility. Refundings are also expensive, and interest rate swaps can be implemented relatively inexpensively.

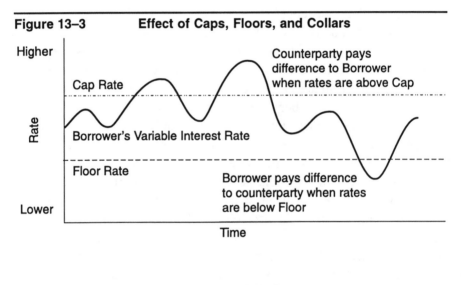

Figure 13–3   Effect of Caps, Floors, and Collars

Cap: Borrower buys a cap so that variable interest exposure will not go above the cap rate.

Floor: Borrower may sell a floor to pay for the cap. Floor makes it so that the Borrower will not benefit if rates go below the floor rate.

Collar: When both a cap and a floor are in place, Borrower's variable interest exposure is collared, meaning it can not go above the cap rate, or below the floor rate.

Swaps can be entered into fairly quickly, and the documentation is relatively standardized. Virtually all swaps use the documentation and terminology developed by the International Swaps and Derivatives Association, Inc. (ISDA), which was formerly known as the International Swap Dealers Association, Inc. The primary document used for swaps is known as the *master agreement*. There is a separate ISDA document entitled *U.S. Municipal Counterparty Definitions* that contains the definitions used by the industry for swap contracts. This second document also sets out forms for the confirmation of a swap transaction. The *confirmation* is a document consisting of a few pages that details all the specifics of that particular swap transaction that are not covered in the generic master agreement.

Another advantage of interest rate swaps is that they can be reversed by entering into a *reverse swap contract*. For example, assume Party A has entered into an interest rate swap where it is obligated to make fixed payments and receive variable payments. Party A can later enter into another swap where it is obligated to make variable payments that coincide with the variable payments that it is receiving under the first swap, in return for a new fixed payment based on current market conditions. While reversing an interest rate swap is quite possible, it is important to remember that the counterparty takes a spread on each side of the transaction, thereby creating inefficiencies in this procedure. Reversing an interest rate swap may be costly, but it also may result in a profit if interest rates have moved in a favorable direction. Swaps are always entered into at current market conditions. As a result, the market will determine whether a profit or loss is realized when an interest rate swap is reversed.

Disadvantages of Interest Rate Swaps

The primary disadvantage of swaps is *counterparty risk*. This is the risk that the counterparty in the transaction will fail to make its payments as required under the swap contract. Most counterparties will be willing to collateralize their position in a swap contract, but the rates on collateralized swaps may not be as favorable as swaps that are not collateralized. Yet collateralization of a swap contract can reduce counterparty risk significantly.

Another risk associated with many swap transactions is *basis risk*. This occurs when the interest rate formula on an interest rate swap contract does not exactly match the interest rate formula on the debt that the party is trying to hedge, or offset. For example, a borrower may have an outstanding VRDB issue that is priced each week by the remarketing agent. If the borrower decides to convert its payment obligation to fixed rate by entering into a swap, it is likely that the only swaps available will be based upon some index that is regularly published and readily available to the public. Currently, the most common of these for a tax-exempt based interest rate swap would be either the J. J. Kenny Index or the Public Securities Association (PSA) Index. Because it is unlikely that the borrower's interest rate will track either of these indexes exactly each week, the borrower will be taking some basis risk in this swap transaction. Conversely, if the borrower has a VRDB issue outstanding in which the interest rate is calculated based on an index, then it may be possible for the borrower to enter into a swap to convert its ultimate payment obligation to a fixed rate with no basis risk at all. This can be accomplished when a swap is available with payments based on the same index as the interest rate on the bonds. There are some structures where basis risk can be completely eliminated, and some where the risk can be significant. Only careful evaluation by a knowledgeable party can determine the extent of basis risk.

Most interest rate swaps are written with terms of 10 years or less, although there are a few counterparties that will write them for up to 30 years. Swaps with maturities beyond 10 years sometimes are referred to as *long-dated swaps*. Some financings have been put together where an interest rate swap is needed throughout the life of the bonds to give the borrower the desired interest exposure, but the swap does not run for the life of the bonds. This situation leaves the borrower exposed to future market risk when either a new swap contract must be found, or the borrower will no longer enjoy the benefit of a swap. Newer financing structures have eliminated this problem either by entering into longer-term interest rate swaps to match the maturities of the bonds, or using an embedded swap structure where the nature of the interest rate exposure on the bonds changes when the swap expires.

The bottom line on interest rate swaps is that they can play an important role in the capital planning for a healthcare institution, but there are certain risks that should be evaluated for each swap transaction. The most reliable way to ensure that the best possible interest rates are achieved in an interest rate swap contract is to competitively bid the swap. Purchasing an interest rate swap from a counterparty without checking other market bids is likely to result in less favorable rates.

When having a financial advisor bid out an interest rate swap contract, the borrower would be well advised to make sure that the financial advisor is independent and has no vested interest in the outcome or the process. In at least one situation, a healthcare institution asked its investment banker (who was also acting as the borrower's financial advisor), to bid out an interest rate swap contract—under the belief that this process would result in the most aggressive bids. The investment banker/financial advisor took bids, but had instructed all potential bidders that a fee of several hundreds of thousands of dollars would have to be paid to that investment banking firm as a fee, and netted out of the swap contract. As a result, the healthcare institution thought that it received competitive bids, but they were all overpriced by the same fee to the investment banker. The healthcare institution had no way of knowing, and probably thought that it had received the best deal the market had to offer. Instead, the financial advisor should have been asked to disclose to the borrower any additional compensation that was to be received from any other source.

▌ Embedded Swap Bonds

Another common use for interest rate swaps is in embedded swap bonds, where the swap is an integral part of the bond. Embedded swap bonds usually offer lower fixed interest rates to a borrower than conventional bonds, although market conditions sometimes reduce the benefit to negligible levels. Figure 13-4 depicts a generic structure for embedded swap bonds that results in a fixed interest rate exposure for the borrower. Most embedded swap bond structures can be explained by the process outlined here. New embedded swap bond structures are sure to develop, but this example will give a basic understanding that should allow a quicker learning of new structures as they are introduced.

Most embedded swap bonds are divided into two distinct periods, the period during which the swap is in effect, and the period after the swap expires. The notional amount of the swap equals the principal amount of the bonds. In this example, the interest rate on the bonds is

Figure 13–4   Embedded Swap Bonds

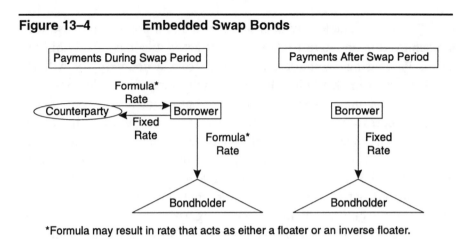

*Formula may result in rate that acts as either a floater or an inverse floater.

variable during the swap period, and it becomes fixed when the swap period ends and continues that way for the remaining life of the bonds. Some structures are used where the swap remains in effect for the life of the bonds, but most swap counterparties will not issue interest rate swaps for more than 10 years.

During the swap period, the borrower pays a formula rate on the bonds. The formula is set according to what is attractive to the market at the time the bonds are sold. The formula rate is floating in this example, and it may react to market changes in any way that the purchaser of the bond wants. The formula rate may float with the market or float inversely to the market (move in the opposite direction that the market moves). It may provide for a single interest rate reset at a future date, or it may float with frequent interest resets until the end of the swap period. It may be leveraged so that it moves in wider swings than the market, i.e., it is more volatile than the market.

When the formula exaggerates the volatility of interest rate swings relative to the market, the instrument is then referred to as a *turbo* bond. The turbo is the multiplier by which market swings are exaggerated. A turbo of two would cause the interest rate to fluctuate with twice the volatility of the market. A turbo of three would cause the interest rate to fluctuate with three times the volatility of the market, and so on. The interest rate formula also may include a cap or a floor to limit its volatility. It may have any combination of these features, and others as well. The formula is specifically developed to give prospective bondholders what they want in terms of interest characteristics. In return, the bondholder is willing to accept a lower interest rate during the fixed rate period after the swap expires.

During the swap period, the swap provides for the borrower to receive the formula rate from the counterparty. This should completely offset the borrower's interest exposure on the bonds during the swap period. The borrower pays a fixed payment to the counterparty during the swap period, equal to the fixed interest rate on the bonds after the swap period. The net result to the borrower is a fixed interest exposure throughout the life of the bonds, at a lower rate than it would have had to pay if it had issued conventional bonds. The lower rate is achievable because the bondholder wants to receive the formula rate during the swap period.

After the swap period, swap payments are no longer made, and the borrower pays the fixed rate on the bonds. The bondholder receives the formula rate on the bonds during the swap period, and the fixed rate for the remaining life of the bonds after the swap period. Many investment banking firms now offer embedded swap bonds under different names. In most cases, the structures of these various bonds follow the structure outlined here, with the differences occurring in the formulas that are in effect during the swap period.

The formula that is most desirable to a potential bondholder will depend upon that bondholder's outlook for interest rates during the swap period. That is why the most desirable formula cannot be determined until the bonds are ready to be sold. Traditionally, official statements describing bond issues tended to describe only the bonds being issued. The advent of these different derivative bonds has made it desirable to describe several different types of bonds in the POS. This allows the borrower to offer a full menu of options on the formula rates of various embedded swap bonds. The purchasers choose which formulas they are willing to pay up for, in terms of a lower fixed interest rate after the swap period. The final OS then describes only the types of bonds that actually are issued. This approach ensures that the borrower will make available to prospective bondholders the formulas they most prefer.

Many embedded swap bond structures contain an additional feature to benefit the bondholders. This feature is an ability to convert the interest formula on any of the bonds to the fixed rate at any time during the swap period. To exercise this option, the bondholder is required, in essence, to buy out the swap at current market conditions in order to convert the interest formula to the fixed rate. The borrower generally is indifferent to this option because it continues to pay the same fixed rate throughout the life of the bonds, regardless of whether the bondholder exercises this conversion option or not. There are some situations, however, where this conversion option on the part of the bondholder may result in unfavorable tax consequences for the borrower. Qualified tax counsel should be consulted before bonds are issued with this conversion feature to determine any possible undesirable consequences.

This discussion of embedded swap bonds has focused on structures that result in a fixed interest exposure for the borrower. Since the term "embedded swap" only refers to the concept that the swap is an integral part of the structure, it is also possible to structure embedded swap bonds where the net interest exposure to the borrower is variable. The most common structure involves issuing fixed rate bonds and simultaneously entering into an interest rate swap agreement to create a synthetic variable rate bond. The advantage of this type of structure is that it does not require any liquidity facility as VRDBs do. It may offer advantages to some borrowers but, again, the borrower must evaluate any potential risks compared to the expected incremental value of using this type of structure.

▌ Dutch Auction Bonds

Dutch auction bonds are a form of variable rate bond that may be used alone, for variable rate financing, or with inverse floater bonds to implement a fixed rate financing. The easiest way to describe Dutch auction bonds is to contrast them with VRDBs. With VRDBs, the interest on the bonds is reset periodically so that the rate always reflects a current short-term rate. The most common format for this reset period is every seven days. In addition to having the interest reset frequently, the holder of a VRDB has the right to put the bond back to the trustee on short notice. The interest rate is reset either by a remarketing agent or by an index. When a VRDB is put, the remarketing agent attempts to remarket the bond to someone else. In the event that the remarketing agent is unable to remarket the bond, there must be a liquidity facility to provide a mechanism to purchase the bond from the bondholder and hold it until it can be resold. VRDBs can be issued for any maturity, but the interest rate always reflects the short-term market because of the short interest-reset period.

Figure 13-5 shows a summary of the comparison of Dutch auction bonds and VRDBs. Dutch auction bonds can have a long-term maturity, like VRDBs, but there is no put option on the part of the bondholder. The rate on a Dutch auction bond is reset periodically, usually every 28 or 35 days, at an auction. The auction process also provides the liquidity for a bondholder to sell the bond so the borrower does not have to provide any liquidity facility. The bondholders are dependent upon the periodic auctions to set the rate on the bonds and to provide a mechanism for selling the bonds.

Figure 13-6 demonstrates how a Dutch auction works. On each auction date, bids are collected from prospective purchasers of the bonds and are ranked from the lowest interest rate to the highest. In this example, there are five bids with the lowest bid being 2.90 percent and the highest being 3.15 percent. The issue size is $20 million. While Bid-

Figure 13–5	Variable Rate Demand Bonds versus Dutch Auction Bonds	
	Variable Rate Demand Bonds	*Dutch Auction Bonds*
Long final maturity	X	X
Rate reset frequently	X	X
Rate reflects current short-term market	X	X
Rate reset by Remarketing Agent	X	
Bondholder has right to put bond	X	
Requires liquidity facility	X	
Rate reset by market at periodic auction		X
Bondholder depends on auction for liquidity		X
Does not require liquidity facility		X

Figure 13–6 Dutch Auction Process
$20 million bond issue

Bidder	Rate	(000) Amount	(000) Allocation
#1	2.90 percent	$5,000	$5,000
#2	2.95 percent	$10,000	$10,000
#3*	3.00 percent	$10,000	$5,000
#4	3.05 percent	$5,000	–0–
#5	3.15 percent	$20,000	–0–

*Clearing bid—interest rate for next period is 3.00 percent

der #1 offered the lowest interest rate of 2.90 percent, that bidder only wanted $5 million of bonds. Likewise, Bidder #2 offered to purchase $10 million of bonds at a rate of 2.95 percent. In the Dutch auction process, the interest rate is set at the lowest bid that will provide offers to purchase all the bonds. In this example, the "clearing bid" is Bid #3 at the rate of 3.0 percent, which will provide enough bids to purchase a total of $25 million in bonds. Since there are only $20 million of bonds available, an allocation process must occur. Bonds are allocated with first priority to the lowest bidder, then the next lowest, and so on until all the bonds have been allocated. The result of this is that although Bidder #3 offered the clearing bid, and desired to purchase $10 million of bonds, Bidder #3 will only be awarded $5 million of bonds because that is all that is available after the orders for Bidder #1 and Bidder #2 have been filled. All bondholders end up receiving the same interest rate until the next auction, and the bid process gives bondholders an incentive to bid aggressively, since the most aggressive orders will be filled first. Bidders #4 and #5 did not receive any bonds because the clearing rate was below the interest rates that they were willing to accept.

Dutch auction bonds have an advantage over VRDBs in that no liquidity facility is required, but the borrower assumes the risk for any problems occurring in the auction process. For example, if the borrower develops any credit problems, potential bondholders may be hesitant to bid for the bonds at the auction, resulting in a failed auction. In this event, the interest rate reverts to a default rate, which usually is significantly higher than what the auction rate would be. The existing bondholders are required to continue to hold their bonds since no one else is willing to buy them, but the borrower is now required to pay the higher default interest rate. Borrowers interested in using Dutch auction bonds for a variable rate financing must be aware that any potential savings due to the lack of a need for a liquidity facility may be offset by the potential risk of a failed auction if there is ever any credit concern on the part of the market. The risk of a failed auction can be alleviated by a borrower when a Dutch auction bond financing is combined with an inverse floater financing to construct a fixed rate bond issue—a financing structure that will be discussed later in this chapter.

Another potential disadvantage of Dutch auction bonds is that they generally require a fairly large issue size. Many institutional investors that typically purchase short-term paper like this are prohibited from purchasing more than 10 percent of any single bond issue. Some are limited to as little as 5 percent of an issue. Many of these investors like to purchase several millions of dollars of an investment at a time. As a result, most underwriters who sell Dutch auction bonds are reluctant to offer to sell an issue of less than $20 million. Some underwriters are hesitant to sell an issue of less than $50 million.

■ Inverse Floaters

The term *floater* applies to any variable rate bond that moves *with* short-term interest rates in the market. This would include VRDBs and Dutch auction bonds. The rate is reset frequently on floaters so that the interest rate on the bonds reflects the current short-term market. The rates on *inverse floaters* are also set frequently, but the rate moves *inversely* to the market, i.e., when short-term rates go up, the rates on inverse floaters go down. Inverse floaters are attractive to investors who believe that short-term interest rates will decline, or at least not increase significantly before these bonds can be sold. Inverse floaters are initially sold at rates higher than current market rates, so there is some cushion for the interest rate to move before the bondholder would have been better off purchasing a different type of bond.

The purchasers of inverse floaters tend to be institutional investors who normally invest in long-term fixed rate bonds. The initial rate on the inverse floaters is set higher than the interest rate that could be obtained on conventional long-term bonds, so the investor is better off if the average rate throughout the life of the inverse floater is higher than what the fixed rate was for the alternative investment of a conventional long-term fixed rate bond. For example, assume that the interest rate for long-term fixed rate bonds is 6.25 percent. If an inverse floater can be issued at an interest rate of 9.00 percent, than a purchaser of that inverse floater will be better off if the rate on that inverse floater averages something greater that 6.25 percent over its life. The 2.75 percent spread between the conventional long-term rate and the inverse floater rate means that for every day the inverse floater is paying 9.00 percent, there can be a day where it is paying a rate as low as 3.50 percent, and the bondholder will be no worse off than if conventional long-term fixed rate bonds had been purchased at 6.25 percent.

This example demonstrates why a bondholder might be interested in purchasing an inverse floater when the expectation is that interest rates will be declining, or that rates will not be increasing significantly for the foreseeable future. The perspective of a borrower, however, is somewhat different. It is unlikely that a borrower would choose to issue inverse floater bonds without some form of hedge to protect the borrower from swings in interest rates. Such a hedge can be obtained in the form of an interest rate swap to create embedded swap bonds, or by combining an inverse floater with a Dutch auction bond to create a fixed rate financing. Figure 13-7 depicts an example of a combined floater/inverse floater financing where an inverse floater is combined with a Dutch auction bond or some other floater to provide such a fixed rate financing.

∎ Combined Floater/ Inverse Floater Financings

The purpose of utilizing this type of financing—as with embedded swap financings—is to provide a long-term fixed interest rate that is lower than what could have been obtained through issuing conventional bonds. For this type of financing, the issue is split in half. One half of the bonds are sold as floaters, and the other half are sold as inverse floaters. In the example depicted in Figure 13-7, the long-term interest rate for conventional bonds is 6.25 percent. For this financing, a target rate is set at 6.00 percent, resulting in a 25 basis point savings for the bor-

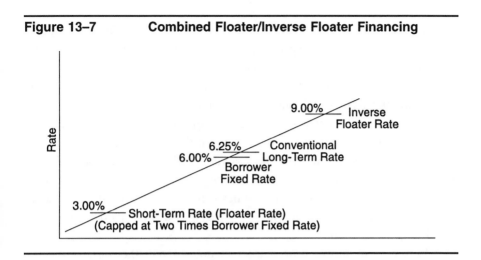

Figure 13–7   Combined Floater/Inverse Floater Financing

rower. To arrive at the 6.00 percent interest rate, the current short-term rate is determined. In this example, the market rate for short-term securities of a comparable rating is 3.00 percent. It is necessary to put a cap on the short-term rate for the floater portion of this financing in order to ensure a fixed rate for the borrower. The cap on the floater bonds is set at two times the borrower fixed rate. In this example, the cap is 12.00 percent. As with most floaters, the half of the bond issue that is sold as floater bonds will always be reflective of the current short-term market each time its rate is reset.

The borrower pays the equivalent of 6.00 percent on *all* the bonds. For every $100 of bonds in this example, the borrower pays a total of $6 in interest. If current short-term rates are 3 percent, the borrower pays 3 percent on $50 of bonds, or $1.50. The inverse holder receives the remainder of $4.50, which is a 9 percent return on the other $50 of bonds. The floater bondholder always receives the current short term interest rate, up to the cap. The interest that goes to the inverse floater bondholders will equal the 6.00 percent that is paid by the borrower, plus the remainder of the 6.00 percent that is available to be paid on the floaters (this residual amount could be a negative number that would result in a return lower than 6.00 percent to the inverse floater bondholder). In this example, there is a 300 basis point (3.00 percent) spread between the 3.00 percent short-term rate and the 6.00 percent borrower fixed rate. This means that the inverse floater bondholders will receive their 6.00 percent plus 3.00 percent for a total of 9.00 percent during this interest rate period. The interest payments to the inverse floater bondholders will change periodically in an inverse manner to the short-term interest paid on the floater bonds. The inverse floater bondholder is able to receive 9.00 percent when the alternative of purchasing conventional long-term fixed rate bonds would pay 6.25 percent. The inverse floater bondholder is willing to take the risk that interest rates will rise, resulting in a decrease in the return on the inverse floater bonds, in return for this premium over the conventional rate. The floater bondholders are purchasing the type of security that they normally purchase. The net result to the borrower is long-term fixed rate financing that is 25 basis points below what the borrower would have paid on conventional long-term bonds.

Figure 13-8 shows how market changes affect the various parties involved with this type of financing. When the bonds were issued, in our example, short-term rates equaled 3.00 percent, the borrower paid a fixed rate of 6.00 percent, and the inverse floater bondholder received an interest rate of 9.00 percent. If short-term interest rates increase to 6.00 percent, then the short-term bondholder will receive 6.00 percent, the borrower will continue to pay 6.00 percent, and the inverse floater bondholder will receive 6.00 percent. If short-term market interest rates increase to 12.00 percent, the rate at which the floater bonds are capped, the short-term bondholder will receive all the interest paid by the borrower for an interest return of 12.00 percent. In this case, the inverse floater bondholder will receive *no interest payment at all*. If interest rates decline from where they were at the time bonds were issued, and short-term interest rates fall to 2.00 percent, the borrower will continue to pay 6.00 percent, and the inverse floater bondholder will receive

Figure 13–8   Combined Floater/Inverse Floater Financing

Effects of Market Changes

Short-Term Rate*	Inverse Floater Rate	Borrower Fixed Rate
3.00 %	9.00 %	6.00 %
6.00 %	6.00 %	6.00 %
12.00 %	0.00 %	6.00 %
2.00 %	10.00 %	6.00 %

*capped at two times the Borrower Rate

10.00 percent. As these numbers indicate, the inverse floater bondholder has the potential of receiving no interest at all on the inverse floater bonds if the interest rate on the floater bonds reaches the cap. As a result, most underwriters will sell this type of security only to sophisticated institutional investors and not to the retail market.

The incentive of higher interest rates to the inverse floater bondholder is available because of the spread between short-term rates and long-term rates. The wider this spread, the more incentive is available for an inverse floater bondholder. As a result, this type of financing tends to be more successful during periods when there is a steep yield curve. A *steep yield curve* means there is a significant difference between short-term interest rates and long-term interest rates at any given point in time. A *flat yield curve* means there is little difference between short-term interest rates and long-term interest rates at a given point in time. An *inverse yield curve* means short-term interest rates are higher than long-term interest rates at that given point in time. Figure 13-9 demonstrates these various yield curves.

Linking Inverse Floater Bonds to Dutch Auction Bonds

There is an interesting opportunity for inverse floater bondholders in the event that prevailing interest rates rise to levels that make the interest return on the inverse floater bonds unattractive. When this financing structure is put together using Dutch auction bonds for the floater, the

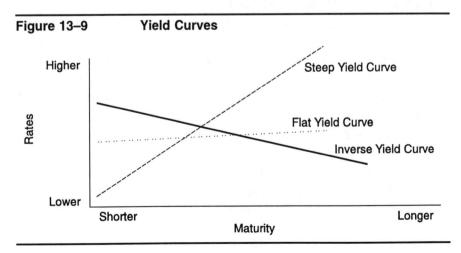

Figure 13–9　　Yield Curves

inverse floater bondholder has the ability to enter the Dutch auction process. For example, in the event that short-term interest rates have increased to 12.0 percent and the inverse floater rate is now 0.0 percent, the inverse floater bondholder can bid a ridiculously low interest rate in the Dutch auction, thereby assuring top priority in any allocation of bonds. Any Dutch auction bond from the same issue that is purchased will offset the yield on an inverse floater bond and will result in a combined yield of 6.00 percent for the two bonds.

This process is called *linking* the bonds. The borrower fixed rate is sometimes referred to as the *link rate*. Some of these bond issues automatically give the inverse floater bondholder the right to purchase Dutch auction bonds without going through the auction process. This means the inverse floater bondholder is always assured of being able to purchase corresponding Dutch auction bonds and linking inverse floater bonds. At the time the bonds were issued, in our example, the inverse floater bondholder received 9.0 percent when the market for conventional long-term bonds was 6.25 percent. The ability to link the inverse floater bonds means the inverse floater bondholder can be assured he will not receive a rate lower than 6.0 percent, as long as he is willing to put up the additional funds necessary to purchase the Dutch auction bonds.

Inverse floater financings offer the advantage to a borrower of a lower fixed interest rate than conventional financings. Variations of these financings that do not use a swap—i.e., versions that use Dutch auction bonds—contain no significant additional risk to the borrower as compared to conventional fixed rate bonds.

While the combination of Dutch auction bonds and inverse floater bonds has only been available to healthcare institutions as a financing vehicle since 1990, these instruments were available to purchasers of bonds several years earlier. This is because a few underwriting firms were purchasing fixed rate bonds and then selling off Dutch auction and inverse floater cash flows from the proceeds of these bonds. This process resulted in a "secondary market" offering of the Dutch auction bonds and inverse floaters.

For example, say an underwriter purchased an entire $100 million term bond issue while under engagement as the senior manager in a negotiated offering. Also, assume the interest rate on the term bonds was 7.0 percent. The underwriter would then place the term bonds in an escrow and sell off *custody receipts* to various investors. One half of these custody receipts would float with the market through a Dutch auction process. The other $50 million of custody receipts would work as an inverse floater by paying the investors that purchased them whatever funds were left over after the floaters were paid. The underwriter might structure these custody receipts so that when they were added together, the net effect was a yield of 6.75 percent. The underwriter would then make a profit equal to the .25 percent per annum on the entire issue, which would equal several million dollars. The investors received securities that behaved relative to the market in the manner they wished, just as if they had been issued that way by the original borrower, but the borrower issued fixed-rate conventional bonds. In this case, the underwriter enjoyed the savings that resulted from using the derivative products, and also received the underwriter's spread for selling the fixed rate bond issue to themselves. The secondary market offering of derivative products has been extremely lucrative for the investment banking firms that have made use of this technique.

▮ Potential Drawbacks to Derivative Financing Structures

There may be at least four potential drawbacks to these derivative financing structures for borrowers. The first is that the versions that utilize interest rate swaps contain counterparty risk, and potentially basis risk. Second, the versions of these financings that utilize Dutch auction bonds require larger issue sizes, usually $40 million or more ($20 million for the Dutch auction bonds and $20 million for the inverse floater bonds). Third, the savings that can be derived from these types of financings are dependent upon market conditions. These structures are more likely to be successful when the yield curve is steeper, and may not offer any benefit in some markets. A fourth potential disadvantage to these structures is that they tend to be more complex than conventional bonds. The complexity may require longer time to prepare the bond issue as well as increased legal fees. However, the savings that can be generated from these types of financings usually make it worth risking all these potential drawbacks. Advice from a good financial advisor who is well versed in these various structures can help healthcare organizations determine which risks are appropriate and which can be avoided—allowing the benefits to be obtained without *any* unacceptable risk.

■ Forward Purchase Contracts

Forward purchase contracts can be used by borrowers to lock in current interest rates for future financings. This might be appropriate when a borrower wishes to advance refund tax-exempt bonds, but is unable to do so for several years due to the tax laws. Another situation where the use of forward purchase contracts might be appropriate is when a borrower knows it will have a need for capital a few years in the future, but feels quite certain that today's interest rates are more attractive than the rates that might be available at that time. In each case, forward purchase contracts will allow the borrower to lock into current market rates.

Forward purchase contracts can be structured using either bonds or interest rate swaps. A *forward bond purchase contract* requires the counterparty to purchase a predetermined amount of bonds, at predetermined interest rates, on a future date within a specified period of time. A *forward swap purchase contract* requires the counterparty to enter into an interest rate swap that will begin predetermined payments, based on a predetermined notional amount and interest rate formula, on a future date within a specified period of time.

A forward bond contract is an agreement for the borrower to sell, and the counterparty to purchase, a set amount of bonds in the future at today's rates. As mentioned above, this can be attractive when a borrower has outstanding bonds that cannot be refunded for several years. The forward bond purchase contract allows the borrower to issue refunding bonds in the future at today's interest rates.

The same net result can be accomplished using a forward swap contract. Under this structure, the borrower assumes it will issue variable rate bonds in the future, when its outstanding bonds become callable. Fixed payments on the swap contract will begin at the time these new bonds are issued, and the variable payments received under the contract will offset the variable payments on the new refunding bonds. The borrower will then be obligated to make fixed payments under the swap contract that will reflect the market rates at the time the forward swap contract was entered into.

Another way to accomplish the forward swap structure is through the purchase of an option on a forward swap. Such an option is known as a swaption. A *swaption* gives the borrower the right to enter into an interest rate swap at some specific point in the future, based on interest rates at the time the swaption is written. In reality, swaptions are not intended ever actually to result in the issuance of a forward swap. Instead, the borrower sells the swaption back to the counterparty on the expiration date at a price determined by the current interest rate environment. The borrower then uses the proceeds to purchase an interest rate swap in the current market that will deliver the benefits of the swap that was negotiated when the swaption was issued. It acts as an insurance policy that pays the additional cost of acquiring a more favorable swap than would normally be available if rates are higher on the expiration date, and provides no benefit if interest rates are lower than they were when the swaption was written.

Use of a swaption locks in current interest rates for use at a later date, which is beneficial if interest rates are higher in the future, but the cost of a swaption can eliminate any benefit of lower interest rates in the future. If interest rates are higher when the borrower is ready to refund its debt, selling the swaption should generate a gain for the borrower that will largely offset the increased cost of refinancing the old debt at higher interest rates than were available when the swaption was written. Conversely, if interest rates are lower than when the swaption was written, the cost of the swaption will largely offset the potential gain that the borrower would have realized from refunding when interest rates were lower than when the swaption was written.

■ Float Contracts

Another form of forward purchase contract that may be attractive to healthcare borrowers is a contract to invest the money that will become available in the various funds of bond issues over time. These instruments are referred to as float contracts. Typically, a fixed rate tax-exempt bond issue will pay out principal once each year, and interest twice each year. The borrower usually is required to deposit funds for these payments into a debt service fund either monthly or quarterly. These funds often are allowed to be invested with no arbitrage rebate requirement, and the borrower attempts to invest them at as high a yield as possible, given the short time until they are needed.

A float contract is an investment vehicle that will guarantee a rate of return on these funds over the life of the bonds. The counterparties that offer these float contracts will pay a borrower an up-front fee for the right to invest the money in the debt service fund as it becomes available over the life of the bond issue. In this situation, the counterparty makes an assumption about future short-term interest rates for the various periods for which funds will be available to invest, and calculates the earnings. Those earnings are then discounted, and the counterparty pays that amount as a fee to the borrower when the contract is closed. Alternatively, the borrower may choose to take the interest earnings over time, rather than as a single up-front discounted payment. In either case, the counterparty has purchased the right to invest those funds in the future, and is expecting to invest them at rates that will generate income greater than the discounted fee paid to the borrower.

If the borrower is to benefit from the sale of the debt service fund earnings, both of the following events must occur. First, the purchase price of the future earnings (the fee paid to the borrower) must be reinvested at a rate higher than the rate the counterparty used to discount the earnings stream. Otherwise, the borrower will never recover the full value of the sale. Second, the borrower only comes out ahead if the actual reinvestment rates that are available for the debt service funds—had the borrower retained them to invest—are lower than the rate received under the contract. If either of these situations does not occur, the borrower might have been better off investing the money held in the debt service fund itself.

Another situation where a float contract may make sense is in a refunding escrow that is funded with open market securities. As discussed in Chapter 12, most refunding escrows can be funded either with SLGS or open market Treasury securities. Using SLGS can often allow the stream of income from the escrow to be tailored to the funding requirements of the refunded bonds, making the escrow 100-percent efficient. This means that money becomes available right when it is needed. However, there can be situations where it is desirable to fund a refunding escrow with open market Treasury securities. It is more difficult to make such an escrow 100-percent efficient because the payments on the Treasury securities are predetermined and cannot be tailored to fit the cash flow requirements of the escrow. Therefore, the portfolio of securities must be set up so that they mature prior to when they are needed to make payments on the bonds. This inefficiency creates the opportunity to use a float contract to obtain some yield on those funds after the securities mature, until they are needed. The exact amounts of money and the periods when they will be available for investment are easily determined once the portfolio of Treasury securities for an escrow has been determined, so a counterparty can bid on the right to invest those funds.

The yields on these float contracts for escrows tend to be significantly lower than the allowable bond yield, but failing to employ a float contract may result in a hidden cost. If a borrower does not use a float contract, the overall yield calculated on the escrow will be higher, because the yield calculation will not take into account periods for which the escrow funds sit uninvested. Reducing the number of days in the yield calculation, while holding the total amount of income received constant, increases the yield. The result is that either the borrower will have to use lower yielding securities in funding the escrow to meet the yield requirement, or less negative arbitrage will be generated in an inefficient escrow. In the latter situation, the borrower will be required to begin rebating sooner any excess earnings from the debt service reserve fund that is being used to earn back all the negative arbitrage.

In other words, failing to use a float contract could result in reducing the amount of income that can be retained from a debt service reserve fund, or any other fund that has moneys to invest. Because of this, even though the return on a float contract for a refunding escrow may offer a low yield, it may offer a greater benefit by allowing other funds related to the same bond issue to be invested at higher yields. The borrower's financial advisor and tax counsel should be able to determine the advisability of using a float contract in these situations.

As with any of these forward purchase structures, float contracts will allow a borrower to lock into current market rates. Borrowers must evaluate the cost of these structures relative to anticipated moves in interest rates. Bidding any of these contracts out on a competitive basis may be the only way a borrower can be sure that the most aggressive offers are received. Depending on the complexity of the variables involved, there can be a wide variance in the purchase prices offered by prospective counterparties on forward purchase contracts. As a result, the borrower typically can enjoy a significant benefit by allowing its financial advisor to bid out forward purchase contracts competitively.

■ Debt Service Reserve Fund Put Agreements

When a bond issue includes a debt service reserve fund (DSRF), the borrower attempts to invest the money held in that fund in such a manner that it will offset the cost of the bonds that funded the reserve, plus recover any negative arbitrage created in any other funds of the bond issue. Since there may be a need to draw on the DSRF to make debt service payments on the bonds, it is unusual for DSRFs to be invested in securities maturing much beyond five to 10 years, even though the maturity of the bonds is 30 years or more. Since the borrower will be paying a 30-year rate on the bonds, and will be investing for a shorter period, the borrower often is not able to obtain a high-enough yield on the DSRF investments to equal the allowable yield on the bonds. The negative arbitrage that arises in any construction fund, refunding escrow, or other fund, is included in the allowable yield calculation for the bonds, thus increasing that yield. When bonds are issued during periods of low interest rates, many borrowers are willing to make the assumption that interest rates will rise to a level in the future where the DSRF will be able to be invested at the allowable yield. The allowable yield slowly increases during periods when the DSRF is invested below the allowable yield, due to the negative arbitrage created in the DSRF itself in that situation.

A DSRF put agreement often can be structured in such a way that it eliminates this investment risk for the borrower, while at the same time providing the liquidity necessary for any draws on the DSRF. These agreements usually are written for a long-term period—anywhere from the first call date on the bonds to the final maturity. The agreement provides that the borrower will invest the DSRF in a qualified investment with a maturity equal to the length of the put agreement. The trustee for the bond issue holds the security and has the ability to put that security to the counterparty, at par, at any time there is a draw on the DSRF and funds are not available to make the necessary payment. When the DSRF is replenished by the borrower after a draw, the trustee will then repurchase the underlying security from the counterparty, again at par.

This instrument allows the borrower to invest in a long-term security, thereby obtaining the yield needed to meet the allowable yield on the bonds, while at the same time providing liquidity to the trustee for any draws on the DSRF through the put agreement. When the DSRF is invested in normal securities, there usually is a requirement in the documents to periodically assess the value of the investments—commonly referred to as "mark to market." If the value of the securities in the DSRF is below a certain level due to rising interest rates or any other reason, then funds must be added to bring the value up to the requirement. Since the DSRF put agreement provides that the trustee may put the securities to the counterparty at par, the need to mark to market is eliminated for the DSRF.

The counterparty is paid a fee to provide this put agreement, which is paid out of the income provided by the security in which the DSRF is invested. For example, assume that a bond issue has an allowable yield of 7.00 percent, and that long-term treasury bonds can be purchased to yield 7.50 percent. It might be possible to enter into a DSRF put agreement where the counterparty will receive 40 basis points out of the income generated from the long-term treasury so the net yield to the borrower is 7.10 percent. The borrower will be obligated to rebate the 10 basis points that is in excess of the allowable yield, but the borrower has locked into a yield for the life of the bond issue that eliminates the investment risk for the DSRF.

Bond lawyers usually require that these put agreements be purchased through a competitive bid process because it is easy for one firm to offer the exact yield needed for the borrower and take the rest of the income as profit. The competitive bid process assures bond counsel that an appropriate fee is being paid to the counterparty for this put feature rather than any excess benefit inuring to the counterparty. The borrower accomplishes its objective as long as any of the bids come in at, or higher than, the allowable yield on the bonds.

Another important aspect in structuring these agreements is that a provision should be made for the borrower to terminate the agreement in the event the underlying bonds are refunded. Many of these agreements have been written where the borrower is obligated to make a penalty payment to the counterparty in the event the agreement is terminated. This should not be necessary since the counterparty's liability disappears when the agreement is terminated. Including provisions that favor the borrower may have an effect on the yields that are received in the bids, but the borrower has nothing to gain on any bid that is higher than the bond yield anyway. Borrowers should structure the terms of the put agreement so that it provides all of the desired flexibility that the borrower wants. If bids are not obtained that meet the allowable yield, then some of the flexibility may be removed to attract higher bids.

▌ Derivative Products—Conclusion

Derivative products can offer significant savings to borrowers, but the added complexity requires careful scrutiny to ensure that the savings are real and worth any potential risk. A borrower's financial advisor must be well versed in the intricacies of the derivative products offered by various firms to be able to help the borrower make an objective and well-informed decision as to whether or not derivative products make sense in any particular situation. The beauty of derivative products is that they tend to be structured for specific market conditions to provide benefits to both borrowers and bondholders. As market conditions change, different derivative products become attractive to potential purchasers, and borrowers must be flexible to offer the appropriate derivative for the market conditions in order to reap the maximum benefits of the lowest possible interest rates.

Counterparties make significant profits by offering derivative products, and make concerted efforts to sell them. When derivative bonds, such as Dutch auction bonds and embedded swap bonds first were introduced to the market, the savings compared to conventional bonds was in the 20 to 30 basis point range. That savings has eroded to about 10 basis points, and disappears altogether in some markets. With embedded swap bonds, it is difficult to know whether the market is dictating the narrower savings, or if the counterparties are skimming some of the benefit. The only way that a borrower can be certain that it obtained the absolute best rates is to incorporate a competitive bid process when purchasing or selling derivative products.

As mentioned in the beginning of this chapter, there has been some negative press regarding derivative products in the financial media. The vast majority of it has dealt with the fact that these are very complex securities and that many of the purchasers of these products may not have realized the volatility or nature of the interest rate swings that can occur with them. The bulk of the risk is taken on by the bondholders of these products, not the issuers. As a result, they should not be sold in the retail market, but only to sophisticated institutional investors. Borrowers should not avoid derivatives just because of the negative press. Instead, each borrower must make its own assessment of the risks relative to the potential rewards of using these products.

14 Fixed-Income Investing

—Robert A. Gottschalk

If it sounds too good to be true, it probably is—cliché, but very germane. Shortcuts and high-risk ventures usually do not pay off, but with a goal, a strategy, and a little common sense, fixed-income investing can be safe and effective. Knowledge and effort create opportunities; shortcuts cause loss of sleep.

There is a tried-and-true plan of action one can use to ensure the success of an investment portfolio. It is not fancy or complex, yet the number of investors who ignore this logical approach is staggering. Successful portfolios begin with realistic goals and objectives, followed by an investment policy that establishes safeguards to protect the investor, while providing enough flexibility to achieve success. Lastly, a well thought out strategy is needed that can meet these objectives while remaining within one's risk tolerances. Most of this chapter deals with the specifics of this plan; however, it might be useful to first look at a snapshot of today's market to understand why this is necessary.

Most conventional fixed-income securities are similar in their make-up. Each has a coupon, maturity date, settlement date, price, and yield. If a fixed-income security is held to maturity, the investor earns the coupon, adjusted for any initial premium or discount expected yield. If, however, the investor chooses to sell the security prior to maturity, the yield actually received could benefit from, or be adversely affected by prevailing market conditions. Certain risks are assumed, but in general, fixed-income securities can be conservative investments. Conventional securities are still predominant; however "fixed-income" does not necessarily translate as "conservative" any more.

The traditional fixed-income market is not so traditional anymore. Not completely satisfied with the opportunities available to investors in conventional fixed-income securities, the marketplace has entered a revolutionary phase. Partly driven by the investor's desire for more yield, and partly by the dealer community's desire to add new income opportunities to their firms, demand began to build for so-called derivative or custom securities in the early 1990s. Financial "engineers" within the securities industry created structures that would perform as desired if a particular external factor, or set of factors, performed in a particular way. Examples: "Would three-month LIBOR (London Interbank Offered Rate) *stay* within a specific range for a given period of time?" "Would French government bond rates *fall*?" The list of alternatives for pricing mechanisms is endless. Investors are offered an above-market yield for accepting the risk of this specified pricing mechanism. If the index performs as the investor expects, he wins. If not, he loses. All these products entail some risk; it is the investor's responsibility to determine what risks he is assuming and if these risks are prudent. An example of such a product and its associated risk is the range note.

A *range note* is an obligation whose interest payment is contingent upon a reference rate (for demonstrative purposes we will use LIBOR) staying within a pre-set range. In other words, for each day LIBOR remains within the range, the investor earns interest. If LIBOR either rises or falls outside this range, no interest is earned. The inducement to buy such a security is an *above*-market interest rate on an obligation of a highly rated credit, such as a federal agency. As an example, in December of 1993, the following specifications were distributed to prospective buyers:

Issuer:	federal agency
Tenor:	1 year
Payments:	quarterly
Principal Repayment:	100%
Coupon:	4.25%
3-Month LIBOR Range:	3.25% – 3.875% (1st six months)
	3.25% – 4.375% (2nd six months)

On December 13, the proposed date of the issue, three-month LIBOR was 3.3125 percent (the average for the preceding 12 months was 3.26 percent). For comparison, the rate on the one-year U.S. Treasury was yielding 3.62 percent at the time, and therefore the *inducement* was a +.63 percent yield to the Treasury. The investor's risk over the one-year life of the issue was that three-month LIBOR would not stay in the prescribed range.

What actually happened? In February 1994, the Federal Reserve began to tighten bank reserves and increase short-term rates. By April 14, three-month LIBOR was 3.94 percent, and therefore outside the range. By May 5, LIBOR was at 4.50 percent. Effectively, then, this obligation was no longer interest bearing. LIBOR stayed above 4.375 percent for the remainder of the term, and the net return for the period was 1.41 percent (4.25 percent for 121 out of 365 days). The inducement of +.63 percent to the U.S. Treasury was not earned for a long enough period to offset the period of time when no interest was earned.

With a market of buyers eager for more yield, *collateralized mortgage obligations (CMOs)* have seen an emergence as well. CMOs are mortgage pass-through securities in which the cash flows are separated into different classes or "tranches." There are a variety of classes available to investors with many different risk characteristics. Some are very sound investments, but others can be extremely risky.

CMO derivatives known as "interest-only" (IO) and "principal-only" (PO) obligations have received a great deal of press during the last couple of years, most of it bad. Buyers of IOs or POs are in essence making large bets on the direction of interest rates. Briefly stated, IOs are mortgage-backed securities that pay the interest on any outstanding balance of the underlying mortgages. Therefore, if mortgage prepayments are slow, the outstanding balance remains high and the IO pays handsomely. If, however, interest rates decline and mortgage prepayments accelerate, interest is earned on a smaller balance and the investor can lose a great deal of value. POs make the opposite bet; they are bought at a deeply discounted price and repaid at par. Thus, the return one receives is based on how fast principal is repaid. If interest rates decline and prepayments accelerate, the PO buyer wins. If rates rise and prepayments slow, POs can be very painful to say the least. The market value of IOs and POs can be *extremely* volatile due to the uncertainty of the underlying cash flows as rates change. For example, from a low in the fall of 1993, long-term rates in general rose about 1.7 percent over six months. The effect on the price of a U.S. Treasury bond was a decline in price of 18 percent, while the effect on the price of PO obligations was a decline of nearly 30 percent. The risk inherent is the extension or reduction of the term—what was bought with an *expectation* of an average life that met certain objectives was radically altered by a decisive shift in interest rates.

"Mortgage derivatives claim victims big and small"

The Wall Street Journal, April 20, 1994

This story in *The Journal* was enlightening from two points: (1) major sophisticated institutional investors among others took the risk and paid the price in the Spring of 1994 for investing in exotic, often mortgage-related, securities; and (2) the dealer community has been somewhat reluctant at times to step in and support (bid) the products they were touting six months earlier.

The article quoted an unnamed, large institutional investor as saying, "You are seeing the ugly side of the street now. The problem is that Wall Street created these bonds. They are the only ones who can price them. And they are not supporting their bonds." Ramin Rouhani, managing director at CDC Investment Management Corp., grouses that "this market doesn't work like a market should" when confronted with a bid range spread of three points (10 times the norm). A final, particularly thoughtful, quote on the subject—"We're not trying to outsmart the smart guys. We're trying to sell bonds to the dumb guys"—is attributed to Michael Vranos, at the time the head of Kidder, Peabody's Mortgage Bond Group.

If price risk were an investor's only concern, that would be one thing, but it is not. Consider credit risk, which is not only relevant to low- or non-rated securities anymore. For example, when the Marriott Corporation planned to restructure into two companies (one burdened with all the debt), its bond prices dropped precipitously in the Fall of 1992. The company noted that, like all public corporations, its fiduciary duty is to stockholders, not bondholders.

"It's our own fault," said Van Kampen Merritt bond fund manager Robert Hickey in the October 7, 1992, *The Wall Street Journal.* "In their rush to buy bonds in an effort to lock in yields, many investors have allowed companies to sell bonds with covenants that have been slim to none."

In addition to insufficient bond covenants, bond investors have had to be concerned with, among other things, the underlying asset quality of certain companies providing *investment contracts,* notably Executive Life and Mutual Benefit Life. Portfolios of so-called "junk bonds,"— viewed as sufficiently safe and no worse than a neutral factor in achieving superior ratings—began to unravel following the Drexel, Burnham Lambert and Michael Milken litigation. The resultant downgrades and defaults put investment contract purchasers at both significant and unexpected risk. In retrospect, relying exclusively on the rating agencies' perspectives was probably a mistake. A review of the insurance companies' investment holdings, listed in the annual report, might have shed some additional light on the risk before the investment contracts were bought.

Anyone who buys anything other than three-month U.S. Treasury bills is taking some risk. The real issue is whether the risk being assumed is carefully and specifically recognized and incorporated into the investment plan. Furthermore, is the risk/reward assessment based on a *neutral* market evaluation rather than on a reaction to *current* market conditions. If A-rated corporate bonds in seven years pay .5 percent more on average over time as compared to the seven-year Treasury, should the fact that, in today's market, the spread is 1.0 percent affect investment *policy*? The answer is no. Might it affect the strategy *constrained* by the policy? Yes. Normally, the better the parameters, the more controlled risk can be taken.

Most investments are made through a securities dealer rather than by private placement or treaty, and securities firms fill an essential role in the process of negotiating prices between buyers and sellers—for both primary and secondary market transactions. Based largely on this role, the industry and its participants project a certain power and allure to those outside the dealer community, including buyers. Securities firms are viewed by many as the authority on certain subjects and as the buyer's advocate.

The reality is that most dealers will do their best to provide what is needed or asked for; however, this should not substitute for the investor's own independent research. In addition, dealers generally understand and support their customers' goals but their mission is to "buy and sell" and not to advise clients, which is a clear conflict of interest.

"You just have to help me out," was the plea of Kathryn Lester, investment manager for the state of West Virginia's consolidated investment fund in 1986 to a Morgan Stanley salesman. A novice in investments, Lester was responsible for a $2.4 billion investment portfolio and turned to Wall Street for an "education." "People assume I know everything, and I don't," she said. Encouraged by the initial results of active trading in a bull market, she forged ahead. When the market turned around in late 1986, losses began to mount, and by 1987 losses rose to $160 million. West Virginia looked around for someone to blame, someone to cover the losses, and found Wall Street. The state contended that Wall Street should have known that what the state was doing was wrong and that it took advantage of Lester's naiveté. Ultimately, all the dealers accused of wrongdoing settled or were fined. Was it the broker's fault that a state employee disregarded the guidelines? Paul Jacobson, a Goldman, Sachs trader, called the suit "extortion on the part of the state" (*Forbes,* October 12, 1992).

■ Portfolio Management Considerations

Focusing on Objectives

Setting objectives regarding investment earnings for specific types of funds to be managed (self-insurance, funded depreciation, and so forth) is where all the work begins; having an investment goal gives purpose to the effort. Clearly understanding and defining the use of the funds, what cash flow is needed, or what sum needs to be there at some point in the future is the basis for determining the other investment steps: policy and strategy. In reality, the investment objectives are normally secondary or a supplement to a larger objective: the corporate strategic approach, such as building a new facility (funded in part by investment earnings), fully funding a pension program (while limiting direct contributions), or providing sufficient operating reserves (without cutting deeply into expenses). Thus, investment goals become a means to an end. The times or situations in which there are no major goals are relatively rare since financial assets are among the more scarce resources, but in this event the discipline of setting investment goals helps to pre-serve the investor's future financial opportunities.

Investment goals must be specific, numerical (nominal or real), with a term limit, and most importantly, achievable. As an illustration of this type of goal setting, imagine the following situation. The most tech-nologically advanced piece of equipment needed in a certain hospital's surgical suites is a "widget." To maintain a competitive advantage, the hospital must purchase it, but three factors need to be considered first: (1) a cost of $1 million; (2) construction and delivery will take 24 months; and (3) the budget is tight and only allows an allocation of $900,000 at this point towards the cost. The alternatives then are to: (1) pass up the opportunity; (2) order the equipment and hope for $100,000 to be freed up in the budget in the future; or (3) set an investment goal and plan to make enough funds available. The goal itself could be: (A) open ended, without specificity, "earn as much as you can;" or (B) tar-get a gross return of 11.11 percent over 24 months (or 5.41 percent annualized, compounded), which will result in the required $100,000. of earnings.

The second objective (B) meets all the tests: specific, numerical, term limit, and achievable. Granted, this is a simple application but the methodology will be the same no matter the amount, term, or other vari-able. If the investment objective is unreasonable—given the investor's open, broadly defined business risk tolerances (e.g., a 15 percent objec-tive in a 6 percent two-year U.S. Treasury note yield market and a low business risk tolerance)—it's probably wise to re-think the purchase or how it's paid for.

Some investment objectives are not as date or amount specific as the situation described above (a pension plan, for example) and require a substitute goal. Instead of setting a two-year time frame for the avail-ability of funds, it becomes a two-year time frame for critical evaluation and reassessment. What is generally accepted as an alternative in lieu of specific goals are market indices. The theory being that if an investor performs as well as the rest of the market then no ground is lost; and, that if historically the indexed basket of investments provided a reason-able real rate of return, then real growth in the investment balance is likely to continue into the future if the portfolio is managed similarly. Indices are developed by securities dealer firms as well as independent analytical companies according to a set of specific criteria. Bond indices, as an example, may be government only, corporate only, a blend, and so forth. They may be short-, intermediate-, or long-term but not all-term since this would dilute its specific measurement value. Once a base period has been established (normally selected based on its market rate neutrality), the "basket" of securities is priced daily or weekly and the gross price is compared to the gross price at the base date. The *difference,* then, is measured against the base price and reflected in the index.

The key to using an index system is choosing the most correct index, which sounds obvious but is occasionally misunderstood. If the investment policy permits the use of Government securities only to maturities of 10 years at most, and if the strategy calls for an average life of seven years, then the long-term corporate or government bond indices are not the correct yardsticks. Rather, the intermediate-term government bond index would apply. A well-chosen index allows for achievable results and effective measurement.

Investment Guidelines

Setting investment guidelines is a step that should occur *after* the investor establishes his/her goals. Risk tolerance should be in direct proportion to the amount of return needed—not a bit more. The two ways that risks are generally classified for fixed-income investing are market risk (or price volatility) and credit risk (or default risk). Related risks include, but are not limited to:

- reinvestment risk,
- timing (or call) risk,
- yield curve (or maturity) risk,
- liquidity risk,
- purchasing power (or inflation) risk,
- exchange rate risk,
- political (or legal) risk,
- event risk, and
- sector risk.

Credit risk and market risk have a dynamic relationship together, and it is very important to understand and respect this relationship.

The issue of market risk, or price sensitivity, by itself can be viewed in two parts: (1) at a point in time, the yield premium required by the marketplace for advancing from one maturity to the next in the same security type, and (2) the yield premium required to change security types. The yield premium then is developed by assessing the appropriate incremental return based on inflation, requisite real rates of return and the returns available on alternative investments.

The graphs in Figure 14-1 show the returns on U.S. Treasury securities and A-rated corporate bonds at December 31, 1993, and on December 31, 1988. Note the different yield spread relationships. Both sets of yield spread relationships primarily reflect maturity risk and provide some insights into the variability of market expectations.

To appreciate the effect on the price of a security due to changes in yields on conventional securities resulting from shifts in interest rates, the simple illustration shown in Figure 14-2 should help.

Price risk becomes an important practical issue normally in two ways: (1) realized losses or gains associated with liquidations to meet other needs, and (2) unrealized losses that have the effect of indirectly impacting future performance.

Realized losses or gains resulting from a sale of securities should be analyzed in much the same way, although most investors tend to view a realized gain as "good" and a realized loss as "bad." The technically correct way to view gains or losses is in the context of the complete return realized over the entire period held $\left(\dfrac{Income \quad {}^{+Gains}_{-Loses}}{Cost} \right)$ and the comparative value of the security sold versus other holdings, for the balance of the period for which performance is to be measured. An example is shown in Figure 14-3.

The consideration of price risk, then, is important. The greater price risk of longer term securities and the normally higher returns available further out on the curve should not be viewed independently. As a practical matter, reviewing price volatility histories and return histories can be very useful in determining a preferred correlation for setting investment guidelines (e.g., does five-year security return/price

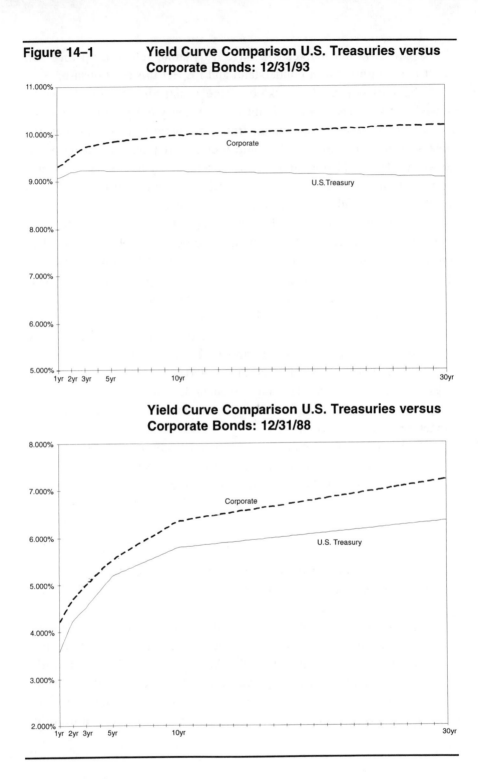

Figure 14–1   **Yield Curve Comparison U.S. Treasuries versus Corporate Bonds: 12/31/93**

Yield Curve Comparison U.S. Treasuries versus Corporate Bonds: 12/31/88

Figure 14–2   Changes in Principal Value Relative to Shifts in Interest Rates

Maturity	Yield 6/30/94	Principal Cost per $1,000,000	Shift in Yield + 100 BP Principal Value per $1,000,000	Change in Principal Value
3 Month	4.22%	$989,588.45	$987,292.33	<$2,296.13>
1 Year	5.48%	$947,511.19	$938,541.32	<$8,969.87>
5 Year	6.95%	$991,672.91	$951,292.13	<$40,380.78>
10 Year	7.32%	$995,107.18	$928,766.73	<$66,250.45>
30 Year	7.61%	$841,471.07	$749,308.75	<$92,162.36>

volatility versus seven-year return/price volatility *better* suit our needs and tolerances?).

Credit risk is a much more subtle subject than price risk, and potentially has a much greater impact on portfolio performance over time. Every investment carries with it *some* credit risk. The goal is to assume only as much credit risk as is necessary to provide the incremental income necessary to achieve the investor's financial goals.

Why buy corporates, *any* corporates, if they pay the same rates as U.S. Treasuries? For most investors there is not a good reason. Fortunately, many of us have access to the reports and ratings of credit agencies like Moody's and Standard & Poor's. These agencies provide an important service that allows investors to, basically, classify risk. Are all A-rated securities the same? Of course not, but at least it gives us a place to start. Will an A-rated credit always be an A-rated credit? Probably not; it's the *dynamics* of the credit markets that provide both opportunity and risk.

Credit guidelines should be based on the ability of the investor to understand and assume risk. Historical relationships of returns between various rating classes can be a very useful starting point; do A-rated securities pay sufficiently more over time than AAAs, and will that offset any real risk of loss? Every investor needs to establish an equilib-

Figure 14–3   Examples of Analyzing Gains and Losses

(1) Total return analysis for U.S. Treasury Notes with varying maturities and six-month horizon as of 6/30/94:

	2 Year	*5 Year*	*30 Year*
Issue	6%–6/30/96	6 3/4–6/30/99	6 1/4–8/15/23
Current Yield	6.17%	6.95%	7.61%

If Treasury Yields Shift	**Six-Month Horizon Yields**		
(a) Security sold with a gain:			
− 50 basis points	7.59%	10.81%	19.81%
(Principal gain per $1 M)	$7,742	$19,821	$53,838
(b) Security sold with a loss:			
+ 50 basis points	4.78%	3.17%	−3.46%
(Principal loss per $1 M)	<$6,178>	<$17,959>	<$47,362>

(2) Which security is the "better" sale?

(A)   U.S. Treasury Note 5-1/8% due **6-30-98** owned at a yield to maturity of 5.125% and a market yield of 12-31-93 of 5.06 % and an *unrealized gain* of $1,800, or

(B)   U.S. Treasury Bill due **6-30-94** owned at yield to maturity of 3.45% and market yield of 12-31-93 of 4% and an *unrealized loss* of $2,850.

Assuming rates held constant or declining: (B), since the breakdown yield for 6 months on (B) is lower than (A), (4% versus 5.06%) which factors in the unrealized gain or loss affect. If rates are *assumed to increase* the "better" sale in spite of the 6-month breakeven analysis is probably the longer-term security.

---

rium point based on the ability to sustain a principal loss and the entice-ment of returns that exceed Treasury securities.

For example, as shown in Figure 14-4, the spreads in yield over time between 10-year A-rated corporates and AAA-rated U.S. Treasury obligations is a dynamic relationship. When spreads widen, investors

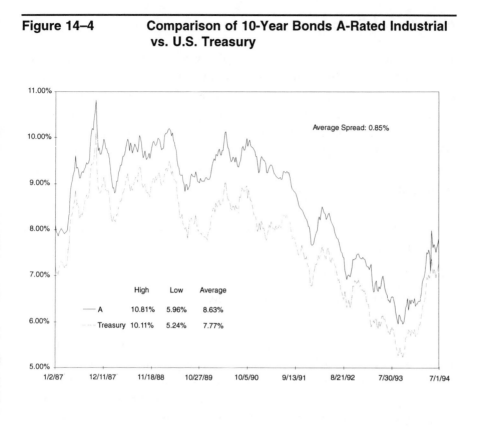

might consider accepting the additional credit risk of an A-rated bond. When spreads narrow, one might be wise to take advantage of the AAA-rated Treasury bond, which offers good relative value.

As has been said, price risk and credit risk together are constantly changing. Using historical relationships between seven- and 10-year Treasuries is important and the historical relationship between A- and AAA-rated corporates is as well. Bringing the two together through sector comparisons and looking at what happens at different stages of the interest rate cycle will add some insights into ways professional managers uncover investment opportunities.

This information, in time, becomes a valuable aspect in setting investment strategy, but for the time being should help in setting the criteria for a solid, effective investment policy.

Investment Policy

The investment policy is a statement of investment philosophy, parameters, and responsibilities. Its purpose is to provide a framework, so that everyone involved—board, senior management, and portfolio management—are all on the same page. While public entities or institutions tend to have extensive, detailed policies to protect the public interest, other institutions, including not-for-profits, tend to have complete yet briefer statements. The length of the policy is not as important as including all the essential parts:

1. the type or types of funds covered, or specifically excluded, by the policy;

2. assigning of specific responsibilities; and

3. setting credit limits and term limits.

Setting in place an investment policy that is a "good fit," or suitable, with the investor's overall approach to business management and goals can provide tremendous assistance in achieving the investment goals. A policy that's too lenient or too restrictive promotes ambiguity in strategy and investment goals that are less likely to be attained. An abridged sample investment policy is shown in Figure 14-5.

Investment Strategies

The investment strategy, or plan, is the tactical approach to achieving the goals through the investment policy. It follows goals and policies, not leads, because it must conform to the restrictive parts of the investment program. Analogously, when planning a vacation, normally the destination and mode of transportation are set before the route is plotted. Strategies can be set to minimize the impact of uncertainty; however, the first consideration is "how much will it affect my results if my strategy is not correct?" The best strategy is the least sensitive to changes in external factors and provides reasonable chance of success in achieving pre-established goals. If the goal is 5 percent nominal annual return over three years, and the choices in strategy offer the following prospects:

Figure 14–5   **Sample Investment Policy**

Scope

This investment policy applies to all financial assets held by the hospital, other than pension fund assets. These funds are accounted for in the hospital's annual financial report and include:

- funded depreciation;

- trustee held project and reserve funds; and

- any new fund created by the hospital, unless specifically exempted by the hospital board.

Investment Objectives

The primary objective of the hospital's investment activities is the preservation of capital. Employing conservative investment practices, the hospital will seek to achieve the highest returns available within the policy guidelines while maintaining sufficient liquidity to meet projected needs.

Authority/Responsibility

The authority for investing funds rests with the hospital's board of directors. The finance committee of the board is responsible for reviewing and approving policy, as well as reviewing performance at least annually. The hospital's finance director is directly responsible for investment management.

Investment Standards

Investments will be limited to high-quality fixed-income securities. The aggregate investment position will maintain an average weighted term to maturity not to exceed three years. Unless specifically exempted due to a particular fund requirement, the aggregate investment position will retain not less than 25 percent of principal in less than 90-day maturities. Unless specifically exempted, the maximum maturity of any investment shall be seven years.

Figure 14–5   Sample Investment Policy (continued)

Quality Investments

Hospital investments will be restricted to the following:

Investment	Maximum Percentage of Portfolio	Maximum Maturity
Direct U.S. Treasury Obligations	100%	7 years
Federal Agency Obligations	75%	5 years
Repurchase Agreements (1)	75%	6 months
Federally Insured Certificates of Deposit	75%	1 year
Secured Certificates of Deposit (2)	75%	1 year
Other Certificates of Deposit (3)	25%	6 months
Banker's Acceptances (3)	25%	6 months
Commercial Paper (3)	25%	3 months

(1)   Direct U.S. Treasury or Federal Agency obligations valued at 102% of investment, delivered to the hospital's safekeeping account.

(2)   Pledge of U.S. Treasury or Federal Agency obligations valued at 100 percent of investment.

(3)   Limited to issuers with the highest Moody's or Standard & Poor's rating.

Investment Controls

Delivery: All negotiable securities will be purchased and/or sold on a "delivery versus payment" basis through the hospital's safekeeping account. Written confirmations, safekeeping reports, and any third-party reports will be verified against the hospital's accounting records.

Other: The finance director will establish and maintain any other investment controls deemed appropriate to ensure the safety of hospital funds.

Approved:

_____
Board Chairman or Finance Committee
Chairman with Board Consent

Date:_____

(a)   3 percent Year 1, 5 percent Year 2, and 7 percent Year 3—for an average of 5 percent

(b)   −10 percent Year 1, 0 percent Year 2, and 25 percent Year 3—for an average of 5 percent the more prudent path clearly is (a).

Two of the more basic fixed-income investment strategies generally employed are the "ladder-type" and the "hourglass-type." The ladder-type investment strategy is implemented by allocating a certain percentage, normally fixed, of investable funds to successive maturities of equal intervals (i.e., 10 percent in 6 months, 10 percent in 12 months, 10 percent in 18 months, etc.). As time passes and increments mature, they are normally reinvested to become the furthermost "rung" on the ladder. This strategy has the effect of establishing a constant average life. If the average two-year Treasury note rate over time meets the earning objectives, then as an example, a laddered portfolio averaging two years will serve to maintain this rate of performance, while providing any needed liquidity from maturities. An example of the performance of a ladder-type strategy is shown in Figure 14-6.

The hourglass-type strategy is implemented by allocating large, usually equally proportionate shares of the investable funds to both long-term *and* short-term securities positions. This has the effect of raising the yield with the higher rates available on the longer-term investments while preserving liquidity with the short-term position. This strategy is a bit riskier than others, such as the ladder-type, due to the concentration of a large portion of the investments in a longer term, with the greater price risk associated; therefore, this strategy's success is more dependent on the direction of interest rates than most others. Correspondingly, this strategy provides a *better* opportunity to achieve *higher* returns if the directions of changes in interest rates are correctly forecast. The effects of an hourglass strategy implemented under rising and falling interest rates are characterized in Figure 14-7.

The selection of the *type* of investment management strategy should be carefully considered in light of the specific goals chosen. The selection should be based on the type of funds, the amount available to invest, the maturity range allowed by policy and the types of permitted investments. Laddering strategies *generally* are more appropriate for construction and self-insurance funds while hourglass strategies can add

Figure 14–6   Application of a Ladder-Type Strategy on a Portfolio

Treasury Bill Maturities	Original Purchase	Reinvestment of 3-Month Bill in 1-Year Bill									
	1/1/92	4/1/92	7/1/92	10/1/92	1/1/93	4/1/93	7/1/93	10/1/93	1/1/94	4/1/94	7/1/94
3 Month	3.93	3.98	4.03	4.09	4.43	4.03	3.38	3.51	3.28	3.40	3.32
6 Month	3.98	4.03	4.09	4.43	4.03	3.38	3.51	3.28	3.40	3.32	3.63
9 Month	4.03	4.09	4.43	4.03	3.38	3.51	3.28	3.40	3.32	3.63	4.68
1 Year	4.09	4.43	4.03	3.38	3.51	3.28	3.40	3.32	3.63	4.68	5.48
Average Yield	4.01	4.13	4.15	3.98	3.84	3.55	3.39	3.38	3.41	3.76	4.28
Average Life (yrs)	0.63	0.63	0.63	0.63	0.63	0.63	0.63	0.63	0.63	0.63	0.63

**Figure 14–7   Hourglass Strategy Holding Period
                            Total Return Analysis**

(1) Rising Rates (12/1/86 to 12/1/88)

Purchase on 12/1/86, $1 million, 30-year U.S. Treasury bonds with YTM (yield to maturity) 7.50 percent, and purchase $1 million in 6-month U.S. Treasury bills with YTM 5.66 percent, then reinvest every succeeding six months at 6.12 percent, 6.46 percent and 7.86 percent, respectively:

2-Year Holding Period Yield	+7.02%
2-Year Total Return	+3.56%

(2) Falling Rates (12/1/88 to 12/1/90)

Purchase on 12/1/88 $1 million 30-year U.S. Treasury bonds, YTM 9.13 percent and purchase $1 million in 6-month Treasury bills with YTM 8.65 percent, then reinvest every succeeding six months at 8.12 percent, 7.85 percent and 8.0 percent, respectively.

2-Year Holding Period	+8.65%
2-Year Total Return	+12.70%

Note: *Holding period yield* equals interest earned

Total return equals interest earned, adjusted for amortization or accretion, plus or minus realized and unrealized gains and losses.

---

value to long-term funded depreciation and fixed-income pension fund investments.

Fundamental to the selection of an investment strategy is the decision whether or not to "match" the investments in maturity and/or interest rate sensitivity to a projected need and/or cost of funds. All too often strategic investment decisions are based on contemporary factors: current market rates, current rate spreads, and current costs. When the markets are at or near extremes, a distortion is created as to what the relationships would *normally* be. For example, at the low point in an interest rate cycle the yield spreads between different securities tend to compress or narrow. Being able to distance the decision on an investment strategy *away* from extremes and towards reasonable expectations is important. This is equally true for consideration of both matched and mismatched positions. In evaluating both benefits and risks, the first consideration should be the purpose of the funds: are they available to invest for a definite period of time without being called away? If there is a finite period (e.g., call date or maturity date on bonds, specified payment dates for other obligations, or targeted funding dates for certain classes of expense), this would serve as an outward boundary for any consideration. The second aspect is the interest rate sensitivity. Investors are motivated to, among other things, produce the greatest amount of return with the least amount of risk. Using historical references as a guide as to the possible outcome of matching versus mismatching may prove useful, as demonstrated in Figure 14-8. The borrower in Example 1 received a positive spread of 1.49 percent over VariFact,™ a tax-exempt 7-day variable rate demand bond index, during this period by investing in a repo that matched market movements. The investment delivered a positive return in all but a very few days during the period. Example 2 shows that a five-year Treasury will probably offer a higher spread above VariFact on any given date, but VariFact may exceed the fixed five-year rate for a significant portion of the time the funds are invested, resulting in a loss to the borrower. Matching the investment to the need avoids this risk.

The decision of whether to match or mismatch investments with a liability and corresponding expense, then, requires careful consideration of two principal issues:

1.　term of the available funds, and

2.　interest rate sensitivities.

To the extent that the probability of achieving the objective through a risk controlled approach (matching) is greater than any incentive to maximize return and increase interest rate risk by mismatching, the appropriate strategy will become clear.

Once the strategy has been decided, the next issue is what investment management style should be considered, with the options being active or passive. The decision should be based on whether or not active management can actually add value or whether a passive strategy is sufficient for the goals to be met. Part of the decision has to be based on the availability and added cost, if any, of having the investments actively managed. *Passive investment management* is the process of evaluating the prospective needs for the funds, laying out an investment

Figure 14–8   One Week Repo versus VariFact Average

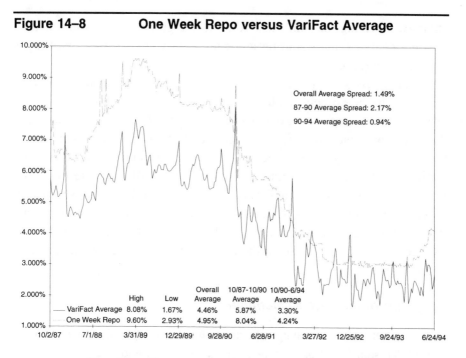

Overall Average Spread: 1.49%

87-90 Average Spread: 2.17%

90-94 Average Spread: 0.94%

	High	Low	Overall Average	10/87-10/90 Average	10/90-6/94 Average
VariFact Average	8.08%	1.67%	4.46%	5.87%	3.30%
One Week Repo	9.60%	2.93%	4.95%	8.04%	4.24%

Five Year Treasury Low versus VariFact Average

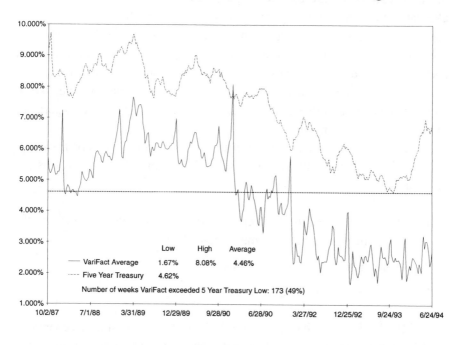

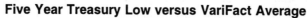

	Low	High	Average
VariFact Average	1.67%	8.08%	4.46%
Five Year Treasury	4.62%		

Number of weeks VariFact exceeded 5 Year Treasury Low: 173 (49%)

strategy, investing the funds according to the guides, reinvesting maturities and coupons, and ignoring any change in values in the investments during the entire cycle.

Active investment management differs from passive in that during the cycle the investment holdings are periodically re-assessed. If the opportunity is presented to exchange one security for another to improve the position of the investments without disturbing the basic integrity of the portfolio, it may be acted on. Active management should not be confused with trading; the goal of trading activity is short-term profits from the frequent buying and selling of securities based on short-term movements in the market. Active management does, however, add some risk to portfolio management. Figure 14-9 shows an example of the differences in yields produced in the active versus passive management of one portfolio.

Selection of a Portfolio Manager

Selecting someone to manage the investment portfolio should be a very careful decision based on a number of factors: 1) an understanding of what the particular needs are and how much to invest; 2) an evaluation of the alternatives for managing funds; 3) an assessment of the skills and experiences of prospective managers; and 4) the costs of having the funds managed. Just as setting goals serves to set the stage for the investment policy framework, so does the investment policy play an important role in the selection of the appropriate management type. The most suitable investment manager is one that understands the goals, has extensive experience in the types of investments allowed, and is cost effective.

The minimum qualifications for investment management responsibilities should be set by the governing board based on the following criteria:

1. Depth and breadth of experience *directly* involved in managing the types of permitted investments considered

2. Formal education on investments

3. Securities industry registrations

After a decision has been reached as to the minimum acceptable qualifications, the board must decide how to go about best selecting a

Figure 14–9   **Active Management versus Passive Management (1 Year) in a Laddered Portfolio 6/30/93 through 6/30/94**

Passive
Holding Structured June 30, 1993

Par	Issue	Coupon	Maturity	Yield to Maturity
$3 M	US Tsy Bills		6/28/94	3.43%
$3 M	US Tsy Note	4 1/8	6/28/95	4.13%
$3 M	US Tsy Note	4 1/4	5/17/96	4.33%

Active Portfolio
Same Holding as Passive Portfolio on 6/30/93

Portfolio Realignment 12/31/93

Par	Issue	Coupon	Maturity	
Sell $3 M	US Tsy Note	4 1/8	6/28/95	Realized Rate of Return 4.72%
Sell $3 M	US Tsy Note	4 1/4	5/17/96	Realized Rate of Return 4.19%
Pur $6 M	US Tsy Bill		3/31/94	Yield to Maturity 3.08%

Re-invest $6 M Proceeds from Maturing Treasury Bills on 3/31/94

Pur $3 M	US Tsy Note	4 1/8	6/28/95	Yield to Maturity 5.00%
Pur $3 M	US Tsy Note	4 1/4	5/17/96	Yield to Maturity 5.49%

Holding Period Yields Comparison

Period	Active	Passive
2nd half 1993	4.11%	3.96%
1st Quarter 1994	3.20%	3.96%
2nd Quarter 1994	4.64%	3.96%
1st Year	4.02%	3.96%
2nd Year	5.32%	4.64%

manager and whether or not it is better to employ a manager on staff versus out-sourcing the job to a professional management company. The benefits of hiring an on-staff manager are the completely dedicated effort and the integrated access of the manager to internal factors such as cash flows. The drawbacks would clearly be the lack of access to information, the costs of market information systems such as Telerate or Bloomberg, and the restricted access to many securities at competitive prices.

Hiring a professional investment management firm that specializes in the kinds of investments allowed has the advantages of multiple individual managers, independent reporting, broader information access, and the potential to access more aggressive bidders due to larger volume. The main disadvantage is the manager's attention being divided among multiple portfolios. The final decision should be based on the associated expectation of achieving the desired results. Figure 14-10 gives a sample of a request for proposal for an investment manager.

■ Beyond Portfolio Management

Reporting

An essential part of the total investment program is that the investment manager reports to senior management and the board of directors on the overall condition of the portfolio. Reporting allows the management and board to monitor and control performance and also allows the investment manager to receive feedback. The frequency of reporting may vary, depending upon the types of assets being managed and the degree of latitude in decision making provided to the investment manager. Reporting on a monthly basis to management, in writing, and quarterly to the board, in a summary form, should provide a sufficient flow of information. The content of the management report should include, at a minimum, an independent pricing of securities holdings and a summary of portfolio statistics, average life (or duration) and average return. Board reports should address policy compliance, a status report on the achievement of goals, and a plan of action for the balance of the period.

1. Is your firm a registered investment advisor under investment advisors Act of 1940?

2. Briefly describe the firm's ownership/affiliation.

3. Is any litigation pending and/or have any legal decisions been reached against the firms or its employees in the past five years? If so, please describe (include any SEC or NASD arbitration settlements).

4. In concert with investment management, does your firm broker/dealer securities or receive any other form of additional compensation for client transactions aside from the direct fee paid by clients?

5. Describe your existing client base for whom you manage short-term fixed-income funds (number of accounts, type, length of relationship, etc.).

6. Briefly describe your firm's investment management philosophy for short-term fixed-income funds.

7. Briefly describe the professional qualifications of your firm for managing short-term fixed-income funds.

8. Provide client return information for the preceding three years. (Realized rates of return—excluding unrealized gains or losses.)

9. What type of account reports do you provide (attach example), and how often are they prepared?

10. Briefly describe the scope of services provided.

11. Briefly describe any additional features, attributes, or conditions that the hospital should consider in selecting your firm for investment management service

12. Describe your proposed fee arrangements.

13. Please provide three references.

When management and the board do not have an adequate procedure in place for reporting and monitoring investment performance, there is exposure. As an example, while many factors besides reporting may have contributed to the recent investment difficulties of the City Colleges of Chicago, the argument can be made that if the board had been monitoring the actions in the context of policies or otherwise, the results might have been different.

"Last September . . . [the district's treasurer] invested almost all of the Chicago Community College District's $100 million in securities backed by principal payments on home mortgages." *(Did this comply with investment policy?)* "Rates on 30-year mortgages had to drop almost one percentage point for the district to obtain higher returns on the bonds than on treasury securities, which aren't as risky." *(Did this comply with investment strategy?)*

"Within weeks...rates began a six month climb. As a result...City Colleges lost millions of dollars."

"The district claimed that [the dealer] misrepresented the risks of the bonds, known as principal-only securities, or POs. It also alleged that the firm knew POs were inappropriate for a taxpayer-supported institution."

"[The firm's] executives...saying they have documents indicating [the treasurer] was authorized to buy the bonds."
Bloomberg Business News, April 7, 1994

Operational Concerns

Last, but certainly not least, are the logistical measures: confirmations, delivery, safekeeping, and statements. They are important because they substantiate the activity, providing a control, or audit mechanism, to ensure the safety of the total process.

The written confirmation of the transaction from the dealer is the first piece of physical evidence of the transaction. The dealer is required to provide a complete description of the security: name, coupon, maturity, and cusip number; and a complete detail of the trade: par value, type of trade (buy or sell), price, extension, accrued interest, delivery instructions, and dates of transaction and settlement.

For control purposes, confirmation should be delivered directly to a securities accounting and control area and not to the individual or area directly responsible for making investment decisions and actions, thereby preserving the integrity of the system.

Delivery of securities may occur either "versus payment" or "free of payment," and delivery may be taken either in a "third party" account or in a "primary" account. *Delivery versus payment* means that the buyer's cash account is not charged for the purchase until the security is presented for payment. Thus, in the event of a delay in delivery or some other problem with settlement, the buyer retains control of its cash position; its risk of not holding either the cash or the investment asset is remote. *Free of payment* delivery is normally a result of the counterparty either maintaining a cash account for the buyer and agreeing to charge the purchase price to the account, where an exchange of securities occurs (as in the case of repo collateral) and both deliveries are free of payment, or where securities serving as collateral exceed the required amount and any excess must be returned.

Safekeeping is provided by most major commercial banks for their clients, in connection with the banks' own safekeeping needs in the Federal Reserve Bank system. Banks are responsible for providing safekeeping receipts and periodic statements of account balances. Both documents are important and should be compared for accuracy to the dealer confirmation, the bank statement of holdings, and the investor's own internal holding reports.

The two major considerations in selecting or retaining a safekeeping bank are *cost* and *service*. Service that allows for the most flexibility in terms of investing, delivering deadlines, statement availability, and personnel availability is desirable; cost should not be the primary concern. Custodial services, provided by the trust departments of commercial banks, encompass all the services provided through bank safekeeping and more. Securities lending, trust accounting, and a professional staff with responsibility for client services are among the benefits. As an example, Figure 14-11 shows the range of custodial services and fees offered through a formal RFP procedure in April 1992.

Figure 14–11	Responses to a Request for Proposal for Custodial Services					
	National Securities Dealer	Regional Bank	Regional Bank	Regional Bank	Local Bank	Local Bank
Security Safekeeping						
Fed. Reserve-Direct	No	✓	✓	✓	✓	✓
Depository Trust Co.	✓	✓	✓	✓	✓	✓
Physical—N.Y.	✓	✓	✓	✓	✓	✓
Security Settlement						
Dlvy. vs. Payment	✓	✓	✓	✓	✓	✓
Free of Payment	✓	No	No	No	No	No
Same Day Settle Cut-Off Time (EST)						
Fed. Reserve	12:00	1:00	11:00	12:00	12:00	10:30
DTC	11:00	2:30	11:00	12:00	1:30	10:30
Physical	11:00	12:00	11:00	12:00	11:00	10:30
Income Collections						
Immediate Credit On All Items	No	✓	No	No	No	No
Wire Transfers						
Cut-Off Time (EST)	5:45	3:00	1:00	3:30	2:00	2:00
Statements						
Transaction	✓	✓	No	No	✓	✓
Frequency	Mo.	Mo.	Mo.	Mo.	Mo.	Mo.
Avail By:	5th Bus. Day	5th Bus. Day	5th Bus. Day	5th Bus. Day	10th Bus. Day	10th Bus. Day
Types:						
Holding	✓	✓	✓	✓	✓	✓
Activity	✓	✓	✓	✓	✓	✓
Other						
Money Mkt. Acct Sweep	✓	✓	✓	No	✓	No
On-line Acct. Access	✓	✓	✓	No	No	Future
Security Lending	✓	✓	No	No	No	No
Annual Fee	.04%	.02%	.015%	.01%	.035%	.05%

15 A Primer on Mergers and Acquisitions in the Healthcare Industry

—Joshua A. Nemzoff

One of the greatest challenges facing the healthcare industry is dealing with the process of market consolidation. For many hospital boards and management teams, a merger, acquisition, or divestiture (all generally referred to as "M&A" transactions) is a once-in-a-lifetime event. Due to the complexity and risk involved in such transactions, millions of dollars can be lost during contract negotiations and due diligence. It is absolutely imperative in today's highly competitive and volatile healthcare industry that hospitals devise an effective merger and acquisition plan. This chapter addresses several concepts relating to M&A transactions in the healthcare industry. They are as follows:

1. components of an effective M&A plan;

2. evaluation and assessment of the consolidation impact;

3. evaluation of the overall impact of shutting down a hospital;

4. examination of out-migration and feeder systems, which are key issues in secondary markets; and

5. examination of the issue of ultimate control of the hospital, which may be the key reason why a hospital will not sell to a competitor.

This chapter also analyzes the M&A process, including the project team, the timing of the acquisition or merger, due diligence, effective negotiations, and key risk areas. In addition, it will offer suggestions in developing the right M&A process and approach.

■ Acquisition Planning and Implementation

Most hospitals do not sell until they get into considerable financial trouble. An acquisition plan is a proactive process that begins by identifying facilities or providers that may or may not be currently for sale—but should be. The acquisition plan determines what the impact will be of consolidation, shutdown, and feeders. It includes an analysis of the anticipated return on investment. Since it makes no sense to attempt to buy a hospital that cannot be purchased, the plan includes the probability of acquisition. It also includes a prioritization of target hospitals—a list that identifies those hospitals in a specific market that your operation should consider buying first. This target list is an essential component of the acquisition plan, which outlines the methodology for pursuing and ultimately acquiring the hospital of your choice as identified by the target list.

■ Evaluation and Assessment—The Valuation Process

The evaluation process (determining the viability of acquiring a hospital) is based on a very simple concept: market share. The larger your market share, the greater the volume of business you will have. The same basic principal holds true for revenues. The greater the volume of your business, the larger your revenue base will be. Combined with effective expense controls and management, a solid revenue base will generate positive cash flow. Cash flow determines value; value determines price; and price establishes what your return on investment from an acquisition will be.

In determining the viability of an acquisition, step one is assessing market share for both your operation and the one you are considering acquiring. Return on investment is the key criterion in this process. Regardless of the purchase price of the facility or provider—whether you assume debt or pay cash—the purchase price and the amount of money that you receive as a result determines your return on investment. Obviously, you do not want to invest in a bad deal that will have a negative or risky return on investment. Cash flow is the essential factor.

In all probability, you have heard and read a great deal about multiples; Earnings Before Depreciation, Interest and Taxes, or EBDIT (pronounced "ebb dit"); and different evaluation techniques. However, the best technique for evaluating a hospital's value is to determine its cash flow and discount that backwards to figure out exactly what you are receiving for the purchase price.

There are two ways to go about analyzing a hospital's value: the free cash method and an EBDIT method. The free cash method is defined as the total amount of cash the hospital is using. It is not solely income, but net cash flow, which includes cash for capital acquisitions, principal payments, and working capital. The EBDIT multiple represents earnings before depreciation, interest, and taxes—basically, a definition of profit. The not-for-profit equivalent of this multiple is income available for debt service.

The average purchase price for a hospital currently is between four and six times EBDIT. This price approximates a 20 to 33 percent discount rate which, given 5 percent cost of capital, results in roughly a 15 to 28 percent return on investment.

These numbers mean that if you are a not-for-profit organization buying a hospital, and the capital cost is 5 percent while the purchase price is four times EBDIT, you will achieve roughly a 28 percent return on investment. This is a solid return and clearly explains why there is a tremendous amount of acquisition activity for hospitals. Should you use the free cash method of assessment, the return on investment drops to roughly 10-20 percent as a result of the involvement of other cash items.

▮ Which EBDIT to Use?

One of the most difficult questions involved in the valuation process is determining which EBDIT method you should utilize in making your decision. For instance, if you are considering purchasing a hospital that historically made $10 million annually, is this the number by which you multiply the EBDIT multiple? Do you buy the hospital for $50 million? What if you conclude that you could effectively manage it and double its revenue to $20 million annually? Do you then multiply five times EBDIT for a considerably larger sum of $100 million? It gets confusing when considering which EBDIT to utilize.

As a guideline, value basically is equal to debt capacity. If you have conducted debt capacity studies, you recall that those studies analyze and determine how much debt you can afford and still allow your facility to operate profitably. Essentially, an evaluation analysis is a similar process. The primary difference is in figuring just how much debt you can afford for the targeted facility.

Once a value has been determined, the actual price offered should be based on one of several circumstances. If you are in a competitive bid situation with three or four competitors (including some for-profit operations) and you bid four times EBDIT, then, in all probability, you will lose. If it is not a competitive bid situation and you bid six times EBDIT, you will pay a price that is too high. Because of this, the circumstances surrounding the actual bidding dictate which of these EBDIT multiples you use. In some cases, you may be wise to offer a price that is lower than the stated range of four to six times EBDIT; in other cases, you may offer a higher price. On average, however, most acquisitions are completed at four to six times EBDIT.

∎ The Impact of Consolidation

One of the most important considerations in any acquisition process is the impact of consolidation. In the healthcare industry, the consolidation impact is what occurs when you have two hospitals in the same market, one of which was recently acquired and which can be managed from an existing facility. On average, hospitals tend to have their overall cost structures running at roughly 40 percent variable costs and 60 percent fixed costs. This average can change based upon the size of the hospital. The selling hospital typically will have this same cost ratio. If you consolidate a hospital (take over the management of the acquired facility), you should be able, at the very minimum, to generate 20 percent savings in its operation.

Where will these savings come from? A great deal of it will come from support staff layoffs—typically from administration, human resources, information systems, the marketing department, and the public relations department. Additionally, you may be able to consolidate some of the out-patient services, such as laboratory and ambulatory surgery. In any case, as you scrutinize the seller's departmental expenses to establish effective expense controls and cuts, you will find there will be numerous opportunities for savings.

The fact that the savings primarily will come from layoffs presents a very difficult human resource issue that nobody enjoys. However, considering that most hospital's operating expenses are 50- to 60-percent labor costs, there is no conceivable way to reach the 20 percent savings without layoffs. Sometimes these layoffs occur immediately after the closing is completed; sometimes they occur three to six months later. Without layoffs, you will be assuming that you can simply manage the hospital better than the previous owner—an assumption that may be dangerous.

The savings do not always occur overnight. It may take 12 to 18 months to generate the targeted 20 percent savings in a newly acquired facility, but the savings discussed here are very real and can be achieved quickly and efficiently. This explains why many of the large for-profit systems are consistently acquiring more hospitals in markets they already dominate. It is not necessarily to create networks to deal with managed care; it can be because they have figured out the positive financial impact of effective consolidation and expense management.

∎ Shut Downs

If you happen to operate in a marketplace where you have the option of shutting down the acquired hospital, the financial picture and strategy change dramatically. The buyer obviously has existing fixed and variable costs. The only additional costs for a shut down are capital costs required for additional capacity to absorb the other facility. However, these capital costs typically are financed. If the buyer has to spend $20 to $30 million in capital costs, these costs generally are not added to the purchase price of the acquired facility. Instead, the debt service is added to the capital costs, which fall into the area of total cost.

The variable costs of the seller are multiplied by the retained volume. This means that if you shut the hospital down, you may only recover 50 to 60 percent of its patients. The rest of them may move to other facilities. When the variable costs are multiplied by the retainage percentage, the result will tell how much variable revenue and variable cost the buyer will receive, and these become the incremental cost.

Since roughly 60 percent of a hospital's total expenses are fixed costs, the key benefit of a shut down is the elimination of these costs. When you shut down a hospital, all its fixed costs disappear.

Shut Down—A Hypothetical Case

To give a clearer idea of what is involved in, and the difference between, shutting down a hospital or consolidating its operations with an existing facility, let us briefly review a hypothetical shut down case.

Assume you are considering the purchase of a 300-bed hospital that you are going to shut down. It is five miles away from your existing facility and has $110 million in revenue and $110 million in expenses. Ten million dollars of this expense is depreciation or interest, so the EBDIT is $10 million. Sixty percent of their costs are fixed, and 40 percent of their costs are variable. You expect to retain 60 percent of their volume after the facility is shut down, and your *capacity cost* is $40 million. This means it is going to cost your operation $40 million to put a new wing on your hospital to service the 60 percent of business from the other hospital when it moves to your facility. The price, using a multiple of five times EBDIT, is $50 million. After you review the situation closely, you decide that $50 million is the right number.

It is at this point that you begin your shut down calculations. The calculations point out that if you are going to get 60 percent of the hospital's volume, you are going to get 60 percent of their revenue, or $66 million. The hospital's fixed costs, which also total $66 million, are eliminated upon shut down. The variable costs multiplied by the 60 percent retainage is roughly $26.4 million. The debt service on $40 million for the new addition at 5 percent turns out to be roughly $2.5 million. So the cash flow of this hospital, which was $10 million as an ongoing operation, is now roughly $37.1 million. The return on investment for the ongoing operation of the facility, based on five times EBDIT, is roughly 25 percent. The return on investment based on shut down is roughly 288 percent.

Although these numbers and assumptions are rough, it is unlikely that the return in a situation with these characteristics would fall below 200 percent. This is precisely why so many hospitals are being shut down; why hospitals in two-hospital towns are trying to shut down the competing hospital; and why a number of companies have bought and then closed hospitals on the very day the acquisition closed. This hypothetical case is just an example of the high return on investment that is available through shutting down a competing hospital.

■ Issues of Importance in Secondary Markets— Out-Migration and Feeders

Out-migration is one of the other key issues in reviewing the process of acquiring hospitals. Small hospitals in secondary markets typically provide primary acute care. The out-migration in these areas can be 50 to 60 percent, and the distance individuals travel can be as much as 40 to 50 miles. Doctors in these hospitals have a tendency to refer patients to other physicians with whom they have a relationship or friendship. If there is a large metropolitan area in close proximity, the referrals typically will go to a number of hospitals. Many hospitals tend to concentrate on their primary service areas when evaluating the potential of attracting new patients, thinking that hospitals there are the primary competition. However, if you have hospitals that are 20, 30, or even 40 miles away that are small, 70- to 100-bed primary care facilities, you may find there is a very substantial impact in buying those hospitals because you are then able to have those patients referred to your hospital as opposed to every other hospital in town. By changing out-migration patterns and putting more of a priority on them, you may find that these feeder hospitals are very inviting targets. The return on investment can be very positive, and if attempts at establishing networks with these smaller hospitals do not work out, you may, out of necessity, have to move into an acquisition mode.

■ Hospital Control—Why Sellers Do Not Sell

The essential reason why hospitals do not sell when they should is very simple: control. Gaining control of the hospital means the clear and substantial dominance of a surviving board of trustees by the buyer. It is not assuming the position of chairman of the board. It is not having the ability to appoint the position of chief executive officer. It is the direct control of the board's actions by the buyer. Without such control, it is extremely difficult to effect a consolidation or a shut down.

The control issue needs to be resolved before you begin the acquisition process. It should not be resolved during the acquisition negotiation or after it. There are literally hundreds of mergers in this country that have been attempted but never consummated, where the control issue was never resolved. Until you resolve the control issue, you simply do not have a solid, plausible deal.

▌ Facility Swaps

The swap process tends to resolve all the control issues. Through an exchange process, control is not an issue. One facility takes control of the other and vice versa. Swapping also resolves the price issue. The negotiations should work as follows: "You pay me five times EBDIT, and I'll do the same."

For these kinds of cash free exchanges of hospital facilities, there are some very serious tax considerations that affect for-profits. These considerations relate to the valuation of those assets on their books. It is clearly a concern for them. Also, if you are going to get involved in a swap, you may have to deal with the fact that you may be swapping hospitals with a healthcare system. There clearly are antitrust implications to be considered when dealing with a system, and there are earnings-per-share implications if you are dealing with a for-profit operation.

▌ The Mergers and Acquisitions Team

Typical M&A transactions involve selling a hospital, acquiring a hospital, or merging two hospitals together, and the organization of an effective M&A project team is critical to the success of these transactions. The project team is very similar in each instance, and a comparable approach to organizing the team is used by many companies, both for-profits and not-for-profits.

Project teams typically should include two board members. These two board members should be actively involved in the process, and kept well informed by both the chief executive officer and the chief financial officer of the facility. There should be a *project director* who serves as the lead negotiator and coordinator for the whole team. Lack of experience in this role can be extremely costly. Also included on the project team are the due diligence and legal teams. This project team structure, as depicted in Figure 15-1, is a fairly simple organization and is designed to produce timely and effective results.

Care must be taken in organizing the project team, particularly in structuring the legal and due diligence teams. Your legal team generally should not consist of your in-house lawyer or a lawyer you hired once for the singular purpose of providing counsel in the acquisition of an MRI Center, or other such project. Instead, the legal team should be made up of professionals who possess expertise in a wide variety of specialty areas that are absolutely imperative for an effective acquisition to take place.

You should have a legal specialist who will serve as *transaction counsel*—an experienced professional in acquisitions who will, essentially, instruct you on how to complete the deal. *Antitrust counsel* should be retained at the very beginning of the acquisition process. If you are buying assets, you must have a *legal specialist in real estate.* Environmental issues are of primary concern, and you will need an *environmental attorney. Tax counsel* will be needed to provide advice on what the exact tax issues are. This area can be extraordinarily complex. You are likely to need *fraud and abuse counsel.* If you do not have

Figure 15-1   The Project Team

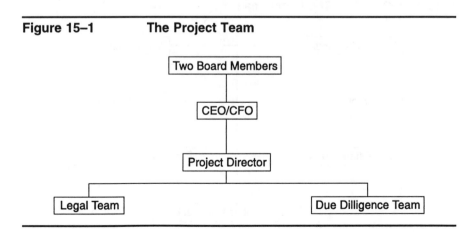

someone who is highly experienced with fraud and abuse to review physician contracts you may be taking over, then you could be assuming an enormous amount of liability that you could avoid. Finally, you will need specialized *labor counsel.* If you are getting involved in assuming pension liabilities, of if you are considering shutting down the acquired hospital, you must have all the above expertise to make sure your interests are covered. One lawyer cannot possibly cover all these areas with the necessary levels of expertise. Figure 15-2 depicts the legal team.

The due diligence team gets even more interesting and complex. This team covers an enormous range of issues. It is not unusual to a have a team consisting of 40 to 60 people to handle due diligence on an acquisition. Of course, you would not have such an extensive team for a $10 million purchase. When the cost of an acquisition rises to $30 to $40 million; however, all due diligence areas must be covered.

It is the role of the project director to coordinate not only the activities of the legal team, but also those of the due diligence team. The director has to ensure that the reports of the legal and due diligence teams are assimilated in the negotiation process.

∎ Timing

The timing of an acquisition is generally a six-month process. It takes approximately two weeks for the initial negotiations. Once these are completed, a letter of intent usually takes another two weeks. After these initial steps are completed, the real work begins.

Figure 15–2   The Legal Team

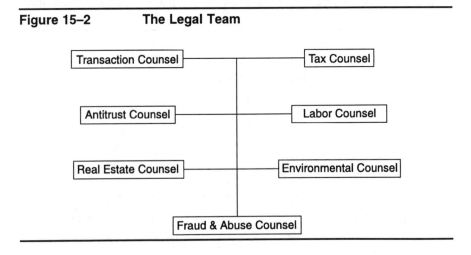

Due diligence takes about two months to complete. Negotiations occur during the entire process, and take about five months. While due diligence is in its process, the purchase agreement is being developed. In fact, the due diligence process leads to the purchase agreement because of its substantial role in the negotiation process. The closing can take one or two months, depending on the circumstances of the purchase.

Figure 15-3 depicts the approximate timetable for completing an acquisition. It is by no means an absolute. Each acquisition has its specific characteristics that either speed up the process or slow it down. The longest period of time spent on an acquisition should be no more than 10 months. If you have the right project team in place before the acquisition process begins, it is reasonable to conclude that you can effect an acquisition within a six-month period—provided the Federal Trade Commission and the Justice Department let you move ahead with it.

▮ Due Diligence

Many professionals believe that the due diligence process is nothing more than reviewing the seller's Medicare cost reports and financial statements, and conducting a building inspection. However, that is not

Figure 15–3   Timing of M&A Process

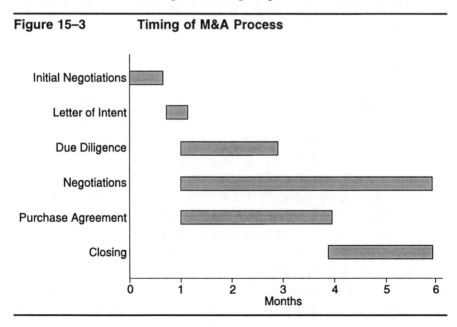

really the primary purpose of the due diligence effort. Due diligence has five goals. The first is *expense analysis*. What is the impact of the acquisition on expenses? The second goal is an *analysis of revenues*. For example, do you have an opportunity to improve the seller's managed-care contracts and increase revenue, or are you going to start losing revenue when you complete the purchase? The third goal is *management assessment*. If you are taking over a hospital, one of the major concerns you need to address is assessing the current management team. Do you want to keep the current team, or do you want to replace them? The fourth objective of the due diligence team concerns the *initial transition plan*. An essential and imperative part of due diligence is that which reveals which departments should be merged and which should be eliminated. This information needs to be completed and agreed upon before the acquisition is finalized.

Finally, one of the key areas of due diligence is to identify hidden problem areas—sometimes referred to as "red flag warnings." An example of this could be the toxic waste dump in the backyard of the hospital. Another such warning could be that the hospital is about to lose a very large managed-care contract. It could be that the building itself has asbestos everywhere. It could be that the hospital does not have an effective information systems operation—it happens to be located in the corporate office and the hospital cannot operate alone. These are examples of issues that a good due diligence effort will reveal.

▌ Negotiations

The negotiation process is completely different from due diligence. It is extremely complex and extremely risky. Inexperienced buyers tend to focus very directly and consistently on due diligence. Experienced buyers tend to focus more on the negotiation process.

The negotiation process consists of both legal and business points, and a strong advocate position is definitely mandatory. If someone tells you they can represent both parties effectively, your response should be: "If you were getting divorced, would you let the same lawyer represent both of you?" The answer, of course, is that you would not.

Acquiring a competitor typically is not a friendly process. Quite frankly, in most instances it is a very difficult situation. No one can represent both the seller and the buyer. It simply will not work. The negotiation process is based upon the letter of intent and on the due diligence process. As a general rule, principals (i.e., board members or management) should never be involved directly in the negotiations. The reason for this is twofold: 1) the principals are too close to the situation; and 2) they represent the court of last resort should negotiations begin to break down. If the key decision makers are in the room when a serious problem develops, there is no one for the two teams to turn to in order to help solve it.

The negotiation process typically involves two lead negotiators on each side: the project director and the transaction counsel. The two must work as a team. The project director covers the business aspects of the deal while the transaction counsel provides legal advice and direction. These two work hand-in-hand, and they should always negotiate together. Having one at the table without the other can mean trouble. Both individuals have imperative roles to play at all times.

■ Risk Factors

The primary risk areas in due diligence are significant. These are the areas where, if you make a mistake, the costs might not simply be $500,000 to $1 million—they are likely to be enormous and potentially devastating. They include Medicare, tax issues, malpractice issues, capital requirements, environmental issues, physician contracts, paid time off, employment guarantees, and market share loss. Each of these alone can be a multi-million dollar issue.

Tax issues in particular can represent multi-million dollar headaches. For example, if you are considering purchasing a hospital from a for-profit company, they might tell you they want to finance the deal as a stock transaction. They may suggest that you buy the stock of their company and convert it later to not-for-profit status. If this situation occurs, you might find that you are going to get slapped with their capital gains tax for converting to not-for-profit, and later find out that the reason they sold the hospital under the financial terms agreed upon is that they did not want to pay the capital gains tax themselves. This is the type of problem that can destroy a deal, or cost you millions of dollars at a later date.

The major risk area in contract negotiations is very simple: having an inexperienced M&A project team. It is imperative that you find professionals who have deep and extensive experience in the art of the acquisition process. If you do not have an experienced team, something is very likely to fall through the cracks that potentially could be devastating, both monetarily and legally. An inexperienced M&A team can prove to be disastrous.

▌ The Wrong M&A Approach

There is at least one right approach to M&A transactions, and many wrong approaches. One element in a wrong approach is consensus building, i.e., trying to get everybody to buy into the acquisition. Typically, every professional on the buyer side will think that the acquisition is an outstanding idea; those on the seller side will have just the opposite opinion. Allowing wide-open negotiations and letting everyone know what is going on is also a step in the wrong direction because it is guaranteed to slow the process to a snail's pace.

Conducting a substantial amount of analysis before you even sign a letter of intent—especially if you do not have a deal yet—can be a waste of time. Inadequate due diligence efforts are also a substantial part of the wrong approach, and having an inexperienced project team poses extreme danger to the success of your effort.

Another aspect of the wrong approach is not getting your board members to buy into the acquisition completely. If you tell one or two members about the acquisition and leave it to them to communicate the plan to the rest of the board members for a vote at a later date, you can cause some very serious problems due to lack of correct and adequate understanding on the part of everyone.

Referring to an acquisition as a merger is a very popular euphemism these days. For instance, when Columbia bought Hospital Corporation of America, it was referred to as a merger throughout the press accounts. However, the new board was made up of four HCA representatives and 11 from Columbia. This was an acquisition, not a merger. By calling a transaction like this a merger, you are risking control issues. Call it an acquisition if that is what it is.

One of the biggest mistakes you can make is guaranteeing jobs. In both shut downs and consolidation, layoffs are inevitable because 50 to 60 percent of a hospital's expenses are labor costs. They are the primary area where savings will be generated. If you guarantee jobs, you eliminate your ability to cut operating costs.

■ The Right M&A Approach

As for the right approach, the initial step is to determine the impact of the acquisition on your market share. That basic analysis drives everything else. If you are not going to be able to maintain market share of the hospital you are purchasing, you are inevitably going to have financial problems at a later date. You must calculate the expected return on investment to make sure the acquisition is a solid and strong business deal. You need to make sure you have a deal before you move ahead with any further analysis. There is no need to spend a great deal of time analyzing a potential M&A transaction when the party on the other end has no intention of being involved in the transaction with you. You must conduct an enormous amount of due diligence once the letter of intent has been signed, but do not waste time and resources conducting a lot of due diligence before it is signed.

Another aspect of the correct approach is to discuss the transaction only with those who absolutely need to have information, and this should be a very, very close and select group. It is not healthy for the intentions of an acquisition or sale to be broadcast throughout the facility. If you have to issue a press release, then work with a professional public relations or investor relations group that knows how to handle it. One thing you will notice in the for-profit sector is that you rarely find out about a deal until it is completed. In the not-for-profit sector, many times one will find rumors circulating the very day the deal is planned. This leads to unfounded rumors that the media will seize upon.

You also need to remove the obstacle of ego. There is a tremendous amount at stake in these transactions. When you are dealing with $50 to $100 million deals, people's livelihoods and their jobs are at stake. Therefore, personal egos and goals cannot be the driving consideration in a transaction of this size.

Do not be afraid to use the *L* word, layoffs. In all probability, there will be layoffs. Although the effect on your personnel can be considerable and negative, you only worsen the situation if you mislead them. If you are structuring a deal where there are not going to be layoffs, chances are you are headed toward trouble anyway.

Finally, put someone who is experienced in charge of the acquisition process as project director. Major transactions can monopolize the time of a CEO or CFO for up to six months if an outside expert is not brought in to run the transaction under their direction. It is also crucial to utilize experienced legal counsel. One of the biggest dangers in these deals is moving ahead without experienced legal professionals.

▎ Conclusion

Selling or acquiring a hospital is an extremely complicated and risky venture that is best handled very carefully. The right M&A approach can result in successful ventures that enable your healthcare organization to cope with the changes being thrust upon it, and the need to adapt to a new environment. Expert planning and execution are the primary keys to successful M&A transactions.

Appendicies

I **Appendix A—Rating Agencies**

I **Appendix B—Municipal Bond Insurance Companies**

Appendix A—Rating Agencies

Fitch Investors Service, Inc.

Fitch opened its doors in 1913 when John K. Fitch established Fitch Publishing Company and brought out The Fitch Bond Book, *the first complete listing of bonds available to investors. Having established its reputation in Wall Street credit circles, the firm saw a need over the following years for differentiating quality in available bonds and in 1922 introduced a system of rating symbols that gauged relative degrees of credit quality. These now-familiar symbols—AAA to D—first appeared in 1923 with the publication of* The Fitch Bond Rating Book.

Fitch's sense of responsibility to investors was evident again during the 1930s when toppling bond prices were having a drastic impact on bank portfolios. Fitch worked closely with U.S. government regulatory officials to create safety guidelines for bank investments.

In 1960, Fitch granted the right to use its rating symbols to Standard & Poor's Corporation and sold to S&P most of its publications and its printing plant. Fitch then concentrated on rating bonds, developing new publications and expanding its rating services to the fixed income community.

Fitch boasts a number of "firsts" in its history: first to rate long-term bank securities and health care debt instruments...first to explain in concrete terms the basis for rating judgments...first to introduce "plus" and "minus" signs with rating symbols. Under new management in 1989, Fitch plans to re-establish itself as an innovator in the financial service industry, adding many more "firsts" to its name.

Fitch is the oldest independently owned rating agency for fixed income securities in the U.S., and up until recently it was also the least visible. We knew when we acquired the company in April 1989 that it was not number one—or even number two—among the five recognized rating agencies. Frankly, it was somewhere at the bottom. But we're changing that.

We're giving the old Fitch a transfusion: new blood, fresh ideas, broader scope. Undercapitalized for so long, Fitch now has the means to institute change and reshape its image. Why are we doing this? Because we believe the credit rating industry has become complacent, not as responsive to clients' needs as it should be. Today's financial environment is vastly different from that of 10 or more years ago. Deregulation has changed some industries irrevocably. Stiffer competition, along with widely fluctuating interest rates and a rapidly changing economy, have played havoc with credit quality—changes have become more drastic and more frequent. Debt structuring and corporate restructuring have reached new levels of sophistication. Yet the rating agencies, Fitch as well as the competition, have remained largely unresponsive to the changes around them. The industry cries for innovation.

At Fitch, our first priority will be to improve rating criteria; our bond ratings will better reflect an issuer's vulnerability to future events. Next, we will support and complement our ratings with more written explanation and research, and finally, we will disseminate rating action more quickly. We want Fitch rating products to be prospective, informative, and pertinent—in short, responsive to today's complex financial needs.

We believe the key to turning Fitch around is good people. From day one we began seeking out the most talented and experienced in the business—people with good track records, with sincerity and integrity, dedicated to improving our service to the financial community—investors, issuers and investment bankers. Fitch employees, from management to the mail room, will have an opportunity to earn equity in the company. Financial incentive is important in attracting the best people.

We want to put Fitch back on the map and if that means the competition has to work a little harder, we like that idea. Everyone, particularly the investors, will benefit.

∎ The Debt Rating Process

The rating of a new issue is the result of an evaluation of its credit risk; it is an assessment of the issuer's commitment to meet the obligations of a specific debt issue in a timely fashion. A rating is a useful tool in investment decision-making. It may also be the basis for relative trading levels. However, it is not an indicator of a bond's price, which may be volatile for any number of reasons. Nor, strictly speaking, is a rating a recommendation to buy, sell or hold.

In assembling information, analysts look at the three C's of credit: character of management, collateral (if any) behind repayment of the debt, and capacity of the issuer to service its debt. This data is then assessed in light of the issuer's positioning in the industry or geographic region, and other factors such as economic, financial market and political considerations. However, this is a highly simplified version of what is, in reality, a complex and exacting process.

An issuer typically seeks two ratings, occasionally three, for various reasons. One rating service may have expertise in a particular area, such as structured finance. An issuer who has split ratings may request a third rating in the hope of strengthening the value of the higher rating. An institutional investor may request a fresh look at a rated security or an evaluation of a small issue not previously rated.

∎ Rating Surveillance

Fitch's job is far from finished once the initial rating is set. Fitch is particularly sensitive to surveillance and is always searching for techniques to improve it. Analysts keep the issuers under constant review, watching the economy, the industry or region and financial press for any development that would impact the credit rating. Takeover threats and leveraged buyouts, changing federal policies and an increasing number of tax referendums make news every day, so this is no small task. An investment grade rating can deteriorate overnight. Too often, investors have suffered because the rating services did not respond quickly enough to such a crisis. At Fitch, if an event should occur that might impact a rating, the issue is immediately placed on the Fitch*Alert list, which serves as an early warning system for investors. Once on the *Alert list, the company undergoes the same sort of scrutiny required for the initial rating, with an intensive investigation of its ability to continue servicing its obligations to investors. As soon as sufficient data are collected, the analyst presents the case once again to the Rating Committee and a revised (or possibly the same) rating is assigned.

∎ Pricing Policy

It is virtually impossible to have a rate schedule that would be fair to everyone since no two financings are ever exactly alike. Each situation is unique in some way, posing different problems and requiring different kinds of expertise. So, although Fitch has a reference schedule, our policy is to approach each issue on an individual basis. Therefore, prices will vary according to the complexity, size and timing of a deal. We encourage clients to come to us on a retainer basis, particularly when they bring a number of deals to market each year. Again, longstanding relationships are of great value and can make the job easier and less costly for both clients and Fitch.

The track record is clear. In a few short years, our ratings have come to mean a great deal more than anyone else imagined. They have major impact; they move markets. *We've responded to changing and emerging market needs.* We've introduced new criteria to analyze increasing complexities in fixed-income securities, and assess market risk uncertainties. *Although what we do is similar to Moody's and S&P in the area of credit risk,* we believe it's different in depth, scope and forward-thinking. Understanding how and why we're different is in your best interest. This brochure highlights our key differences and advantages, mindful that new ideas and developments are occurring here every day. *Fitch credit ratings cover municipal, structured and corporate financings. Fitch market risk ratings cover CMOs, mutual funds and derivatives,* and their investment performance under different interest rate conditions. *Investors drive the demand for ratings.* Life insurance companies, banks and trust companies, pension funds, mutual funds, investment advisors, individual investors and Federal and State regulators rely on Fitch ratings in making their investment and regulatory decisions. *We're here to inform investors.* We're here to respond to your needs, help you understand the impact of changes and trends in the market; enable you to make better decisions. For every hour other agencies spend with investors, our goal is to spend three to four. *Seasoned, entrepreneurial people are the engine of our success.* They've worked in, been exposed to and fully understand the market and investors' problems. And, since Fitch employees have a personal stake in the Company, they treat clients differently, work harder and work with enthusiasm. *The rating process isn't a black box.* We don't punch a lot of numbers into a computer and get an answer. It requires the participation of the issuer with the rating agency. It's a relationship with full disclosure and constructive dialogue between all parties. *Our policy is to provide credit ratings upon request.* We don't rate everything under the sun: issuers ask for a Fitch rating, because of its value to investors. This insures investors that each rating is independent, objective and well thought out. We put our credibility on the line with every one.

Setting a new standard for rating agencies is to everyone's benefit. Let us show you what service really means.

■ Products

Fitch's primary business is the analysis of fixed income securities. Our primary service is the assignment of credit ratings (AAA, AA, etc.) to publicly offered securities. These include straight corporate debt, municipal bonds, convertible debt, and preferred stock. We also assign ratings to issuance programs including commercial paper, deposit notes and medium-term notes, as well as the claims paying ability of insurance companies.

Ratings provide a guide to investors in determining the credit risk associated with a particular security. The ratings represent Fitch's assessment of the issuer's ability to meet the obligation of a specific debt issue or class of debt in a timely manner.

Specifically, Fitch provides three levels of credit analysis: Public Credit Ratings, Private Credit Ratings (aka: Private Placement Ratings), and Private Credit Opinions.

Public Credit Ratings

Public Credit ratings involve full scope analysis. A complete analysis of the debt issue is done by the assigned analysts who then make a recommendation to the Rating Committee. The Rating Committee, by consensus, determines the rating assigned. The rating is disclosed to the general public via press release. A detailed credit report is prepared and sent to our subscriber list before the sale if the debt is not a secondary market rating. For new-issue ratings, copies of our reports are provided to the investment banking or advisory firm prior to the sale. Public Credit ratings are periodically reviewed to reflect updated credit information.

Private Credit Ratings (aka: Private Placement Ratings)

Private Credit Ratings involve the same detailed level of analysis as Public Credit Ratings with some exceptions. The ratings are not disclosed to the public. A credit report may be prepared but it is solely for the use of the party requesting the rating. In most cases, the rating is not surveilled.

Private Credit Opinions

Private Credit Opinions involve a review of an obligor's creditworthiness with regards to a proposed debt financing. Opinions are done on a private basis and are solely for the internal use of whomever requests the opinion. Opinions do not include a detailed review of all information, or the completion of all procedures, which are necessary to reach a final rating. Only the general category of rating is conveyed, i.e., no plus, neutral or minus indication is given. The opinion is not surveilled.

■ Health Care Rating Process

Introduction

Municipal health care bonds generally are revenue bonds issued on behalf of an underlying obligor, such as a hospital, nursing home, or continuing care retirement community. For ease of understanding, such a health care entity is henceforth referred to as an "obligor."

Rating Request

Rating requests are typically received from an investment banker or a financial advisor on behalf of the obligor. Requests also may be received directly from the obligor or from the actual issuer of the bonds. Generally, Fitch will look to the source of the rating request to act as the primary contact throughout the rating process.

Fees

Fitch's rating fees depend on the analytical time involved, the travel expenses incurred, and the size and complexity of the issue being rated. Since financings vary from issue to issue, each requires differing areas of expertise. The all-inclusive fee is normally established upon receipt of the minimum required information and before the site visit. There is no ongoing fee for expenses incurred by Fitch in the surveillance and maintenance of an outstanding bond rating. Fees range from $4,000 to $100,000.

Timing

We encourage the primary contact to involve Fitch in the financing process as soon as practical. In most cases, this will allow Fitch to better serve the obligor and facilitate the financing schedule. The information requirements should be sent to Fitch five to seven working days before the site visit; in this way, discussions at the site visit can concentrate on issues of greatest credit importance. As soon as possible after the site visit (three to seven days), a rating committee will assign a rating. Fitch recognizes that last minute rescheduling is not unusual and every attempt is made to work within the financing schedule.

Required Information

To begin its analysis, Fitch requires details of the proposed financing, five years of audited financial statements and utilization data, interim financials and utilization information, a financial feasibility study (if available), and all pertinent legal documents.

Site Visit and Management Meeting

Site visits are an integral part of the analytical process. With few exceptions, a site visit and management meeting are required. We expect to meet with various representatives of the obligor. These representatives may include members of the board of trustees, the president or administrator, medical staff representative, the chief financial officer, and the director of nursing. Other participants of the financing team may also be contacted, i.e., the auditor, financial feasibility study consultant, bond counsel, etc.

Rating Committee

After the site visit has been completed, the assigned Fitch analysts will prepare a report for the rating committee. The obligor's management representative and other members of the financing team may receive follow-up phone calls to resolve any outstanding issues.

The rating is assigned during a formal meeting of the rating committee. The rating committee is comprised of the members of the Health Care and Higher Education Group and other staff members of the public finance department.

Ratings may be appealed. The interested parties are given the opportunity to present any additional information to the rating committee. The rating committee will then reconvene and make a final determination of the rating.

Published Reports

After a rating is assigned, it is communicated to the primary contact for the obligor. The rating is also released to the public via a press release.

A comprehensive credit report is also published. Depending on the financing schedule, we strive to have this report available at the time the preliminary official statement is mailed, i.e., before the negotiated pricing or competitive bid date.

Fitch encourages potential investors to call with any credit questions.

Surveillance

It is imperative that Fitch continues to receive updated information from the obligor so that the outstanding rating reflects current information.

The information needed to maintain ongoing surveillance is not as detailed as that required for initial rating. In most instances, duplicate copies of information that is routinely prepared by management for the board of trustee's meetings will suffice. At a minimum, this information should include interim financial statements, utilization data, information regarding major capital expenditures, and any material changes in management or services.

Periodically, an abbreviated credit report is published. Any time we change a rating, a published report is issued. These updates are part of our service to investors and facilitate a better secondary market in the bonds. Although Fitch does not require face-to-face update meetings, we strongly encourage them and will request a meeting if the circumstances warrant.

■ Rating Information Requirements—Hospitals

The following is an outline of information Fitch needs for its rating process. Applicants should discuss and provide information on the primary obligor for the bonds being rated. If an obligated group is involved, discuss and provide information for the obligated group members on both a separate and combined basis. If a feasibility study and/or a preliminary official statement is available, it should already address many of the items listed below.

This listing of information requirements is not meant to be all encompassing. Our needs vary and depend on the structure of the issue being rated as well as the particular credit characteristics of the borrower. Participants to the bond financing should be willing to share any other data determined to be useful in rendering our credit opinion.

I.   FINANCING PLAN

1. Description and timetable; include the following detail, based on the purpose of the financing:

   a. If a construction project:

      (i)   The percent of project costs being financed with bond proceeds

      (ii)   The amount, source and timing of any equity contribution

      (iii)   Certificate of Need application and approval letter and copies of any other approvals needed and secured

      (iv)   Guaranteed Maximum Price information; include a copy of the draft construction contract

      (v)   Experience of architect and degree of completed drawings

      (vi)   Experience of general contractor

   b. If refunding:

      (i)   Reasons for refunding; e.g., legal, economic or both

      (ii)   Purpose of refunded bonds; status of any related project and a copy of the Official Statement/Prospectus related to such prior issue

  c. If financing prior or future capital expenditures, indicate type of equipment and timing

  d. If acquisition:

      (i)   Reasons for sale/purchase

      (ii)   Results of any independent valuation study

      (iii) Third party reimbursement ramifications

      (iv) Working capital needs

2. Statement of Sources and Uses of Funds

3. Debt Service Schedule

4. The Preliminary Official Statement/Prospectus

5. All legal documents to be executed and related opinions under which the Bonds will be issued: Master/Trust Indenture, Bond Indenture, Loan/Lease Agreement, Guaranty Agreements, Escrow Agreement, etc.

II. GENERAL DESCRIPTIVE INFORMATION

1. Brief history of the organization

2. Development of physical plant, size, major construction projects and improvements

3. Description of services

4. Existence of any educational programs, interns/residents and college/university affiliations

5. Corporate legal structure, with brief description of each entity

III. MANAGEMENT AND STAFF COMPLEMENT

1. Board of Trustees:

  a. For each member, provide profession or occupation, board position, current term and total years of service

  b. Brief description of appointment process, standing committees and governing powers

2. Management: Resume for each of the senior executive personnel and heads of major departments; if managed via contract, a summary of contract

3. Medical Staff:

  a. Number of active, associate and courtesy staff members for each of the past five fiscal years

  b. Average age of the active staff

  c. Board certification and board eligibility status

  d. Admissions by age groups

  e. The top ten admitters and list for each: admissions, age, and specialty

  f. Location of physician offices

      g. Types of practices (solo, partnerships, etc.)

      h. Admitting privileges to other hospitals

      i. Recruitment policies

      j. Current vacancies

  4. Nursing:

      a. Composition of staff (RN's, LPN's, NA's)

      b. Turnover rate/vacancy rate

      c. Recruitment policies

      d. Salary structure versus competitors

  5. Other:

      a. Existence of or attempts to bring in unions; any strikes, work stoppages

      b. Average number of full time equivalents (FTEs) for last five fiscal years, current year and budgeted

IV. SERVICE AREA

1. Market and demand analysis that defines the facility's primary and secondary service areas

2. General socio-economic data of service area (city, county) including description of population trends, major employers, unemployment rates, income levels, etc.

3. Market share data:

      a. For each hospital in the service area, based on the most current data available as compared to three to five years previously, list:

         (i) Licensed/operated beds

         (ii) Admissions (or discharges)

         (iii) Patient days

         (iv) ALOS and occupancy rates

         (v) Rooms rates

         (vi) Distance from subject facility

         (vii) Percent share of the market based on admissions and patient days

      b. Also include descriptions of each competitor's unique services and any future plans (expansion, new services, etc.)

4. List of other health care competitors/providers (HMOs, PPOs, free standing urgi-centers, etc.) in the service area

V. OPERATIONS

1. Accreditation/licensing status and results of last accreditation survey

2. Brief list of insurance policies and coverage limits; provide a list of all outstanding claims and pending lawsuits

3. Top 10 DRGs; indicate profit or loss on each

4. List of all participating HMOs and PPOs; briefly describe reimbursement agreements

5. Capabilities of management information systems.

VI. UTILIZATION DATA

1. Inpatient statistics by major service (medical-surgical, pediatrics, obstetrics, etc.) for each of the last five fiscal years:

    a. Licensed and available/staffed beds

    b. Admissions (or discharges)

    c. Patient days

    d. ALOS and occupancy rates

Newborn data should be separate

2. Outpatient statistics for each of the last five fiscal years by major service: ER, clinic, same day surgery, etc.

3. Year-to-date inpatient and outpatient statistics with comparisons to last year and budget

4. Medicare and total Case Mix Index for each of the last five fiscal years

VII. FINANCIAL DATA

1. Audited financial statements for each of the last five fiscal years

2. Auditor's management letters issued in each of the last five fiscal years, along with any of management's responses

3. Year-to-date financial statements with comparisons to last year and budget

4. For this fiscal year: full year (original) budget with revisions (if applicable)

5. For last fiscal year: full year budget

6. For next fiscal year: full year budget

7. Room charges for the last five fiscal years

8. Payor class mix, based on;

    a. Percentage of revenue

    b. Percentage of admissions

    c. Percentage of patient days
       for each of the last five years; categories to include Medicare, Medicaid, Blue Cross, HMO/PPO, commercial, self-pay and other, and should add up to 100%

9. Demand and financial feasibility study projections

10. Long range plan and three to five year capital budget

11. List of all short and long term debt (including any debt which is guaranteed by the Hospital), indicating original amount, outstanding balance, security features, maturity dates and applicable legal provisions

12. Lines of credit, security features and history of use

13. Cash management policies

VIII. SURVEILLANCE

After an initial rating is assigned, Fitch requires certain ongoing information to assure that the rating reflects the obligor's current status. The information includes, but is not necessarily limited to, certain items listed under the headings of Operations, Utilization Data and Financial Data. The frequency of update could be as often as monthly.

▌ Investment Grade Bond Ratings

Fitch investment grade bond ratings provide a guide to investors in determining the credit risk associated with a particular security. The ratings represent Fitch's assessment of the issuer's ability to meet the obligations of a specific debt issue or class of debt in a timely manner.

The rating takes into consideration special features of the issue, its relationship to other obligations of the issuer, the current and prospective financial condition and operating performance of the issuer and any guarantor, as well as the economic and political environment that might affect the issuer's future financial strength and credit quality.

Fitch ratings do not reflect any credit enhancement that may be provided by insurance policies or financial guaranties unless otherwise indicated.

Bonds that have the same rating are of similar but not necessarily identical credit quality since the rating categories do not fully reflect small differences in the degrees of credit risk.

Fitch ratings are not recommendations to buy, sell, or hold any security. Ratings do not comment on the adequacy of market price, the suitability of any security for a particular investor, or the tax-exempt nature or taxability of payments made in respect of any security.

Fitch ratings are based on information obtained from issuers, other obligors, underwriters, their experts, and other sources Fitch believes to be reliable. Fitch does not audit or verify the truth or accuracy of such information. Ratings may be changed, suspended, or withdrawn as a result of changes in, or the unavailability of, information or for other reasons.

AAA Bonds considered to be investment grade and of the highest credit quality. The obligor has an exceptionally strong ability to pay interest and repay principal, which is unlikely to be affected by reasonably foreseeable events.

AA Bonds considered to be investment grade and of very high credit quality. The obligor's ability to pay interest and repay principal is very strong, although not quite as strong as bonds rated 'AAA'. Because bonds rated in the 'AAA' and 'AA' categories are not significantly vulnerable to foreseeable future developments, short-term debt of these issuers is generally rated 'F-1+'.

A Bonds considered to be investment grade and of high credit quality. The obligor's ability to pay interest and repay principal is considered to be strong, but may be more vulnerable to adverse changes in economic conditions and circumstances than bonds with higher ratings.

BBB Bonds considered to be investment grade and of satisfactory credit quality. The obligor's ability to pay interest and repay principal is considered to be adequate. Adverse changes in economic conditions and circumstances, however, are more likely to have adverse impact on these bonds, and therefore impair timely payment. The likelihood that the ratings of these bonds will fall below investment grade is higher than for bonds with higher ratings.

Plus(+) Minus(-) Plus and minus signs are used with a rating symbol to indicate the relative position of a credit within the rating category. Plus and minus signs, however, are not used in the 'AAA' category.

NR Indicates that Fitch does not rate the specific issue.

Conditional A conditional rating is premised on the successful completion of a project or the occurrence of a specific event.

Suspended A rating is suspended when Fitch deems the amount of information available from the issuer to be inadequate for rating purposes.

Withdrawn A rating will be withdrawn when an issue matures or is called or refinanced, and, at Fitch's discretion, when an issuer fails to furnish proper and timely information.

FitchAlert Ratings are placed on FitchAlert to notify investors of an occurrence that is likely to result in a rating change and the likely direction of such change. These are designated as "Positive," indicating a potential upgrade, "Negative," for potential downgrade, or "Evolving," where ratings may be raised or lowered. FitchAlert is relatively short-term, and should be resolved within 12 months.

Credit Trend Credit trend indicators show whether credit fundamentals are improving, stable, declining, or uncertain, as follows:

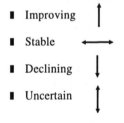

- Improving
- Stable
- Declining
- Uncertain

Credit trend indicators are not predictions that any rating change will occur, and have a longer-term time frame than issues placed on FitchAlert.

▮ Speculative Grade Bond Ratings

Fitch speculative grade bond ratings provide a guide to investors in determining the credit risk associated with a particular security. The ratings ('BB' to 'C') represent Fitch's assessment of the likelihood of timely payment of principal and interest in accordance with the terms of obligation for bond issues not in default. For defaulted bonds, the rating ('DDD' to 'D') is an assessment of the ultimate recovery value through reorganization or liquidation.

The rating takes into consideration special features of the issue, its relationship to other obligations of the issuer, the current and prospective financial condition and operating performance of the issuer and any guarantor, as well as the economic and political environment that might affect the issuer's future financial strength.

Bonds that have the same rating are of similar but not necessarily identical credit quality since rating categories cannot fully reflect the differences in degrees of credit risk.

BB Bonds are considered speculative. The obligor's ability to pay interest and repay principal may be affected over time by adverse economic changes. However, business and financial alternatives can be identified which could assist the obligor in satisfying its debt service requirements.

B Bonds are considered highly speculative. While bonds in this class are currently meeting debt service requirements, the probability of continued timely payment of principal and interest reflects the obligor's limited margin of safety and the need for reasonable business and economic activity throughout the life of the issue.

CCC Bonds have certain identifiable characteristics which, if not remedied, may lead to default. The ability to meet obligations requires an advantageous business and economic environment.

CC Bonds are minimally protected. Default in payment of interest and/or principal seems probable over time.

C Bonds are in imminent default in payment of interest or principal.

DDD, DD and D Bonds are in default on interest and/or principal payments. Such bonds are extremely speculative and should be voted on the basis of their ultimate recovery value in liquidation or reorganization of the obligor. 'DDD' represents the highest potential for recovery on these bonds, and 'D' represents the lowest potential for recovery.

Plus(+) Minus(-) Plus and minus signs are used with a rating symbol to indicate the relative position of a credit within the rating category. Plus and minus signs, however, are not used in the 'DDD', 'DD', or 'D' categories.

▎ Short-Term Ratings

Fitch's short-term ratings apply to debt obligations that are payable on demand or have original maturities of generally up to three years, including commercial paper, certificates of deposit, medium-term notes, and municipal and investment notes.

The short-term rating places greater emphasis than a long-term rating on the existence of liquidity necessary to meet the issuer's obligations in a timely manner.

F-1+ Exceptionally Strong Credit Quality. Issues assigned this rating are regarded as having the strongest degree of assurance for timely payment.

F-1 Very Strong Credit Quality. Issues assigned this rating reflect an assurance of timely payment only slightly less in degree than issues rated 'F-1+'.

F-2 Good Credit Quality. Issues assigned this rating have a satisfactory degree of assurance for timely payment, but the margin of safety is not as great as for issues assigned 'F-1+' and 'F-1' ratings.

F-3 Fair Credit Quality. Issues assigned this rating have characteristics suggesting that the degree of assurance for timely payment is adequate, however, near-term adverse changes could cause these securities to be rated below investment grade.

F-5 Weak Credit Quality. Issues assigned this rating have characteristics suggesting a minimal degree of assurance for timely payment and are vulnerable to near-term adverse changes in financial and economic conditions.

D Default. Issues assigned this rating are in actual or imminent payment default.

LOC The symbol LOC indicates that the rating is based on a letter of credit issued by a commercial bank.

Moody's Municipal Department Rating Hospital Revenue Bonds

The Rating Process

▮ Introduction

It is within Moody's Municipal Department that ratings are assigned to short-term and long-term tax-exempt debt instruments, including hospital revenue bonds. Many hospital revenue bonds are rated on the basis of credit substitution if they have bond insurance or a bank letter of credit. This brochure describes the rating process for hospital revenue bonds which are secured solely by hospital operations.

A bond rating is a measure of relative credit worthiness. As credit analysts, we look to historical trend data to assist us in making evaluations about future performance. However, since ratings involve judgments about the future and are used by investors as a means of protection, we also look at the "worst" potentialities in the "visible" future rather than solely at an institution's past record and present status. Therefore, a rating reflects statistical factors as well as an appraisal of long-term risks, including the recognition of many non-quantifiable factors.

The discussion which follows serves two explanatory roles. The mechanical process used to reach a rating decision is outlined and the key analytic factors employed in the process are described.

Initial Contact and Required Documentation

Typically, a hospital's underwriter, financial consultant, or the public entity issuing bonds on the hospital's behalf informs Moody's that it is requesting a rating. This contact occurs a few weeks before the expected sale of the bonds. Hospitals usually may not in their own name issue bonds bearing interest exempt from taxation. However, public bodies (state or local authorities, counties, cities, etc.) are able to do so on behalf of health care institutions. Virtually all tax-exempt hospital revenue bonds rated by Moody's are issued by a public entity with a hospital responsible for meeting all debt service requirements under the terms of various legal agreements.

The hospital's financing advisor or the firm which will underwrite the bond sale sends the documents associated with the sale to Moody's. These include the preliminary official statement, the feasibility study (if prepared), legal agreements such as a trust indenture, mortgage or lease, management letters, and recent annual financial reports. Many of these documents are only in draft form at this stage. Upon receipt of this information, one or two Moody's hospital analysts are assigned to review the materials. Preliminary research is undertaken concerning both the hospital's service area and competing hospitals. The analysts will follow the bond offering from these initial phases through the rating assignment.

Visits and Meetings

Analysts normally spend a day or two conducting an on-site visit of the hospital. They view all facilities and tour the service area. A formal meeting is held with members of the hospital's board, top administrative personnel, bond counsel, the feasibility study consultants, community leaders, and the hospital's financial advisors. If such a visit is not required, a meeting is usually held at Moody's office in New York City with the hospital representatives.

Credit Report Preparation and Presentation to Rating Committee

A detailed credit report is written in which debt factors, legal security, financial matters, hospital services, utilization, and the area demographics and economy are evaluated. (A discussion of these factors follows under the heading "Analysis of Hospital Revenue Bonds.") A supervisor reviews the report and discusses the rating recommendation which the analyst(s) then presents to the Rating Committee. After a thorough discussion, a consensus is reached and a rating is assigned.

The Rating Committee consists of senior officers of the Municipal Department. Members serve on a rotational basis, and consistency is stressed. Accordingly, a hospital revenue bond rated **A** is considered to be of comparable credit quality to a general obligation bond rated **A**.

Release of Rating

The hospital (through its financial consultant or underwriter) is immediately informed of the rating. Very occasionally the rating is formally appealed. If new information is provided, the rating will be reviewed. This appeal process may or may not lead to a change in rating.

Once a rating is assigned, it is within the public domain and is included in a number of Moody's publications, including the weekly *Bond Survey*, the monthly *Bond Record*, and in Moody's *Municipal & Government Manual*. The credit report is published and sent to subscribers within a day or two of assignment of the rating. A courtesy copy is provided to the hospital.

Rating Reviews

All Moody's ratings are reviewed on a regular basis for as long as rated debt remains outstanding. Annual financial reports of the hospital's operations, data concerning completion of new facilities, utilization statistics, and other information must be supplied on a timely basis. Failure to do so can result in rating withdrawal. The sale of additional bonds (even if insured or backed by a letter of credit) prompts a complete rating review, although a meeting may not be needed.

■ Analysis of Hospital Revenue Bonds

The basic analytic factors considered in the assignment of ratings for hospital revenue bonds are discussed below. Although the same factors are evaluated in analyzing different situations, no set formula is used. The same item deemed significant in analyzing the debt position of one hospital could be of minor importance in relation to another hospital.

Debt Factors

An evaluation is made of the actual issuer of the debt, usually an authority, a county, or some other public entity. The unit's past experience, if any, in servicing hospital debt is considered. There should be no legal or administrative impediment which could bring into question the issuer's ability to meet its specified responsibilities. The magnitude of the hospital's debt is measured, and various debt ratios are computed for comparative analysis. The size of the debt load is considered in light of prior, present, and future borrowing needs.

Prompt debt retirement is a favorable credit factor; bonds should be retired during the useful life of the project being financed. At the same time, net revenues available to pay bond principal and interest should comfortably cover those requirements. Typically, if historic net revenues provide at least 1.00 times coverage of the projected maximum annual debt service requirement, a definitive rating will be assigned. If such coverage is lacking, a conditional rating most likely will be assigned. The conditional aspect of a rating remains in place until after project completion and satisfactory financial operations thereafter are demonstrated. If a hospital plans to retire its debt unusually rapidly or unusually slowly, a full explanation should be provided. Moody's also evaluates the reasonableness of interest rate assumptions on new debt. If debt service projections are based upon an unrealistically low interest rate, it may be necessary to stretch the debt, reduce the principal amount, or accept lower coverage.

The use of bond proceeds is examined carefully. Moody's will rate hospital revenue bonds only if all approvals (certificate of need, etc.) have been received. The certificate of need and the feasibility study should demonstrate the appropriateness of the project. The timeliness of the project is also evaluated. Construction which responds to a definite need within its service area allows a hospital to maintain or improve its competitive edge. Construction which is long overdue is less risky but may indicate that management lacks foresight. A building project can interrupt service delivery. Moody's considers this problem in terms of both utilization and revenue generation. The construction timetable should be reasonable. Moody's always wants to know if any project funding is to be derived from sources other than bond proceeds. A hospital contribution often shows a strong commitment and the ability to generate revenue. A successful fund-raising drive also can indicate management's objectives and community support. If investment earnings flow to a construction fund, interest rate assumptions should be realistic. Normally, interest requirements during construction are capitalized, and the debt service reserve fund is fully funded initially.

Future financing plans are carefully considered in the rating process. The imposition of additional debt is not necessarily a negative factor as it may be required for project completion.

The absence of any further plans may lead to the conclusion that the hospital will be unprepared for future developments. The additional bonds test should provide both protection to the bondholder and adequate flexibility for the issuance of parity debt.

▌ Bond Security Provisions

A financially strong hospital serving a prosperous service area may receive a low bond rating if its debt is poorly secured. Accordingly, an analysis is always made of all legal documents pertaining to the bond sale. These documents include the bond resolution, trust indenture, lease and sublease (or mortgage), and guaranty agreements. The strengths of the legal protections provided are determined. The flow-of-funds provisions are analyzed, including how any drawdown of the debt service reserve fund would be replenished. The additional bonds test should be neither so lenient as to dilute security nor so restrictive as to prove inhibiting. A rate covenant should be realistic and compare favorably with both historic performance and projected results. Investments by the trustee should be restricted to high quality securities. The analyst will also examine the hospital's ability to transfer assets, issue guarantees, and enter into merger or consolidation agreements. Legal documents (for example those which allow for the issuance of variable rate demand obligations) should not be so flexible as to weaken overall bondholder protection.

Financial Factors

In considering financial factors, the analyst determines if the hospital is in a strong position to incur debt. Changes in gross revenue, operating and maintenance costs (O & M), and net revenue are looked at closely. Sharp increases in O & M are of concern unless operating and other revenues have grown correspondingly. An aberration resulting from capital expenses financed from available current revenues may be treated positively.

Operating revenues should exceed operating expenses, but other sources of revenue (such as gift giving) are also examined. These sources of revenue most often are better applied toward capital items or one-time expenses, particularly if they are non-recurring or difficult to project. The status of accounts receivable is important on its own merit and speaks to the quality of management. Hospitals earning high credit ratings do not have serious problems collecting monies owed them, nor do they have an increasing trend of days in accounts receivable. Additionally, the higher-rated hospitals are successful in collecting reimbursements promptly. Margins of comfort for the bondholder are viewed as being diminished if a hospital continues to operate under a break-even fiscal policy.

Among the more important documents examined is the feasibility study. Its forecasts are compared closely with recent historical results to determine whether the assumptions used are reasonable and projections attainable. When goals seem unachievable, the individuals who prepared the study are questioned about their findings. While the feasibility study typically covers a forecast period of five years, Moody's rating is applicable for the life of the bonds based on information at a given point in time.

Certain states have rate review commissions which regulate the level and frequency with which hospitals may increase rates. In other states the imposition of such restrictions is a distinct possibility. Although rate adjusting constraints rarely work in a hospital's favor, they need not be a negative factor, particularly if they have been in place for an extended period and a hospital has not suffered from them. On the other hand, a hospital will be looked upon negatively if it has not raised rates as needed when it had the ability to do so. Moody's carefully examines how well a hospital has coped with Medicare's transition to a prospective payment system (PPS).

Other financial matters of concern include malpractice insurance and litigation. A hospital should carry adequate insurance for malpractice claims and other risks at a reasonable cost and should not be faced with a malpractice suit or other pending litigation which could have a severe impact upon its financial condition.

The Hospital

A unique feature of hospitals vis-a-vis the tax-exempt bond market is that they exist in a competitive environment. City residents do not have a choice of providers of water and sewer services but they do have a choice of which hospital to use.

Moody's compares a hospital with its direct competition (and nationally) in relation to such matters as physician recruitment, attraction of patients, financial results under prospective payment, and average length of stay. The economy of the hospital's service area is also an important rating consideration. A hospital in an area facing secular decline rather than cyclical problems may have that trend reflected in its rating. Population increases are generally deemed favorable unless they reveal demographic shifts to which the hospital cannot adjust. Normally a large facility or a hospital system offering a wide range of services is in a better position than a small, acute-care institution. A deteriorated plant with code deficiencies is a matter of concern.

Although analyzing the quality of management is difficult, this examination is a vital part of the rating process. As has been mentioned above, certain financial characteristics serve to measure management success or failure. An active policy-setting board of trustees which provides continuity is a favorable component; frequent turnover within the top management team is not.

Utilization trends are examined with the same care as financial trends. Increasing utilization is not, in and of itself, a positive sign. Analysis of changes in patient composition and the types of services being provided are examined in depth. The offering of services on an outpatient basis and of ambulatory surgery, and their level of utilization, are important considerations. Other trend criteria measured and compared include: admissions, patient days, percent occupancy, and emergency room visits. The hospital's accreditation history is reviewed. If full accreditation is lacking, the reasons should be provided. A hospital's educational affiliations and/or research facilities enhance the hospital's overall reputation.

The nature of the medical staff is also examined. Favorable attributes include a young age of the leading admitting doctors, a low rate of turnover, minimal reliance upon a few physicians for the bulk of admissions, and a high percentage of board certified or board eligible doctors.

A hospital's record of labor relations is important, particularly if a hospital has had a series of labor problems and is about to become unionized. Unionization, wage scales, pensions, and labor relations generally are areas in which hospitals are measured against their competition.

Appropriate corporate reorganization can help a hospital's credit position if assets are shielded, reimbursement posture is improved, or if better investment practices can be implemented. Likewise, mergers and/or the creation of a system could lead to favorable rating consideration. Economies of scale, more professional management, easier physician recruitment, and a linkage of services producing referrals are among the advantages which can be gained. However, neither corporate reorganization nor the creation of a system guarantees a higher rating. Corporate reorganization can result in a new hospital system ill suited to meet the needs of its participants. Such a development detracts from overall credit quality.

The analytic factors mentioned above form the basis for rating most hospital revenue bonds. However, every bond issue is examined carefully, separate and apart from all others.

Questions concerning the rating process are welcome and should be addressed to:

Municipal Department
Moody's Investors Service
99 Church Street
New York, New York 10007
Telephone: (212) 553-0300

∎ Key to Moody's Municipal Bond Ratings

Aaa

Bonds which are rated Aaa are judged to be the best quality. They carry the smallest degree of investment risk and are generally referred to as "gilt edge." Interest payments are protected by a large or by an exceptionally stable margin and principal is secure. While the various protective elements are likely to change, such changes as can be visualized are most unlikely to impair the fundamentally strong position of such issues.

Aa

Bonds which are rated Aa are judged to be of high quality by all standards. Together with the Aaa group they comprise what are generally known as high grade bonds. They are rated lower than the best bonds because margins of protection may not be as large as in Aaa securities or fluctuation of protective elements may be of greater amplitude or there may be other elements present which make the long-term risks appear somewhat larger than in Aaa securities.

A

Bonds which are rated A possess many favorable investment attributes and are to be considered as upper medium grade obligations. Factors giving security to principal and interest are considered adequate, but elements may be present which suggest a susceptibility to impairment some time in the future.

Baa

Bonds which are rated Baa are considered as medium grade obligations; i.e., they are neither highly protected nor poorly secured. Interest payments and principal security appear adequate for the present but certain protective elements may be lacking or may be characteristically unreliable over any great length of time. Such bonds lack outstanding investment characteristics and in fact have speculative characteristics as well.

Ba

Bonds which are rated Ba are judged to have speculative elements; their future cannot be considered as well-assured. Often the protection of interest and principal payments may be very moderate, and thereby not well safeguarded during both good and bad times over the future. Uncertainty of position characterizes bonds in this class.

B

Bonds which are rated B generally lack characteristics of the desirable investment. Assurance of interest and principal payments or maintenance of other terms of the contract over any long period of time may be small.

Caa

Bonds which are rated Caa are of poor standing. Such issues may be in default or there may be present elements of danger with respect to principal or interest.

Ca

Bonds which are rated Ca represented obligations which are speculative in a high degree. Such issues are often in default or have other marked shortcomings.

C

Bonds which are rated C are the lowest rated class of bonds, and issues so rated can be regarded as having extremely poor prospects of ever attaining any real investment standing.

Con.(...)

Bonds for which the security depends upon the completion of some act or the fulfillment of some condition are rated conditionally. These are bonds secured by (a) earnings of projects under construction, (b) earnings of projects unseasoned in operating experience, (c) rentals which begin when facilities are completed, or (d) payments to which some other limiting condition attaches. Parenthetical rating denotes probable credit stature upon completion of construction or elimination of basis of condition.

Those bonds in the **Aa, A, Baa, Ba** and **B** groups which Moody's believes possess the strongest investment attributes are designated by the symbols **Aa1, A1, Baa1, Ba1** and **B1**.

Suspension or withdrawal of a rating may occur if new and material circumstances arise, the effects of which preclude satisfactory analysis; if there is no longer available reasonable up-to-date data to permit a judgment to be formed; if a bond is called for redemption; or for other reasons. Withdrawal of a rating usually results from a definable situation such as failure to submit information on a timely basis. Suspension usually occurs when ambiguity prevails. Until the situation is clarified, the unit's rating will remain suspended.

Excerpts from Moody's Investors Service

An Issuer's Guide to the Rating Process[1]

Public Finance Department

■ Introduction

Founded nearly a century ago to analyze the securities of U.S. railroads, Moody's Investors Service today is the world leader in credit research services. Thousands of issuers, issuer intermediaries, and investors around the world rely on Moody's for credit ratings that are accurate, consistent, and comprehensive.

In 1909, John Moody introduced the rating system that has become an international standard, with the well-known symbols ranging from Aaa to C to indicate levels of credit quality.

Moody's began rating tax-exempt municipal debt in 1918. Today the Public Finance Department maintains over 40,000 ratings on the short- and long-term obligations of about 20,000 issuers in the United States and Canada—states, provinces, cities, counties, school districts, Canadian Crown corporations, and a wide range of other municipal entities. Moody's rates in excess of 90% of the municipal market's rated long-term volume annually.

This guide has been published in the hope that the reader will gain a better understanding not only of the rating process, policies, and procedures used by the Public

---

1 Copyright © 1993 by Moody's Investors Service, Inc. Publishing and executive offices at 99 Church Street, New York, NY 10007.

Finance staff at Moody's, but also of the overriding principles of thoroughness, accuracy, and impartiality that drive our work. It is not intended as a primer on analytic criteria or methods. Detailed discussions of Moody's analytic criteria are available in a number of other publications, depending on the nature of the debt. For example, *Moody's on Revenue Bonds: The Fundamentals of Revenue Credit Analysis* and *Moody's on Airports: The Fundamentals of Airport Debt* are comprehensive guides to Moody's rating methodology. Our Perspective line of publications, which includes *Perspective on Structured Finance, Perspective on Bond Insurance, Perspective on Municipal Issues, Perspective on Asset-Backed Finance, Perspective on Canada*, and *Perspective on Health Care Finance*, features periodic policy pieces on rating criteria and issues or trends of significance to the debt markets.

Moody's Role in the Capital Markets

A Moody's credit rating is an independent opinion about the future. It is an assessment of the ability and willingness of an issuer of debt, as well as its legal obligation, to make full and timely payments of principal and interest on the debt security over the course of its maturity schedule. The rating scale represents a consistent framework for ranking and comparing the relative risks of many debt issues.

Moody's long history of accuracy in its judgments has earned the confidence of thousands of institutional investors, securities traders, brokers, and others who find the rating system to be a quick, efficient, and trustworthy guide in contributing to countless investment decisions. Not only do investors use these ratings in selecting investments, but they also examine Moody's underlying analysis for statistics, trends, and opinions that assist their own internal analytic efforts. It should be understood that assignment of a rating does not constitute a recommendation to buy, sell, or hold a security. Ratings are designed exclusively for the purpose of grading bonds according to their credit qualities and do not take into consideration factors such as the direction of future market price or the risk parameters of the investor. A decision to invest in a given bond may be governed by its yield, its maturity date, or other factors for which the investor may search, as well as on its credit quality—the only characteristic to which the rating refers.

The credibility Moody's has earned with investors can, in turn, be beneficial to issuers in achieving cost-effective debt issuance.

Generally, ratings can help issuers by broadening the market for their securities to investors who otherwise might be unaware of the opportunity, by improving the terms of the issue itself, and by stabilizing market access in times of stress.

Organization of Moody's Public Finance Department

There are more than 300 associates in Moody's Public Finance Department, representing a diverse group of professionals. In addition to analysts, the largest segment of our employees, the department is staffed with experienced professionals in the areas of operations, information and technology, legal analysis, and marketing.

Most of Moody's analysts have attended graduate school, studying a wide range of disciplines which include public policy analysis, finance, law, urban planning, and economics. The majority of our analysts come to Moody' with experience in a field related to government or finance. Active participation in professional societies is encouraged and supported. Our analysts are well known throughout the public finance community, and their expertise is frequently tapped for speaking at seminars and conferences, as task force members, and on a wide range of public finance-related issues.

The analytic staff is organized into four major rating areas: regional ratings; structured finance, not-for-profit institutions, and financial guarantors; state ratings; and Canadian ratings.

Regional Ratings

Regional ratings analysts are assigned to a specific geographic region of the country, and generally follow all local issuers within a given state or group of states in that region. These analysts review virtually all debt issued by the assigned municipal entities regardless of underlying security (i.e., general obligation bonds, revenue bonds, lease financings, etc.). This organizational framework allows analysts to develop expertise on local statutes, financial reporting practices, tax and debt limits, local economies, political issues, and management as well as other factors underpinning the creditworthiness of specific municipalities and related enterprises.

To complement this regional structure and add depth and a national perspective to our coverage of key analytic issues, Moody's has introduced several enterprise revenue specialty groups corresponding to the major categories of revenue bond issuance nationwide. Each group includes a cross section of analysts with specific expertise in analyzing the given enterprise system; they are available to assist the regional analyst assigned to a particular revenue bond issue. The industries represented are public power; water and sewer; solid waste/resource recovery; airports; ports; mass transit; and toll roads. Other groups have been formed to address special financing structures, such as commercial paper/variable rate demand obligations (VRDOs), and state revolving funds and other types of pool financing. An in-house legal analysis group, staffed by attorneys who are also experienced credit analysts, is available to assist our analysts with credit issues of a legal nature.

▮ Structured Finance, Not-for-Profit Institutions, and Financial Guarantor Ratings

The analysts in the structured finance, not-for-profit institutions, and financial guarantors groups are responsible for the following types of ratings: those that are credit supported or asset backed, those for health care and higher education facilities, and those that carry bond insurance. Analysts assigned to the credit-supported ratings group research and analyze debt issues that possess some type of credit enhancement or substitution, e.g., letters of credit, liquidity facilities, and a variety of derivative products. The credit-supported ratings group also assigns ratings to refunded issues. The asset-backed finance group is primarily responsible for assigning ratings to mortgage revenue bonds issued by state and local housing finance agencies. Student loans, asset sales, FHA-insured issues, mortgage insurance funds, and bonds backed by the Government National Mortgage Association (Ginnie Mae) are also evaluated by analysts in this group. The health care analysts assign ratings to bonds issued by tax-exempt hospitals, health maintenance organizations (HMOs), and nursing homes. Our higher education analysts evaluate debt issued by colleges, universities, and other institutions of higher learning. Finally, Moody's bond insurance group analysts are responsible for the claims-paying ratings assigned to the municipal bond insurance companies that Moody's rates, and for ensuring that the procedures are followed by which the claims-paying rating is substituted for the underlying security of an issuer's bonds. Analysts in the structured finance, not-for-profit institutions, and financial guarantors groups frequently have experience in related sectors, such as health care, housing finance, banking, or law.

Investor Services and Strategic Business Development

In addition to the primary areas of credit analysis, the Public Finance Department contains two groups of professionals dedicated to serving Moody's primary customer segments: investors and issuers. Our investor services group provides rating information, portfolio services, subscriptions to *Municipal Credit Reports* and other public finance publications, as well as any other services associated with investor relations. In addition, sales, marketing, and product design and publication functions are also performed within the investor services group. The strategic business development group focuses on services and products for issuers and issuer intermediaries, while also taking responsibility for all staff development and training.

Product Resources

Our product resources staff provides extensive support to all of our analytic efforts and makes possible the publication of the broad range of products the public finance market regularly receives. The group comprises an information center, database and data analysis specialists, systems development personnel, and production and graphics staff. Information management and technology play a vital role in serving our clients.

Framework for Credit Analysis

At Moody's, we have been evaluating the complexities of public finance for almost 75 years and our role in the public finance marketplace has not changed: Moody's provides investors with comprehensive information about public sector debt and, most important, with an independent, objective assessment of the relative creditworthiness of those debt obligations—a credit rating. Although the subtleties of the public finance market change continually, the fundamental need to provide investors with an appropriate assessment of credit risk remains the same. Investors must have a concise way to gauge the risk that an obligor will be unable or unwilling to pay its debt according to the terms of a specific bond issue. This fundamental concept of municipal credit risk analysis applies equally to general obligation debt, special tax bonds, lease obligations, and enterprise revenue bonds.

Our rating process looks at past performance and trends as well as at estimated future prospects. It is a process that employs proven methodologies and criteria but also recognizes the unique credit characteristics of each issue that we rate. Our analysis encompasses qualitative as well as quantitative criteria; therefore, adequate, relevant, and reliable data must be provided to Moody's in order for us to maintain our standards in making rating decisions.

A Moody's credit evaluation is not a snapshot of one brief period in an issuer's existence. Most often, our evaluations are done in the context of what has taken place over the last five to 10 years. The public finance analysts at Moody's emphasize real-time current information within the context of a continuing flow of data. And with the many thousands of ratings that we maintain across the United States, Moody's has extensive familiarity and expertise with every facet of municipal finance—the successes as well as the problems.

Our ability to provide the broadest rating services available in the public finance market rests on our large pool of highly skilled analysts with expertise in all areas of municipal credit analysis. A superior technical and informational support team, which uses powerful analytic workstations, broad comparative data bases, a comprehensive library, and the latest in production and distribution facilities, enables Moody's to offer clients comprehensive and timely ratings and analysis in a variety of formats including our *Municipal Credit Reports*, detailed comparative reviews and research publications, and our electronic distribution networks.

▮ The Rating Process

Applying for a Rating

The rating process for a debt issue begins with a request for a rating, which may be made in writing or by telephone, by the issuer, its financial advisor, or the underwriter. A formal written application is not necessary. Ideally, the request should be made well enough in advance of the expected sale date to provide sufficient time for credit analysis, face-to-face meetings or on-site visits when necessary, as well as the timely release and publication of the rating. Application two to four weeks in advance is desirable, although it is understood that market conditions may dictate a much narrower time frame. The rating process could be longer for first-time issuers, particularly if a meeting or on-site visit is requested. Repeat issuers, on the other hand, may find that there will be some efficiencies that allow us to accommodate a tighter schedule. The Public Finance Department rates securities on request, for a fee. Information about our fees can be obtained prior to beginning the rating process by calling our Customer Service Department at (212) 553-0901.

Information Requirements

The credit analyst will look both to historical trends and current conditions, in addition to prepared projections, when making evaluations about future performance. A credit rating for long-term debt reflects analysis of objective statistical factors and an appraisal of potential long-term risks that include the recognition of many non-quantifiable variables. In order to assess both these quantifiable and non-quantifiable factors, a variety of documents must be examined. Credit ratings for short-term instruments are derived from an appraisal of somewhat different credit factors and our informational requirements are therefore different, as is the rating scale (MIG ratings). An issuer's long-term and short-term debt ratings are distinct; one cannot be inferred from the other.

In conjunction with the request for rating, all pertinent documents should be submitted to Moody's. Preliminary drafts of documents are acceptable at this stage. Moody's typically requires the following:

▮ The preliminary official statement

▮ Audits or annual financial reports for at least the last three fiscal years

▮ The most recent budget for operations

▮ The capital budget (or planning document)

▮ The bond counsel opinion addressing the debt's legal status

▮ All legal documents relating to the security for the debt

Other supporting documents may also be needed depending on the type of debt issue. For example, for a school district bond, Moody's would need information on enrollment trends; for a resource recovery system revenue bond, engineering studies dealing with operating projections and project feasibility should be submitted; for a tax anticipation note, the need for cash flow data is critical. Entirely different information requirements exist for the many structured finance ratings that we provide. All information must be current. A detailed listing of the specific information required for the most common types of debt that we rate can be found in the appendix of this publication.

Confidentiality

As part of the rating process, issuers often provide Moody's with information not in the public domain. It is Moody's practice to protect the confidentiality of that information while using it to make accurate rating decisions.

The Analyst's Role

Our public finance analysts perform the research and analysis needed to determine the creditworthiness of the debt issue. To reach a rating recommendation, the analyst evaluates all information presented by the issuer, and relies heavily on Moody's own historical files and computerized public finance data base. This data base, which is one of the most comprehensive of its kind in the municipal finance industry, includes a wide range of demographic and labor market data about localities across the nation and selected financial information.

Moody's has also developed medians of performance for a variety of financial, operating, and debt statistics that help in evaluating the credit strength or weakness of a particular issuer in relation to others of similar size and type. These medians, which are updated annually, are available upon request.

During the course of a rating review, analysts place emphasis on areas of special or heightened analytic concern. Issuers and their representatives are kept informed of these concerns, and are given every opportunity during the rating process to respond to analysts' questions and provide additional relevant credit information.

∎ Meetings and On-Site Visits

The rating process for many of our ratings includes a meeting between the issuer and Moody's analysts. A meeting with the issuer provides us an opportunity to discuss issues not easily communicated through documents, thereby augmenting the analyst's research. Equally important, meetings also permit the analyst to become familiar with local officials, as management capability can be a key rating factor. While rarely an absolute necessity, rating meetings are most beneficial under the following circumstances:

∎ This is the issuer's first bond issue to be rated by Moody's.

∎ The debt issue is particularly large and complex.

∎ Significant changes (positive or negative) have occurred in an issuer's underlying credit factors.

∎ Moody's has not met with representatives of the issuing entity for an extended period.

Meetings are held either at Moody's offices in New York City or San Francisco or on site. Holding the meeting on site is appropriate if an area and/or facility tour is deemed essential by Moody's and the issuer, or if key persons cannot come to Moody's.

About one month prior to the date of the bond issue sale is the ideal time to telephone Moody's either to request a meeting or to discuss whether one should be scheduled. Meetings typically take place about two weeks before the date of sale.

What is discussed in detail at a rating meeting varies depending upon the most critical areas of concern for a particular debt issue. For this reason, the following guidelines can help an issuer be best prepared to communicate the most critical points to our analysts.

■ Prepare an agenda that will lead to discussion of the issue's credit strengths and weaknesses.

■ Send documents to Moody's well in advance of the meeting date.

■ Talk to our analysts before the meeting to determine informational needs. Specific items might be requested in light of unique circumstances associated with a particular bond issue.

■ Key officials should attend, if available, particularly those most familiar with financial operations and debt policy.

There is no one perfect formula for the ideal meeting. For the analyst, a productive meeting is one where all critical ratings issues—whether administrative, legal, financial, economic or debt-related—are addressed. The key is ensuring the flow of relevant information. Meetings are most valuable when they provide the analyst with supplemental information that cannot be obtained through a review of the documents.

If an on-site tour is appropriate, one or more analysts may participate. Analysts are most interested in a balanced and accurate view of the issuer. A tour itinerary should, therefore, highlight both the issuer's strong points and problem areas. Important projects previously financed, those under construction, and likely future needs should be covered. If a visit is associated with a revenue bond rating, a tour of the enterprise system's facilities is usually recommended.

Rating Committee and Rating Decisions

When data collection and analysis have been completed, the analyst presents the rating recommendation for a senior staff member's sign-off. The prepared analysis and supporting materials are then presented to a departmental rating committee, which consists of senior members of the Public Finance Department serving on a rotational basis. These committees vary in size and committee sessions vary in duration, depending on the nature of the rating scenario under consideration. The ultimate rating decision rests with this rating committee, which evaluates the information presented, reaches a consensus, and then officially assigns the rating.

Rating Dissemination

With the assignment of a rating by the rating committee, the analytic process is concluded. The analyst then calls a designated representative of the issuer and, if different, the party who applied for the rating to notify them of the rating decision. The analyst typically notifies the issuer or its financial advisor by telephone, followed by official written notification. The newly-assigned rating will not be publicly released until the issuer or its authorized representative has been contacted. Once that occurs, the rating becomes public information.

After the rating is released to the issuer, Moody's expends considerable effort to ensure the broadest possible dissemination of the issuer's rating to the public finance market. Ratings are delivered via electronic vendor services such as the Bloomberg System and Munifacts, allowing for real-time delivery of all our rating decisions. Moody's Rating Desk makes the rating available to the public by telephone enquiry. *A Municipal Credit Report* is produced and distributed to investor clients, detailing the issue's credit factors, and the rating is also published in other Moody's publications, such as the *Bond Record*. If the debt issue is likely to be of very high public interest, Moody's issues a press release to alert various national and appropriate local newspapers and national wire services.

Rating Appeals

At times during the preparation of a credit rating, it becomes apparent that the rating will not reach the level expected or sought by the party requesting the rating. In fact, the analyst may plan to recommend a rating downgrade.

It is always Moody's intent that the rating process be clear to issuers and that our judgments be sound and fair. We therefore strive to ensure that issuers and their intermediaries are made aware at an early stage in the analytic process of all issues that may ultimately affect the outcome of the rating decision. Dialogue through each step of the rating process is intended to provide issuers with an adequate opportunity to respond to our concerns so that they are not surprised by the rating eventually assigned. Particularly when the likely rating outcome is a downgrade or a rating other than that anticipated by the issuer, our thoughts on the credit will be shared prior to finalization of the process to be sure that we have all relevant input from the issuer and that our approach to the rating is well understood.

Nevertheless, occasions may arise where fundamental disagreement exists between the issuer and Moody's over the rating conclusion that has been reached. On such occasions it is possible for the issuer to appeal the rating decision prior to its public release. It is Moody's policy that a full and fair hearing of the views of all parties to a transaction be part of the formal rating process, however, rather than part of a separate appeal process after the rating has been assigned. We have found that an open and candid approach during the rating process has actually resulted in a reduction in the need for appeals. In those instances where an issuer does not concur with Moody's rating conclusion and can provide additional information that was not previously considered in support of its position, a review of the rating will be undertaken. The views of the issuer and the new information will be reviewed by Moody's analysts and rating committee members and a final rating decision will be made.

Rating Surveillance

At Moody's the rating process does not end with the sale and closing of a municipal finance transaction. Rating currency is a critical facet of Moody's service to issuers and to the investing public and, therefore, the Public Finance Department regularly reviews outstanding ratings to confirm their accuracy. The process for updating an outstanding rating parallels that which occurs at the time of the debt sale. We review similar information (excluding documents specifically related to a sale, such as an official statement or legal opinion), drawing on extensive in-house files and data bases, and follow the same steps in assigning a rating. The analyst will contact the issuer to discuss developments that have occurred since the debt rating was last reviewed. If appropriate, the analyst may arrange for a meeting at Moody's or on site. Upon completion of our review, we utilize the broadest channels for dissemination, including a brief synopsis of the rating rationale which is available to our investor clients via electronic vendor services.

There are a variety of reasons why an issuer's outstanding debt rating may come up for review. These "triggers" include a sale of new debt by the issuer; current events that can affect an issuer's credit fundamentals; the need to verify that an action that was expected to occur some time after the initial rating was assigned has actually occurred (e.g., a necessary rate or tax increase was passed); and finally, just the passage of time, which can have an effect on an issuer's credit position. The issuer can facilitate the monitoring of its rating by sending Moody's annual audits and budgets and keeping us informed about significant events that have a bearing on credit position. Every effort is made to obtain this critical information. If an issuer fails to provide it, withdrawal of the rating may result.

Rating Withdrawals

Withdrawal of an existing rating can occur under a variety of circumstances. It should be noted that a rating withdrawal or its ultimate reinstatement is always at the discretion of the rating committee. The most common reasons for a rating withdrawal include:

■ The debt has matured or has been called and redeemed.

■ A letter of credit securing a debt instrument has expired in accordance with its terms.

■ In the case of a **VMIG** rating, the liquidity support for a demand feature of the debt instrument has expired, or the debt has been converted to a fixed interest rate without a demand feature, so that a **VMIG** rating is no longer applicable.

■ The debt has been refunded and Moody's has not been asked to review the rating on the refunded bonds, or Moody's has reviewed the rating and found it ineligible for a refunded (#Aaa) rating.

■ Debt with an equal or related claim on pledged revenues has been sold and no rating has been requested for the new issue.

■ In the course of seeking annual update information that we request for surveillance purposes, Moody's has not been provided with sufficient information to reach a rating decision. Such a circumstance will result in a withdrawal due to inadequate information.

Rating Suspensions

A rating suspension may occur if new and material circumstances arise, the effects of which preclude satisfactory analysis. Suspension usually occurs when ambiguity prevails. By contrast, withdrawal of a rating usually results from a definable situation such as failure to submit required information on a timely basis. Until the situation is sufficiently clarified to determine the appropriate rating, the issuer's debt rating will remain suspended. Reinstatement or revision of the rating is at the discretion of the rating committee.

Absence of a Rating

Where no rating has been assigned to a debt issue, it may be for reasons unrelated to the quality of the issue. Should no rating be assigned, the reason may be one of the following:

I An application for rating was not received or accepted.

I The issue or issuer belongs to a group of securities that are not rated as a matter of policy.

I There is a lack of essential data pertaining to the issue or issuer.

I In the case of short-term debt, the debt issue was not judged to be of investment grade.

Inquiries

Moody's makes every effort to keep abreast of developing trends and structures in the Public Finance marketplace. We welcome inquiries from issuers and their intermediaries, and encourage you to contact us when you have a question about the rating process or wish to discuss issues regarding municipal finance. Please refer to our most recent staff card for the name and telephone number of the appropriate manager who can respond to any questions you may have on the areas discussed above.

I Special Rating Policies and Procedures

Ratings on Credit-Supported Debt

Numerous municipalities and not-for-profit entities now access the capital markets by issuing debt securities fully supported by highly-rated third parties. For a broad segment of borrowers, public financing is not possible without access to the supported market.

Other borrowers desire the financing flexibility that structured transactions make possible. Historically, issuers have favored bond insurance and bank letters of credit as forms of credit substitution. The types of support employed in third-party structures are numerous and varied, however, and also include corporate guarantees, irrevocable revolving credit arrangements, guaranteed investment contracts, and escrowed securities.

For issuers that obtain insurance from one of the municipal bond insurance companies that carry a claims-paying rating from Moody's, we have procedures in place by which the insurer's claims-paying rating is substituted for the rating that would otherwise be derived from the underlying security provided by the issuer. The assignment of the insured rating takes place after we have received an executed insurance policy, which generally is in a standard format pre-approved by Moody's. Our analysts review the policy covering the issue and the structure of the transaction to verify that our rating criteria for full and timely payment of debt are met. Upon completion of this review and verification, the insurer's claims-paying rating is assigned. Separately, we also analyze the underlying credit quality of the insured issue in order to update investors regarding any outstanding parity debt, as well as for our evaluation of the insurer's risk portfolio. Standard procedures for surveillance and dissemination of credit information apply to insured issues.

For investors, third-party credit support is intended to substitute the credit risk of the support provider for that of the weaker debt issuer. Effective credit substitution requires more than incorporation of strong third-party credit support, however. In rated transactions, effective substitution is achieved by the combination of a strong credit support provider with structural mechanisms and protections designed to overcome various legal risks (particularly bankruptcy) associated with the issuer or borrowing beneficiary. Full credit substitution should insulate the investor completely from the risks associated with the issuer or borrower.

Moody's is actively engaged in rating credit-supported debt and our rating approach reflects the dynamic nature of this segment of the market. Thus the approach continues to evolve, accommodating market needs as well as legal and regulatory developments and the nuances of individual transactions. In view of the differences among the individual types of support instruments, and of the various legal structures, underlying relationships, and other circumstances, specific rating assessments are necessarily done on a case-by-case basis. Issuers and intermediaries are encouraged to contact Moody's directly for specific information on credit-supported issues, or to discuss new supported-debt concepts.

Ratings on Refunded Bonds

Moody's has been rating refunded municipal bonds for over two decades. Municipal issuers choose to refund their outstanding debt for a number of reasons, most often to take advantage of a lower interest rate environment.

To effectively refund an outstanding issue of bonds, an issuer sets up an escrow account with an independent escrow trustee and, with the proceeds of the refunding bond sale and/or the deposit of other available funds, purchases securities that will mature in times and amounts sufficient to pay principal, interest, and any corresponding call premium on the bonds to be refunded. The securities are deposited in the escrow account and held by an independent third party—the escrow agent or trustee—for the benefit of the refunded bondholders. If structured correctly, the refunded bonds will be fully secured by the monies and investments deposited in the escrow account and the issuer will have no future monetary obligation with respect to the refunded bonds. The securities deposited in the escrow account are U.S. Government Treasury or agency securities. The refunded bonds are thus secured indirectly by U.S. Government obligations and can be rated by Moody's based on the quality of the government securities and the integrity of the escrow structure.

Moody's assigns **#Aaa** ratings to those series of advance-refunded bonds that reflect the highest quality and stability of the pool of escrowed assets, as well as the protections inherent in the legal structure of the escrow agreements.

Since Moody's assigns a **#Aaa** rating only if the refunded bonds are secured by direct U.S. Government securities (or direct obligations the principal and interest of which are unconditionally guaranteed as to full and timely payment by the U.S. Government), the refunded bondholders are not exposed to the normal fluctuations in credit quality associated with most types of investments.

The Public Finance Department now has a specialty group within the structured finance, not-for-profit institutions, and financial guarantor ratings group to analyze and rate refunded bonds. Please contact them for questions you may have regarding refunded debt.

■ Preliminary Indicators

As its name suggests, a preliminary indicator is an early indication by Moody's of the credit quality of a debt issue as structured or conceived. The preliminary indicator policy was instituted by Moody's to assist the issuer in deciding whether to apply for a definitive rating, to obtain credit enhancement, to restructure an issue to improve marketability or credit quality, or to postpone or cancel a sale. The indicator presents a preliminary assessment, which may be determine with less stringent information requirements than is the case with regular ratings.

The indicator may take one of three forms:

■ **Basic** The issuers will be informed whether or not the issue is "investment grade" (defined as **Baa** or above).

■ Assignment of MIG Ratings to Near-Term Maturities of Long-Term Issues

At the request of our issuer clients and to better serve their marketing objectives in the issuance of long-term debt, Moody's now permits the assignment of short-term (MIG) ratings to specific near-term maturities of long-term debt. For detailed information on this change in application of the MIG rating system, please refer to the appendix.

■ Conditional Ratings

Bonds for which the security depends upon the completion of some act or the fulfillment of some condition are rated conditionally and designated with the prefix "Con." followed by the rating in parentheses—e.g., **Con. (A)**. These are bonds secured by: (a) earnings of projects under construction, (b) earnings of projects unseasoned in operating experience, (c) rentals that begin when facilities are completed, or (d) payments to which some other limiting condition attaches. The parenthetical rating denotes the probable credit stature upon completion of construction or elimination of the basis of the condition.

■ **Rating category-specific** Moody's will inform the issuer whether the debt falls within a particular rating category, e.g., **A-A1, Aa-Aa1**, etc.

■ **Rating specific** The issuer will learn exactly what the assigned rating would be, e.g., **A1, MIG 3**, etc.

The issuer or its financial intermediary decides which "degree of specificity" is desired at the time of application.

Generally, requests for indicators will be accepted from issuers, borrowers through conduit debt issues, or their financial intermediaries (financial advisors and underwriters with whom the issuer or borrower has an ongoing relationship). Applications for an indicator will not be accepted from parties not representing issuers or borrowers (e.g., funds holding the debt or bond insurers) without the agreement of the issuer/borrower to provide information as requested.

Indicators are available for new unrated debt issues that come to market using new legal documents, or for complete refundings of previously issued rated debt using new legal documents. Indicators are not available for debt issues that are on a parity with issues that already carry a Moody's rating. If an issuer has publicly stated that a rating has been applied for (in an offering statement that has already been distributed or through other means), then the issue is not eligible for a rating indicator.

There is no specific time frame attached to the expiration of an indicator or its conversion to a definitive rating. Upon request by the applicant, any indicator once assigned can be converted to a definitive rating but will require the submittal of all credit information normally required in the standard rating process. Changes over time in credit quality, as well as a material change in the structure of a transaction from that to which the indicator was assigned, may lead, however, to a change in the rating ultimately assigned.

As is the case with our standard ratings, dissemination of the indicator is made both orally and in writing to the issuer, designated issuer intermediary, or other applicant. The indicator is not disseminated to other parties by Moody's. No *Municipal Credit Report* or other analytic information will be released to any party, nor will the analyst discuss the indicator with an outside party (e.g., bond insurer) except with the express approval of the applicant.

No application for an indicator for a potential new parity issue can be accepted unless all outstanding rated parity debt is currently credit substituted, e.g., LOC-supported, insured, etc. Applications for indicators for outstanding unrated debt will be granted or denied on a case-by-case basis. Moody's reserves the right to assign a definitive rating without request, based upon the indicator if, in our judgement, the indicator process is improperly used by the issuer or its intermediaries.

▌ Hospital Revenue Bonds

Primary Documents

Official statement or prospectus

Notice of sale (if public sale)

Legal opinion

Relevant legal documents including, but not limited to, the master trust indenture (if applicable), trust indenture and loan agreement

Annual audited financial statements for the past five years and unaudited year-to-date interim statements (with figures for prior year's comparable period)

Historical inpatient and outpatient utilization for the past five years and year-to-date interim figures (with figures for prior year's comparable period)

Financial feasibility study, if available, or management's own utilization and financial projections

Management letters (a.k.a. accountant's letter of recommendation) for past five years

Sources/uses of funds for proposed debt

Support Documents (for information not contained in any of the aforementioned documents)

Description of hospital and its services

Description of corporate organizational structure

Physician staff information (i.e., number of total staff; number of active staff; number of active staff that are board certified; number of admissions attributed to, and age of, the 10 leading admitting physicians; deletions and additions to active staff for past five years; average age of active staff)

List of competitors and relevant utilization information; include market share analysis, if available

Number of full-time equivalent employees for past five years

Medicare case mix index

Percent of gross patient revenues for past five years by payor type

Schedule of annual principal and interest payments for new and outstanding debt

■ Letter-of-Credit-Backed Issues

Primary Documents

Official statement or prospectus

Notice of sale (if public sale)

Legal opinion

Trust indenture

Resolution or bond ordinance

Letter of credit and reimbursement agreement

Loan or lease agreement

Bank counsel enforceability opinion (foreign and domestic)

Preference (bankruptcy) opinion

Bond purchase agreement

Support Documents (as applicable, for information not contained in any of the aforementioned documents)

Remarketing agreement

Tender agent agreement

Pledge and security agreement

Guaranty agreement

Mortgage and/or collateral documents

Standby bond purchase agreements

Interest rate swap agreement

Guaranteed investment contract

■ Refunded Bonds

Primary Documents

Escrow agreement or letter of instructions (in draft form if the refunding closing has not occurred, otherwise an executed copy)

Primary legal instruments for both the refunded and refunding bonds (i.e., trust indenture, resolution, bond ordinance)

Official statements for both the refunded and refunding bonds

A verification report attesting to the sufficiency of funds in the escrow, which must be prepared by either a certified public accountant or some other person or entity acceptable to Moody's

Escrow agent's attestation of the securities purchased and held in the escrow account

Defeasance opinion (if available)

Preference opinion (if applicable)

Section 362(a) opinion (if applicable)

Notes: In order to facilitate the rating process, Moody's recommends that we receive the refunded documents in draft form prior to the refunded closing date. Early receipt enables us to work with the issuer and other parties to ensure that the provisions of the escrow meet our criteria, thereby eliminating the need to supplement the documents after the closing date.

▌ Assignment of MIG Ratings to Near-Term Maturities of Long-Term Debt Issues

At the request of issuers and to better serve their marketing objectives in the issuance of long-term debt, Moody's now permits the assignment of short-term (**MIG**) ratings to specific near-term maturities of long-term debt. Traditionally, Moody's ratings scales have been used to indicate a credit judgment on the entirety of either a long-term or short-term debt issuance. The alphabetic rating scale has historically been used for long-term issues and, in recognition of the differences between short- and long-term credit risk, separate and distinct **MIG** ratings were used for short-term obligations.

Our recent change to the application of the **MIG** rating system provides for the use of a **MIG** rating to denote the credit standing of an individual maturity of a long-term debt offering. Our revised analytic approach allows us to separate and analyze for rating purposes a specific near-term maturity or maturities of a long-term offering, while examining and rating the entire long-term issue.

The use of and applicability of the **MIG** rating system for this purpose is governed by strict analytic criteria. In order to be eligible to obtain a **MIG** rating on a near-term maturity of a long-term debt issue, at least one of the following three criteria must be met:

▌ An evaluation of overall credit strengths leads to a determination that funds have a high likelihood of being on hand for payment.

    This determination will be made through a rigorous examination of financial operations in order to ascertain that there is a high level of predictability of budgeted revenues and expenditures and of cash flows.

▌ An examination of revenue streams or dedicated monies for debt service, including among others: specific taxes with payment priority assigned to debt service; or debt service reserve funds invested in high-quality, liquid investments giving assurance of debt repayment.

▌ An examination reveals broad general levels of liquidity such as endowment funds or other borrowable resources, giving a high level of confidence that the payment of the near-term maturity is assured.

In addition, the issuer must have requested and be eligible for a long-term debt rating for the entire issue. A **MIG** rating request for a specific maturity is optional on the part of the issuer or its intermediary and will be provided initially as a preliminary indicator. A preliminary indicator request for a **MIG** rating will be accepted from secondary market applicants only with the consent and cooperation of the issuer. If the preliminary indicator is acceptable to the issuer or intermediary, it is then converted to a definitive rating. The assignment of a **MIG** rating to a part of a long-term borrowing is intended to address only the maturity or maturities in question. Neither the ability to assign a **MIG** rating to a near-term maturity nor the level of the rating provided is directly tied to the long-term credit quality of the issuer. Under some circumstances, an issuer with distinctly weak long-term credit characteristics may be able to achieve the highest level **MIG** rating; conversely, the inability to assign a **MIG** rating to a near-term maturity does not necessarily imply a negative view of an issue's long-term credit characteristics. There should be no inference of **MIG** credit standing to those long-term issues for which a **MIG** component was not requested or included.

▌ Key to Moody's Municipal Ratings

Moody's ratings provide investors with a simple system of gradation by which the relative credit qualities of debt instruments may be noted.

There are nine basic rating categories for long-term obligations. They range from **Aaa** (highest quality) to **C** (lowest quality). Those bonds within the **Aa, A, Baa, Ba** and **B** categories that Moody's believes possess the strongest credit attributes are designated by the symbols **Aa1, A1, Baa1, Ba1** and **B1**. Advance-refunded issues that are secured by escrowed funds held in cash, held in trust, reinvested in direct non-callable United States Government obligations or non-callable obligations unconditionally guaranteed by the U.S. Government are identified with a # (hatchmark) symbol, i.e., **#Aaa**.

There are four rating categories for short-term obligations that define an investment grade situation. These are designated as Moody's Investment Grade or **MIG 1** (best quality) through **MIG 4** (adequate quality). Moody's assigns the rating **SG** to credit-supported financings that have been identified as speculative quality investments. The **SG** designation applies to short-term debt instruments and tender features that derive full credit support from a financial institution whose short-term debt is rated **NP** (Not Prime) by Moody's Corporate Department.

Similar to our short-term **MIG** ratings are Moody's commercial paper ratings. Moody's assigns "Prime" ratings to commercial paper, ranging from **P-1** at the high end to **P-3** at the low end. Commercial paper issues not considered by Moody's to fall within these investment-grade categories are rated **NP**.

In the case of variable rate demand obligations (VRDOs), a two-component rating is assigned. The first component represents an evaluation of the degree of risk associated with scheduled principal and interest payments, and the other represents an evaluation of the degree of risk associated with the demand feature. The short-term rating assigned to the demand feature of VRDOs is designated as **VMIG**. When either long- or short-term aspect of a VRDO is not rated, that piece is designated **NR**, i.e., **Aaa/NR** or **NR/VMIG 1**.

Issues that are subject to a periodic reoffer and resale in the secondary market in a "Dutch auction" are assigned a long-term rating based only on Moody's assessment of the ability and willingness of the issuer to make timely principal and interest payments. Moody's expresses no opinion as to the ability of the holder to sell the security in a secondary market "Dutch auction." Such issues are identified by the insertion of the words "Dutch auction" into the name of the issue.

▌ Definitions of Long-Term Bond Ratings

Aaa

Bonds that are rated Aaa are judged to be of the best quality. They carry the smallest degree of investment risk and are generally referred to as "gilt edge." Interest payments are protected by a large or by an exceptionally stable margin and principal is secure. While the various protective elements are likely to change, such changes as can be visualized are most unlikely to impair the fundamentally strong position of such issues.

Aa

Bonds that are rated Aa are judged to be of high quality by all standards. Together with the Aaa group they comprise what are generally known as high-grade bonds. They are rated lower than the best bonds because margins of protection may not be as large as in Aaa securities or fluctuation of protective elements may be of greater amplitude or there may be other elements present which make the long-term risks appear somewhat larger than in Aaa securities.

A

Bonds that are rated A possess many favorable investment attributes and are to be considered as upper-medium-grade obligations. Factors giving security to principal and interest are considered adequate, but elements may be present which suggest a susceptibility to impairment some time in the future.

Baa

Bonds that are rated Baa are considered as medium-grade obligations; i.e., they are neither highly protected nor poorly secured. Interest payments and principal security appear adequate for the present but certain protective elements may be lacking or may be characteristically unreliable over any great length of time. Such bonds lack outstanding investment characteristics and, in fact, have speculative characteristics as well.

Ba

Bonds that are rated Ba are judged to have speculative elements; their future cannot be considered as well assured. Often the protection of interest and principal payments may be very moderate, and thereby not well safeguarded during both good and bad times over the future. Uncertainty of position characterizes bonds in this class.

B

Bonds that are rated B generally lack characteristics of the desirable investment. Assurance of interest and principal payments or maintenance of other terms of the contract over any long period of time may be small.

Caa

Bonds that are rated Caa are of poor standing. Such issues may be in default or there may be present elements of danger with respect to principal or interest.

Ca

Bonds that are rated Ca represent obligations which are speculative in a high degree. Such issues are often in default or have other marked shortcomings.

C

Bonds that are rated C are the lowest rated class of bonds, and issues so rated can be regarded as having extremely poor prospects of ever attaining any real investment standing.

■ Definitions of Short-Term Loan Ratings

Short term issues or the features associated with **MIG, VMIG** or **SG** ratings are identified by date of issue, date of maturity or maturities or rating expiration date and description to distinguish ratings from each other. Each rating designation is unique with no implication as to any other similar issue of the same obligor. **MIG** ratings terminate at the retirement of the obligation while a **VMIG** rating expiration will be a function of each issue's specific structural or credit features.

MIG 1/VMIG 1

This designation denotes best quality. There is present strong protection by established cash flows, superior liquidity support or demonstrated broad-based access to the market for refinancing.

#MIG 2/VMIG 2

This designation denotes high quality. Margins of protection are ample although not so large as in the preceding group.

MIG 3/VMIG 3

This designation denotes favorable quality. All security elements are accounted for but there is lacking the undeniable strength of the preceding grades. Liquidity and cash flow protection may be narrow and market access for refinancing is likely to be less well established.

MIG 4/VMIG 4

This designation denotes adequate quality. Protection commonly regarded as required of an investment security is present and although not distinctly or predominantly speculative, there is specific risk.

SG

This designation denotes speculative quality. Debt instruments in this category lack margins of protection.

Standard & Poor's Ratings Group

▮ How to Obtain a Health Care Revenue Bond Rating[1]

S&P's Municipal Healthcare Finance Group maintains ratings on more than 3,000 issues. Recently, S&P has experienced an increase in the number of inquiries about the rating procedures for healthcare bonds. Following are answers to some of the most frequently asked questions about S&P's rating process for non-profit hospital issues. For further details, please call (212) 208-1805.

Typically, what documents are required for a healthcare bond rating?

- ▮ Five years of audited financial statements for obligated group;
- ▮ Most recent year audited statements for system if different from obligated group;
- ▮ Management letters if available;
- ▮ Interim financial statements with prior year comparisons;
- ▮ Utilization statistics for five years and interim period with prior year comparisons;
- ▮ Projections of payor mix, utilization, and financial statements with underlying assumptions through first full year after project completion, or for three years for a refinancing;

■ Official statement, including descriptive information about the institution, competition, market share, medical staff characteristics, management, reimbursement, local economics and demographics, and other relevant factors;

■ Legal documents including trust indenture, bond resolution, lease or loan agreement;

■ Sources and uses of funds; and

■ Debt service schedule (including all outstanding debt).

For multi-hospital systems, both consolidated and individual audited statements are usually required. Utilization by facility is also necessary in most cases. For all ratings, please submit two copies of the documents listed above.

How long does it take S&P to complete a rating?

On average, S&P completes its rating process one week after receipt of full documentation. If *all* of the standard information is not received one week prior to the initial rating meeting, or if major features of the financing are modified during the rating process, it will take longer for the analyst to compete the analysis.

Shorter turnarounds are possible in certain cases where S&P has recently affirmed a rating.

My hospital fits most of the 'A' ratios published in S&P's annual ratios report, but we received an 'A-'. This seems unfair. Why didn't we get an 'A' rating?

Both qualitative and quantitative factors lead to a rating. Financial analysis is just one aspect of the review. A very competitive service area, project risk, poor local economy or weak medical staff might explain why a hospital is rated below what its ratios would seem to indicate. Conversely, the absence of competition and a growing economy can sometimes compensate for lower cash levels or thinner margins. Also, the ratios are just medians and the sample size for most categories is very small.

Does S&P require an independent feasibility study?

No. However, an independent feasibility study is in a hospital's best interest, especially if a project is being financed and the hospital does not demonstrate historic pro forma coverage. Internally prepared feasibility studies are suitable for hospitals that show historic pro forma coverage or for refinancings.

What kind of assumptions should a hospital include in projections about future reimbursement levels?

S&P expects forecasts to reflect the most likely levels for reimbursement, which may often be a continuation of current methods. If a change in reimbursement levels is likely, S&P expects management to use the most conservative assumptions. Sensitivity studies may be useful in cases where a change in reimbursement levels is expected. For example, many teaching hospitals provide information that measures the impact of the Medicare indirect medical education adjustment factor being reduced, even though the current rate is 7.7%. In other cases, hospitals that received large increases in Medicare reimbursement last year have provided sensitivity studies showing lower levels in the future, since it seems likely that both federal and state governments will be unwilling to continue paying currently high Medicaid rates. S&P looks favorably on management that anticipates potential changes, quantifies the financial impact, and outlines a responsive strategy.

How does S&P evaluate HMO/PPO contracts?

Revenues derived from such contracts can range from a few percent to almost 40% in some service areas. S&P is interested in the size and nature of each major HMO contract. S&P is also interested in the relationship between the hospital's costs and contract payments.

Our hospital is in the midst of merger discussions with another institution, and we are concerned about confidentiality during the rating process. Does S&P disclose all information received from issuers?

S&P is required to keep all such information confidential and is accustomed to reviewing strategic plans and other sensitive information. Management should advise S&P of any confidential matters so that we can be clear about what may and may not be discussed publicly.

Our hospital plans to issue additional debt next year but we do not yet have details regarding the project. How should we address this at our upcoming rating meeting?

S&P must be informed of planned future debt financings. In this case, since the financing is expected relatively soon, we would require some basic information about the issue, such as:

- a description of what the money will be used for,
- an estimate of annual debt service, and
- whether the hospital will make an equity contribution.

For projects that are planned for several years in the future, S&P would be interested in more general information. Failure to disclose plans for additional debt reflects poorly on management and could jeopardize ratings.

Does S&P require a site visit?

S&P meets with hospital managers in our New York and/or San Francisco offices, as well as on-site at hospitals throughout the country. For new ratings, existing ratings where management has changed, or where a large project is planned we would prefer an on-site visit. If we have visited the hospital recently, or the size of the issue is relatively small, or if hospital management has plans to be in New York or San Francisco, we would meet in S&P offices. In these cases, slide projectors and VCRs are available to assist hospital representatives with their presentations. Refinancings for predictably stable ratings would not require a trip, and in some cases, a meeting is unnecessary.

How long should a rating meeting last?

Two hours is a good goal to set. If the analysts have received the documents in advance, the meetings can be well focused and efficient. For complex project financings or other unique bond issues, meetings tend to be longer. If we visit the hospital, a 30-minute tour of the facility is useful. In cities where S&P is unfamiliar with competitor hospitals and the local economy, a service area tour may be requested. This is decided on a case-by-case basis.

How much does it cost to get a healthcare bond rating?

For fee information regarding healthcare or other municipal issues, please call (212) 412-0355.

Nancy Rubini
(212) 208-1812

∎ Health-Care Analysis in a Changing Environment[2]

"It is important for S&P to understand the relations a provider has with primary-care physicians, as well as with the rest of the medical staff."

One of the questions investors, investment bankers, and health-care providers ask most frequently is, "How has S&P changed the way it analyzes health-care providers, given the possibility of national health-care reform?" Irrespective of national reform, S&P has fine-tuned its analytical approach in recognition of the market-driven changes in health care that already are occurring.

Increased competition among providers, industry consolidation as evidenced by mergers and alliance formation, and increasing managed-care contracting—a key element of the managed-competition model of health reform—reflect the forces that are reshaping health care. In response to these private sector reforms, certain areas of S&P's traditional health-care analysis have risen in importance over the past several years. Therefore, its health-care analysis already incorporates many anticipated elements of the managed-competition model of reform, whether it occurs on a national or regional basis. The areas discussed below now contribute more heavily to ratings than they have in the past.

S&P continues to emphasize both qualitative and quantitative factors in determining the rating of a health-care entity. However, in today's more competitive health-care market, an examination of the provider's competitive position—including its market position and share, relationships with key market constituents, and cost structure—is essential to predict success in an increased managed-care environment.

Competitive Profile

Assessing an institution's overall market share, market share for key services, and competitive position in its primary and secondary service areas has become an increasingly important area of focus for S&P as an indicator of credit strength. Management's ability to assess its institution's strengths and weaknesses and to develop sound strategies to enhance the institution's competitive position is crucial to continued success. In meetings with S&P, management teams should be prepared to discuss these topics in detail, with the understanding that S&P will respect the confidentiality of the discussions.

As managed-care contracts provide incentives to shift care from inpatient to outpatient settings, as well as to continue to reduce overall length of stay, S&P's analysis has taken a broader view of utilization. Number of outpatient procedures, number of same-day surgeries, observation days, and general trends in outpatient volume are examined, in addition to the traditional inpatient volumes, to accurately focus on facility utilization and competitive position. To the extent that utilization is flat or declining, S&P is interested in a hospital's ability to control resource consumption and preserve cash flow.

Relations with Key Market Constituents

S&P recognizes that relationships with other providers, physicians, and insurers have changed dramatically over the past several years. Some health-care providers have fully integrated the acute-care, primary-care, and insurance product into much larger, more complex health-care entities to control all critical system components. Many more are moving in this direction. Therefore, S&P will ask management to highlight these key relationships during a rating presentation.

Managed-care contractors increasingly are pushing providers to deliver a full continuum of care, including primary care and ambulatory surgeries, as well as the traditional acute-care services. They are looking for an institution to provide this care on a regional basis. An institution may follow several paths to achieve this level of comprehensive services: it may decide to develop its own vertically integrated network or forge alliances with other health-care providers to achieve the same goal. As managed-care contractors become more selective and demand one-stop shopping convenience, stand-alone acute-care providers in competitive markets are in danger of being locked out of managed-care contracts unless they develop or align with other providers that offer a full array of services.

Mergers, acquisitions, and affiliations are expected to continue, and most management teams have actively considered some of these alternatives. If the strategic plan does not address how the provider is working with or looking at other health-care entities, S&P will pursue this point with management.

"At the core of health-care reform initiatives is the issue of cost. Low-cost, efficient providers that offer quality care will be more successful in winning and retaining contracts."

Given the increased power of primary-care physicians to direct patient flow and resource utilization in a managed-care environment, it is important for S&P to understand the relations a provider has with primary-care physicians, as well as with the rest of the medical staff. Strained medical staff relations or the lack of involvement of physicians in the governing and planning process will likely spell disaster in the long run for the provider—particularly in markets with high managed-care penetration shifting toward capitation.

The establishment of physician hospital organizations or similar structures is viewed positively if it enhances physician loyalty and establishes appropriate financial incentives. Additions to staff, traditionally an area of focus, has shifted to include an emphasis on recruitment of primary care physicians.

Managed-Care Contracting

Payor mix remains a rating consideration. The growth of managed-care contracts and the potential for increased financial risk has resulted in a more in-depth discussion of how an institution handles the many facets of this business.

The managed-care market penetration and type of contracting arrangements in place (per diem vs. capitation) are used as a gauge to determine how much emphasis is appropriate. As a rule, if managed-care represents 10% of an institution's revenues, or if capitation is the prevailing contract type, S&P will look more closely at this component.

Starting with the macro perspective, S&P compares the institution's level of managed-care contracting with the market's overall profile. The type of contracting arrangement also is critical in determining the amount of emphasis that is placed on this topic. Other areas of focus are: knowledge of the local managed-care market, managed-care provider solvency, the hospital's contracting objective and strategy, understanding managed care's actual and potential impact on the hospital's performance, and an assessment of the contracting process.

In recognition of the unique nature of this contracting process, many providers are hiring personnel with direct insurance industry experience. Development of an appropriate information system that integrates financial and clinical information is important in monitoring the profitability of the managed-care contracts and managing resources.

Cost and Quality

At the core of health-care reform initiatives is the issue of cost. Low-cost, efficient providers that offer quality care will be more successful in winning and retaining managed-care contracts than other providers. In a capitated managed-care environment, low-cost providers will be rewarded, while others will feel increased financial pressure. Therefore, it is important that fixed costs be included in this profile, as well as variable costs. Institutions that are highly leveraged and have little operating flexibility may find profitability is limited and may have trouble maintaining managed-care contracts. Typically, S&P asks how the provider's costs compare with others and is interested in any initiatives undertaken to control or reduce costs of providing services. A discussion of operating flexibility to make further cost reductions also is helpful.

Equally important is the quality debate. S&P is frequently asked whether it factors quality into the rating. To date, because there is no standardized measure of "quality" for the health-care industry, it is difficult to base a rating assessment on this issue. However, S&P includes quality proxies—such as level of board-certified physicians, the history of malpractice claims paid, and accreditations—in its analysis.

Financial Performance

Financial position and performance remain important elements, particularly cash levels. S&P expects third-party payments to continue to decline with the move to capitation and continued pressure on Medicare and Medicaid budgets. Therefore, a high concentration of governmental payors remains a rating concern.

Institutions that have accumulated healthy cash positions while adequately maintaining plant will be better able to withstand these reduced payments, to make additions to plant as needed, and to fund certain new business initiatives that might be necessary. However, if business fundamentals are not sound, currently food financial performance and position will not be sufficient to offset these long-term concerns.

Refinements Continue

The health-care environment will continue to evolve based on federal, state, and private sector initiatives. It is likely that national reform, once passed by Congress, will be phased in, giving health-care providers time to adjust to the new incentives. In addition, the managed-competition model now being developed in the private sector is the likely choice for reform.

These expectations are implicit in S&P's approach to analyzing health-care credits. In the absence of an immediate massive overhaul, as might occur with a single-payor system, that could dramatically alter the foundation of analysis, S&P's rating approach will continue to adjust to reflect ongoing changes in the health-care industry.

Joan Pickett
(212) 208-1818

Excerpts from Standard & Poor's Municipal Finance Criteria 1994

∎ Introduction

Role of Ratings

Over the years, Standard & Poor's Corp. credit ratings have achieved wide investor acceptance as easily usable tools for differentiating credit quality. Issuers range from public corporate utilities such as Commonwealth Edison Co. to conglomerates such as ITT Corp. To these are added municipal issuers such as New York City and Anchorage, Alaska, foreign governments such as Japan and Finland, and foreign corporations such as Nippon Telegraph & Telephone Public Corp. and Imperial Chemical Industries PLC of England. Issuers sell bonds with varying security pledges and seniority, and also issue debt that is insured, structured, or complex in various other ways. Ratings published by S&P provide a single scale to compare among this array of different debt instruments.

The value of a rating emanates from the validity of criteria and reliability of judgment and analysis of S&P's professional staff. S&P's criteria are regularly communicated through *CreditWeek Municipal, CreditWeek* and *CreditWire*—S&P's electronic ratings dissemination service. The credibility of ratings also requires objectivity. S&P's objectivity results from not investing for its own account, not serving as an underwriter, financial advisor, or manager of funds, and being independent of the issuer's business.

S&P operates with no government mandate, subpoena powers or any other official authority. As part of the media, S&P simply has a right to express its opinions in the form of letter symbols. Recognition as a rating agency relies on investors' willingness to accept its judgment.

Investors' Use of Ratings

To use credit ratings properly, one should first understand what a rating is and is not. The rating performs the isolated function of credit risk evaluation, which is one element of the entire investment decision-making process.

A credit rating is not a recommendation to purchase, sell, or hold a particular security. A rating cannot constitute a recommendation as it does not take into consideration other factors, such as market price and risk preference of the investor. Moreover, because S&P receives confidential information from issuers, S&P believes it would be improper to recommend the purchase or sale of rated bonds. Rating agencies that do publish "market" recommendations may forego management contact, relying exclusively on publicly available data.

A rating is not a general-purpose evaluation of an issuer. For example, an issuer's 'AA' rating may be based primarily on a specific security or third-party support underlying the obligation.

Although many probing questions are asked the issuer at various stages of the rating process, S&P does not perform an audit, nor does it attest to the authenticity of the information provided by the issuer and upon which the rating may be based. Ratings can be changed, withdrawn, or placed on CreditWatch as a result of changes in, or unavailability of, information.

Ratings do not create a fiduciary relationship between S&P and users of the ratings; there is not legal basis for the existence of such a relationship.

Issuer's Use of Ratings

It is commonplace for municipal issuers to structure financing transactions to reflect S&P's credit criteria so they qualify for higher ratings. However, the actual structuring of a given issue is the function and responsibility of an issuer and its advisors. S&P is the recipient and user of materials prepared by those in a position to attest to such materials' accuracy and completeness. Although S&P will react to a proposed financing, publish papers outlining its criteria for that type of issue, and interpret and make evaluations available to an issuer, underwriter, bond counsel, or financial advisor, S&P does not function as an investment banker or financial advisor. Adoption of such a role ultimately would impair the objectivity and credibility that are vital to S&P's continued performance as an independent rating agency.

■ S&P's Municipal Credit Services

S&P's credit evaluations encompass a range of services of use to both debt issuers and investors. Generally, S&P offers these services only at the request of an issuer or investor. Where S&P has a request from an investor, S&P provides a rating or other service only with the cooperation of the debt issuer since, in the municipal market, S&P believes, that debt issuers remain the chief source of accurate and timely information needed to maintain a current and accurate credit assessment. The following are the chief credit services offered by S&P on municipal securities

These services are governed by S&P's policy on the release of ratings. Once a rating request is made, it may be withdrawn only prior to the meeting of the rating committee. Even where a request is withdrawn, S&P reserves the right to comment on any issue sold in the public market if, in S&P's judgment, market interest warrants such comment.

Public Rating Services

■ **Published Ratings:** This is S&P's standard rating service for municipal debt issues sold publicly. It provides a published rating, as well as surveillance on rated issues, credit reports detailing the basis for the rating, and dissemination of the rating, credit reports, and related information over *Creditwire*, S&P's electronic information network, and in *CreditWeek Municipal, CreditWeek, Municipal Ratings Handbook*, and other S&P publications.

■ **Published Underlying Ratings (SPURs):** This is a rating assessment of the stand-alone capacity of an issue to pay debt service on a credit-enhanced debt issue, without giving effect to the enhancement that applies to it. These ratings are published with the designation SPUR to distinguish them from the credit-enhanced rating that applies to the debt issue, and are provided with surveillance for as long as the SPUR rating is outstanding.

Private Rating Services

■ **Preliminary Ratings:** These ratings are provided on debt issues before they are sold in the public markets. S&P also provides preliminary ratings to assess a credit-enhanced issue's underlying capacity to pay, but these ratings, unlike SPURs, are valid only on the date they are issued and are published only at the request of the debt issuer. To maintain the integrity of the rating process, S&P will convert a preliminary rating to a public rating when and if the issue sells in the public market.

■ **Private Placement Ratings:** Same as preliminary ratings, but applied to issues sold in the private placement and limited distribution markets.

Other Services

■ **Credit Opinions:** For financings on which issuers or investors wish to evaluate rating potential without a subsequent obligation to request a rating, S&P provides credit opinions. These are not ratings, but are broad indications of what credit strength a proposed financing provides. Credit opinions are restricted to the following: noninvestment grade, borderline noninvestment/investment grade, investment grade, and high investment grade. Credit opinions are not ratings, since they are based on limited information, and should not be represented as such. Credit opinions do not obligate the issuer to request an S&P rating.

■ Rating Definitions

Long-Term Debt

An S&P corporate or municipal debt rating is a current assessment of the creditworthiness of an obligor with respect to a specific obligation. This assessment may take into consideration obligors such as guarantors, insurers, or lessees.

The debt rating is not a recommendation to purchase, sell, or hold a security, as it does not comment on market price or suitability for a particular investor.

The ratings are based on current information furnished by the issuer or obtained by S&P from other sources it considers reliable. S&P does not perform an audit in connection with any rating and may, on occasion, rely on unaudited financial information. The ratings may be changed, suspended, or withdrawn as a result of changes in, or unavailability of, such information, or for other circumstances.

The ratings are based, in varying degrees, on the following considerations:

1. Likelihood of default—capacity and willingness of the obligor as to the timely payment of interest and repayment of principal in accordance with the terms of the obligation;

2. Nature and provisions of the obligation;

3. Protection afforded by, and relative position of, the obligation in the event of bankruptcy, reorganization, or other arrangement under the laws of bankruptcy and other laws affecting creditors' rights.

Investment Grade

AAA Debt rated 'AAA' has the highest rating assigned by S&P. Capacity to pay interest and repay principal is extremely strong.

AA Debt rated 'AA' has a very strong capacity to pay interest and repay principal and differs from the highest rated issues only in small degree.

A Debt rated 'A' has a strong capacity to pay interest and repay principal although it is somewhat more susceptible to the adverse effects of changes in circumstances and economic conditions than debt in higher rated categories.

BBB Debt rated 'BBB' is regarded as having an adequate capacity to pay interest and repay principal. Whereas it normally exhibits adequate protection parameters, adverse economic conditions or changing circumstances are more likely to lead to a weakened capacity to pay interest and repay principal for debt in this category than in higher rated categories.

Speculative Grade

Debt rated 'BB', 'B', 'CCC', 'CC', or 'C' is regarded as having predominantly speculative characteristics with respect to capacity to pay interest and repay principal. 'BB' indicates the least degree of speculation and 'C' the highest. While such debt will likely have some quality and protective characteristics, these are outweighed by large uncertainties or major risk exposures to adverse conditions.

BB Debt rated 'BB' has less near-term vulnerability to default than other speculative issues. However, it faces major ongoing uncertainties or exposure to adverse business, financial, or economic conditions which could lead to inadequate capacity to meet timely interest and principal payments. The 'BB' rating category is also used for debt subordinated to senior debt that is assigned an actual or implied 'BBB-' rating.

B Debt rated 'B' has a greater vulnerability to default, but currently has the capacity to meet interest payments and principal repayments. Adverse business, financial, or economic conditions will likely impair capacity or willingness to pay interest and repay principal. The 'B' rating category also is used for debt subordinated to senior debt that is assigned an actual or implied 'BB' or 'BB-' rating.

CCC Debt rated 'CCC' has a current identifiable vulnerability to default, and is dependent upon favorable business, financial, and economic conditions to meet timely payment of interest and repayment of principal. In the event of adverse business, financial, or economic conditions, it is not likely to have the capacity to pay interest and repay principal. The 'CCC' rating category also is used for debt subordinated to senior debt that is assigned an actual or implied 'B' or 'B-' rating.

CC Debt rated 'CC' typically is applied to debt subordinated to senior debt which is assigned an actual or implied 'CCC' debt rating.

C The rating 'C' typically is applied to debt subordinated to senior debt which is assigned an actual or implied 'CCC-' debt rating. The 'C' rating may be used to cover a situation where a bankruptcy petition has been filed, but debt service payments are continued.

CI Debt rated 'CI' is reserved for income bonds on which no interest is being paid.

D Debt rated 'D' is in payment default. They 'D' rating category is used when interest payments or principal payments are not made on the date due even if the applicable grace period has not expired, unless S&P believes that such payments will be made during the grace period. The 'D' rating also will be used upon the filing of a bankruptcy petition if debt service payments are jeopardized.

Plus(+) minus(-) The ratings from 'AA' to 'CCC' may be modified by the addition of a plus or minus sign to show relative standing within the major rating categories.

c The letter 'c' indicates that the holder's option to tender the security for purchase may be canceled under certain prestated conditions enumerated in the tender option documents.

p The letter 'p' indicates that the rating is provisional. A provisional rating assumes the successful completion of the project financed by the debt being rated and indicates that payment of debt service requirements is largely or entirely dependent upon the successful timely completion of the project. This rating, however, while addressing credit quality subsequent to completion of the project, makes no comment on the likelihood or the risk of default upon failure of such completion. The investor should exercise his own judgment with respect to such likelihood and risk.

L The letter 'L' indicates that the rating pertains to the principal amount of those bonds to the extent that the underlying deposit collateral is federally insured, and interest is adequately collateralized. In the case of certificates of deposit, the letter 'L' indicates that the deposit, combined with other deposits being held in the same right and capacity, will be honored for principal and pre-default interest up to federal insurance limits within 30 days after closing of the insured institution or, in the event that the deposit is assumed by a successor insured institution, upon maturity.

Continuance of the rating is contingent upon S&P's receipt of an executed copy of the escrow agreement or closing documentation confirming investments and cash flows.

N.R. Not rated.

Debt obligations of issuers outside the United States and its territories are rated on the same basis as domestic corporate and municipal issues. The ratings measure the creditworthiness of the obligor but do not take into account currency exchange and related uncertainties.

Bond investment quality standards: Under present commercial bank regulations issued by the Comptroller of the Currency, bonds rated in the top four categories ('AAA', 'AA', 'A', 'BBB', commonly known as investment-grade ratings) generally are regarded as eligible for bank investment. Also, the laws of various states governing legal investments impose certain rating or other standards for obligations eligible for investment by savings bank, trust companies, insurance companies, and fiduciaries in general.

Rating Outlooks

An S&P rating outlook assesses the potential direction of an issuer's long-term debt rating over the intermediate to longer term. In determining a rating outlook, consideration is given to any changes in the economic and/or fundamental business conditions. An outlook is not necessarily a precursor of a rating change or future CreditWatch action.

Positive indicates that a rating may be raised.

Negative indicates that ratings may be lowered.

Stable indicates that ratings are not likely to change.

Developing means ratings may be raised or lowered.

N.M. means not meaningful.

Notes

An S&P note rating reflects the liquidity factors and market access risks unique to notes. Notes due in three years or less will likely receive a note rating. Notes maturing beyond three years will most likely receive a long-term debt rating. The following criteria will be used in making that assessment:

■ Amortization schedule—the larger the final maturity relative to other maturities, the more likely it will be treated as a note.

■ Source of payment—the more dependent the issue is on the market for its refinancing, the more likely it will be treated as a note.

Note rating symbols are as follows:

SP-1 Strong capacity to pay principal and interest. An issue determined to possess a very strong capacity to pay debt service is given a plus (+) designation.

SP-2 Satisfactory capacity to pay principal and interest, with some vulnerability to adverse financial and economic changes over the term of the notes.

SP-3 Speculative capacity to pay principal and interest.

Commercial Paper

An S&P commercial paper rating is a current assessment of the likelihood of timely payment of debt having an original maturity of no more than 365 days. Ratings are graded into several categories, ranging from 'A' for the highest-quality obligations to 'D' for the lowest. These categories are as follows:

A-1 This designation indicates that the degree of safety regarding timely payment is strong. Those issues determined to possess extremely strong safety characteristics are denoted with a plus sign (+) designation.

A-2 Capacity for timely payment on issues with this designation is satisfactory. However, the relative degree of safety is not as high as for issues designated 'A-1'.

A-3 Issues carrying this designation have an adequate capacity for timely payment. They are, however, more vulnerable to the adverse effects of changes in circumstances than obligations carrying the higher designations.

B Issues rated 'B' are regarded as having only speculative capacity for timely payment.

C This rating is assigned to short-term debt obligations with a doubtful capacity for payment.

D Debt rated 'D' is in payment default. The 'D' rating category is used when interest payments of principal payments are not made on the date due, even if the applicable grace period has not expired, unless S&P believes such payments will be made during such grace period.

Variable-Rate Demand Bonds

S&P assigns "dual" ratings to all debt issues that have a put option or demand feature as part of their structure.

The first rating addresses the likelihood of repayment of principal and interest as due, and the second rating addresses only the demand feature. The long-term debt rating symbols are used for bonds to denote the long-term maturity and the commercial paper rating symbols for the put option (for example, 'AAA/A-1+'). With short-term demand debt, S&P's note rating symbols are used with the commercial paper rating symbols (for example, 'SP-1+/A-1+').

▌Organization

S&P traces its history back to 1860. Today it is the leading credit rating organization and a major publisher of financial information and research services on U.S. and foreign corporate and municipal debt obligations. S&P was an independent, publicly owned corporation until 1966, when all of S&P's common stock was acquired by McGraw-Hill Inc., a major publishing company. S&P is a wholly owned subsidiary of McGraw-Hill and is independent of any investment banking firm, bank, or similar institution. In matters of credit analysis and ratings, S&P operates entirely independent of McGraw-Hill. S&P has two operating groups: S&P's Ratings Group, which conducts all ratings activities, and S&P's Information Group, which provides investment, financial and trading information, data, and analyses—primarily on equity securities. Each group operates separately from the other.

S&P has been assigning ratings to corporate bonds since 1923, municipal bonds since 1940, and commercial paper since 1969. It has outstanding ratings on bonds and preferred stock issues of some 2,000 domestic and foreign corporations, and 12,966 municipal, state, national, and supranational entities. In addition, there are commercial paper ratings on more than 1,900 issuing entities. S&P's public ratings are published in several of its print and electronic services and are disseminated through the general and financial news media.

S&P's Ratings Group now has eight offices—New York, London, Tokyo, Paris, Stockholm, Melbourne, Frankfurt, and San Francisco. The London and Tokyo offices were opened in the mid-1980s as the ratings business expanded internationally. Additional steps to pursue a global strategy were taken in 1990 with the acquisition of Australian Ratings Pty. Ltd. (Melbourne, Australia), Insurance Solvency International Ltd. (London, England), and 50% of Agence D'Evaluation Financiere (Paris, France) renamed S&P-ADEF. Also in 1990, S&P acquired the remaining 50% interest in Nordisk Ratings AB, a rating agency in Sweden. In 1992, S&P took an interest in a rating agency in Madrid, serving the Spanish market.

▋ Issuer Meeting

Issuers frequently inquire about what takes place during a meeting with S&P and how best to prepare for it. The chief purpose of the meeting is to establish a forum in which S&P and the issuer can exchange information.

This discussion takes place either in S&P's New York headquarters or at the issuer's location. The S&P analysts involved become familiar before the meeting with the issuer's preliminary official statement and supporting documents.

Normal procedure at the meeting is for the issuer to make a 10-15 minute introductory statement highlighting the more important features of the submitted documents. S&P then poses questions designed to clarify or supplement the data already advanced.

S&P (and hopefully the issuer) tries to allocate time toward the end of the meeting for discussion of any relevant points not covered routinely by the agenda. One caveat: S&P prefers that the key public officials and not only a few necessary representatives participate. If more information is necessary, S&P can follow-up by phone.

▋ CreditWatch and Outlooks: Gauging Future Ratings

Because S&P's CreditWatch and its rating outlooks are both indicators of a rating's potential direction, users of S&P's data sometimes ask how the two gauges relate to each other.

CreditWatch

CreditWatch is used to indicate potential rating changes that may be contemplated in the near future. Unless otherwise noted, a rating decision usually will be made within 120 days of an issue being placed on CreditWatch.

An issue is placed on CreditWatch with "positive" or "negative" implications, depending on whether an upgrade or a downgrade is being considered. Listings usually are triggered by such events as litigation, court rulings, or voter tax initiatives, or by significant deviations from expected trends, such as a severe shortfall of projected revenue or significant changes in short-term borrowing trends. Where possible, S&P indicates about when it will affirm or change ratings, as well as the likely new rating category if it is determined that the rating should change.

Developing implications. In very rare cases, when significant developments are pending that could result in a higher or lower rating, depending upon their final resolution, a CreditWatch listing with "developing" implications can occur.

When an issue is placed on CreditWatch with "developing" implications, S&P states specifically under what circumstances the rating would be expected to rise and under what circumstances it would be expected to fall. A listing with "developing" implications is exceedingly rare for a municipal issue since, in most cases, the likely direction of the potential rating action is clearly "positive" or "negative."

Placement of an issue on CreditWatch does not mean a rating change is inevitable. Also, since S&P continuously monitors all of its ratings, the CreditWatch list is not intended to include all issues under review. Thus, rating changes can occur without an issue first having been placed on CreditWatch.

Rating Outlooks

CreditWatch was established in 1981, with the launch of S&P's CreditWeek. Building on the success and acceptance of CreditWatch, S&P in 1990 began indicating "rating outlooks" as an additional means of showing potential direction of ratings. Outlooks are intended to indicate potential rating direction over an intermediate term—up to several years.

Every credit is assigned an outlook of positive, negative, or stable, and the likelihood of a rating change for an issue with a positive or negative outlook is not as strong as it is for debt listed in CreditWatch. Current events or trends, however, when developed over time, may lead to consideration of a higher or lower rating over 12-36 months.

An outlook might be revised when voter initiatives call for reduced taxing power for a city government but implementation may be delayed for months or years, either because of litigation, legal ambiguities, or the implementation timetable. More frequently, however, negative or positive outlooks reflect current or recent financial situations that by themselves are not enough to warrant a rating change but may eventually lead to a change if the trend continues.

Most outlooks are stable. It is interesting to note that most municipal debt ratings by S&P carry stable outlooks—perhaps 5% or less of S&P's individual debt ratings are listed on CreditWatch or are changed in a given year. This reflects the traditional stability and credit quality enjoyed by state and local governments and is a hallmark of municipal bonds.

Economic factors tend to change slowly over time; those issuers that exhibit economic volatility, perhaps due to a tax base concentrated in a single industry or taxpayer, are likely to have this volatility already reflected in their ratings. Financial operations can be volatile from year to year, but most local governments have succeeded in maintaining their financial position within a "band" of fund balance levels and avoiding deficit fund balances.

A short period of negative financial operations, leading to drawdowns of fund balance, may result in a negative outlook designation; swift financial deterioration and deficit fund balances, however, are more likely to lead to placement on CreditWatch, or directly to a lowered rating, if the deterioration is accompanied by increased issuance of short-term cash-flow debt or deficit bonds.

In noting the stability of municipal credit over time, S&P acknowledges that credits and ratings can sometimes change relatively quickly—one need only look at the fiscal crises in California in 1991-1992, or in Massachusetts in 1989-1990, to see how quickly finances can deteriorate when left unattended by budget makers. CreditWatch and rating outlooks are S&P's best means for "calling the turns" in credit ratings when municipalities' best laid plans go awry.

Revenue Bonds

■ Health-Care, Higher Education, and Other 501(c)(3) Financings

This section outlines the criteria used to rate not-for-profit health-care providers, higher education entities, and other separately incorporated 501(c)(3)institutions.

Both tax-exempt and taxable bond issues for not-for-profit entities are rated by the municipal finance department. Ratings on government-owned entities, such as a county hospital or a community college secured by the full faith and credit of the municipal entity, are based on G.O. criteria with input on industry trends from the revenue area.

Additionally, rating criteria for public universities are outlined in this section and contrasted with those of the private university sector. Rating criteria for these not-for-profit entities are presented together, since the analysis is similar in many respects. The analysis of bonds issued by these entities differs significantly from most other revenue bonds in that not-for-profit institutions function in a highly competitive environment. Typically, these corporations issue debt secured by a specific revenue stream through a state or local financing authority, which provides access to the capital markets.

As a matter of policy, S&P will not rate religious organizations. However, S&P rates debt issued by religiously sponsored organizations if the borrower is a separate legal corporation with an independent board, has separate audited financial statements, and does not rely on donations from the sponsoring entity. While it is not policy to rate start-up facilities, S&P will rate corporations resulting from mergers or consolidations, provided sufficient historical operating and financial information on the predecessor organizations and forecasted information are provided. There is no size limit on the entities S&P will rate, although smaller institutions generally exhibit significantly greater vulnerability in a number of respects.

S&P's rating criteria for these not-for-profit corporations examine both the quantity and quality of the revenues pledged. This analysis focuses on five broad areas that will be discussed more fully in the sections that follow. In general, these areas are: legal structure, demand, service area characteristics, institutional characteristics and market position, management, and financial factors and debt structure.

■ General Health-Care Criteria

The continuing emphasis on containing health-care costs and increasing efficiency of health-care providers has resulted in a number of different health-care entities seeking access to the capital markets. As a result, S&P's rating criteria have been expanded to cover a number of not-for-profit health-care providers in addition to single-site hospitals and multihospital systems (*see below*).

S&P Rated Health-Care Providers

S&P's health-care group rates a broad spectrum of health-care providers, including but not limited to:

- ■ Single-site hospitals—including rehabilitation, children's, and psychiatric institutions;
- ■ Multihospital systems;
- ■ University/teaching hospitals;
- ■ University faculty practice plans/medical specialty practices;
- ■ Health Maintenance Organizations (HMOs);
- ■ Cancer centers; and
- ■ Continuing care retirement communities and nursing homes.

While each type of not-for-profit health-care provider has unique areas of analytical focus, the framework for all is similar. S&P continues to emphasize qualitative and quantitative factors in determining the rating of a health-care entity. However, in today's more competitive and continually evolving health-care environment, an examination of the provider's competitive position—including its market position and share, relationships with key market constituents, and cost structure—is essential to predict success in an increased managed care environment. In response to private sector reforms, these areas of S&P's traditional health-care analysis have risen in importance over the past several years.

Rating Procedure

To conduct a comprehensive analysis of a health-care provider, S&P requests that basic documentation be submitted that focuses on the key areas of legal structure, demand and service area characteristics, institutional characteristics and competitive profile, management and administrative factors, and financial factors. An independent feasibility study is not required by S&P to rate a health-care financing. However, such a study may be in the institution's best interest, especially if a project is being financed and the hospital's ability to cover long-term debt is dependent upon completion of the project and addition of new services. Internally prepared financial projections, including a summary of all pertinent assumptions, is acceptable for hospitals that show historical pro forma coverage or for refinancing.

While a site visit is not required to obtain a rating, it is typically part of the rating process, particularly for a first-time issuer and in cases of large capital projects or recent management changes. In place of a site visit, management may choose to meet in S&P's New York or San Francisco offices. Refinancing for predictably stable ratings do not require a trip and, in some cases, a meeting is unnecessary.

Legal Review

S&P evaluates the legal provisions of a health-care bond issue based on the credit strengths and weaknesses of the health-care obligor. Legal provisions alone cannot prevent operating and financial performance declines, interruptions of debt service payments, events of default, and the risk of overall credit deterioration. Consequently, while weak or liberal provisions can cause a lower rating to be assigned, strong legal covenants will not lead to a rating higher than that of the obligor. It is credit quality that determines the degree of influence legal provisions bear on a bond's rating.

Legal covenants should provide adequate protection to bondholders while allowing hospital management sufficient operating flexibility to respond to changing business conditions. S&P, however, will assess any action taken by a hospital in the future that affects its credit quality, even if such action is addressed in the legal documents, and will adjust the rating accordingly.

Basic Documentation Requirements

To rate a health-care provider, S&P requires that the following information be supplied:

- Five years of audited financial statements for obligor(s)
- Most recent year audited statements for system if different from obligated group
- Interim financial statements with prior year comparisons
- Management letters, if available
- Utilization statistics for five years and interim period with prior year comparisons
- Projections of payor mix, utilization, and financial statements with underlying assumptions through first full year of project completion, or for three years for a refinancing
- Official statement, including descriptive information about the institution, competition, market share, medical staff profile, management, reimbursement, local economy and demo graphics, and other relevant factors
- Legal documents, including trust indenture, bond resolution and loan or lease agreement
- Sources and uses of funds
- Debt service schedule, including all outstanding issues

For multihospital systems, both consolidated and individual audited statements usually are required. Utilization by facility is also necessary in most cases.

Demand and Service Area Characteristics

As managed care contracts provide incentives to shift care from inpatient to outpatient settings, as well as to reduce the overall length of stay, S&P's analysis has taken a much broader view of utilization. Number of outpatient procedures, number of inpatient and outpatient surgeries, observation days, and other general trends in outpatient volume, in addition to the traditional inpatient volumes, is examined to accurately assess demand for a provider's services and competitive position. To the extent that utilization is flat or declining, S&P is interested in a provider's ability to control resource consumption and preserve cash flow. Population trends, unemployment rates, local wealth levels, and major employers are analyzed to determine their impact on health-care utilization and payor profile. Additionally, the population profile is important in determining the type of services needed. Typically, an older population is likely to require more intense inpatient services than a younger population, which may be most effectively treated on an outpatient basis. The types and levels of services provided are important analytical considerations affecting the institution's competitive and financial position. For example, major teaching hospitals, regional referral centers, and large medical centers draw patients from broader regional bases, providing some insulation from local economic cycles. This information feeds into S&P's assessment of demand for the institution's services, its market position relative to the needs of the population and to the competition, and the evaluation of the institution's strategic plans. The reimbursement and planning environment also is an important service area characteristic, which frequently affects financial results. Several states have rate-setting and planning regulations, such as certificate of need, in an attempt to control health-care costs and expenditures. Therefore, an understanding of the unique features of a state's reimbursement and health planning environment is an important element in understanding a provider's fiscal well being.

Institutional Characteristics and Competitive Profile

The competitive environment, always an important element, has become even more so with the continued growth in managed care contracting and overall heightened competition for patients on both an in-patient and out-patient basis. An in-depth understanding of the provider's market share over time for key services, centers of excellence, and competitive position in its primary and secondary service areas has become an increasingly important area of focus for S&P as an indicator of credit strength.

A special designation, such as sole community provider, can be a significant institutional consideration recognizing a unique role the provider plays. Often this translates into a financial advantage, as the provider receives increase reimbursement.

S&P reviews the size of the provider's medical staff, the average age of the staff, and level of board certification and admission dispersion among the top admitters. The ability to attract and retain new doctors is another useful indicator. Additions and deletions to staff, traditionally an area of focus, has shifted to include an emphasis on recruitment of primary care physicians. Given the increased power of primary care physicians to direct patient flow and resource utilization in a managed care environment, it is important for S&P to understand the relations a provider has with primary care physicians, as well as with the rest of the medical staff including an understanding of practice patterns and loyalty of the medical staff to the institution. The establishment of physician hospital organizations or similar structures is viewed positively if it enhances physician loyalty and establishes appropriate financial incentives. Not only have relationships with physicians changed, but S&P recognizes that relations between other providers and insurers have also changed. It is important to highlight these key relationships during the rating process, particularly since affiliation agreements and network formation have become frequently adopted competitive strategies

Management and Administrative Factors

One of the best indicators of management's ability is the provider's track record. However, given the competitive operating and reimbursement environment, the past may not always be a predictor of future results. Therefore, S&P's analysis of management seeks to determine whether the management team exhibits the depth and experience to provide leadership, deal effectively with the medical staff, budget effectively, monitor and control financial and personnel resources, define the hospital's role, and develop a dynamic strategic plan to maintain a competitive position. Management's ability to assess its institutions strengths and weaknesses and to develop sound strategies to enhance the institution's competitive position is crucial to continued success. In meetings with S&P, management teams should be prepared to discuss these topics in detail. The provider's management, information, and capital budgeting systems should be adequate for the size, type, and complexity of the institution. Management information systems have become an essential tool for successful negotiations with managed-care providers. S&P discusses with management the types and frequency of monitoring and reporting to the staff and to the board of trustees. Another area of discussion is risk management and the hospital's history with malpractice claims and settlements. The role of the board and their interaction with the management team continue to be areas of analytical focus. The board's size, composition, structure, and activity are noted, with particular consideration given to their participation in setting strategic and financial policies.

Financial Factors

Financial position and performance—particularly cash levels—remain important elements of S&P's analysis. However, if a provider's business fundamentals are not sound, currently good financial performance and position may not be sufficient to offset longer-term business concerns. For example, a very competitive service area, risk associated with construction of a major project, a weak local economy, or a weak medical staff profile might explain why a hospital is rated above or below what its financial profile might otherwise indicate. Conversely, the absence of competition and a growing economy sometimes can compensate for lower cash levels or thinner margins. S&P's financial analysis highlights income statement, balance sheet, and cash flow statement trends. One bad year is not necessarily a negative factor, unless it is determined to the beginning of a permanent shift in financial performance.

Income statement analysis focuses on revenue growth, payor mix and profitability by payor, and overall profitability. Given continued efforts to control health-care expenditures at both the federal and local levels and the shift to managed care from traditional indemnity coverage, financial results will continue to be under pressure in the near term. Given the growth in managed care contracting, S&P will ask management about its managed care contracting strategy, to explain managed care's actual and expected impact on financial performance, and to discuss the contracting process.

S&P is interested in measuring an institution's financial flexibility or its ability to meet its debt service requirements even under stressful conditions. Some benchmarks of financial flexibility are the ratio of fixed costs to variable costs, and full-time equivalents to adjusted occupied bed. Low-cost providers with a favorable payor mix and market dominance will have a clear advantage. Competitive pressures may constrain high-cost providers from raising prices, even though they may be suffering financially. Typically, S&P will ask how the provider's costs compare with other providers and is interested in any initiatives undertaken or underway to control or reduce costs of providing services.

Key income statement indicators are operating and excess margins, historical pro forma debt service coverage, and debt burden. The balance sheet analysis focuses on leverage, liquidity, and cash flow. Key balance sheet ratios are days' cash on hand, cash flow to total debt, the cushion ratio, and debt to capitalization. In general, due to the diminishing pricing flexibility and the continued increase in regulatory and reimbursement pressures, the level of cash reserves consistent with a particular rating category has increased while the debt to capitalization ratio has decreased.

■ Health-Care Systems

S&P's revised definition of a health-care system includes vertically integrated systems that may or may not have multiple hospitals, as well as traditional multihospital systems. The previous definition, which required three acute-care hospitals exhibiting some degree of geographic and financial dispersion, has become less applicable in this era of health-care reform. The new definition includes systems that have multiple business lines, even if geographic dispersion is lacking.

The number of systems, particularly those rated in the 'AA' category, continues to rise. System ratings generally are higher than ratings for single-site facilities because of the financial and nonfinancial synergies that may accrue to systems.

S&P's approach to rating health-care systems is similar to that used for single-site facilities. In both cases, creditworthiness depends on certain qualitative, quantitative, and legal factors. However, a system's credit standing can be enhanced by geographic, financial, and product line dispersion. When rating systems, S&P evaluates the extent to which these credit enhancing qualities exist. The strength of the obligated group, as defined in the master indenture, is particularly important. Key rating considerations also include the system's structure, management's administrative philosophy, and any economies achieved through consolidation of financial and management resources.

Obligated Group

The first step in the rating process is to evaluate the obligated group that covenants to repay the debt issue. The obligated group might not include all the entities in the system. For example, the initial obligated group often excludes leased and managed facilities, ventures not related to health care, and for-profit corporations. Similarly, the group often excludes businesses that are unable to refinance existing debt or those that might diminish the group's creditworthiness.

S&P then assesses any management plans that would change the obligated group's strength. Potential acquisition, divestiture, and diversification strategies are particularly important. Plans to divest an important revenue-producing entity or absorb a losing operation can affect the obligated group's financial strength. Many systems also guarantee the debt of weaker institutions, either as a diversification strategy or to buoy an affiliated institution in distress. As a result, S&P examines the downside risk of guarantees. S&P also evaluates potential transfers of cash or other assets out of the obligated group. Sheltering assets may be attractive for some purposes but often weakens the balance sheet.

Finally, S&P reviews the system's activity outside the obligated group. Health-care systems often have the opportunity to engage in health-related services and alternative delivery systems, as well as speculative nonhealth-related projects. Although these activities may take place in subsidiaries excluded from the obligated group, S&P evaluates the scope of such ventures and assesses their impact on the system's creditworthiness.

System Composition

The primary focus of health-care ratings is the obligated group. However, the system's underlying components also are important. Answers to the following questions are critical to system evaluation:

- In a system where members are geographically dispersed, are their economic and competitive markets favorable?

- How far along the vertical integration spectrum is the system, relative to its markets?

- What are the bed size, geographic location, and market position of the group's major acute-care players?

- Is the system constrained by any regulatory, competitive, reimbursement, or economic environments?

- Are the scope and types of services varied throughout the system?

In addition, S&P evaluates each entity's percentage contribution to net revenues, assets, and profits, financial and admission trends, payor mix, and overall profitability. These factors demonstrate the degree of financial, geographic, and risk dispersion in the system. Positive rating factors associated with systems include management expertise, access to capital, economies of scale, pricing flexibility, and the use of corporate personnel, centralized cash management, and insurance and pension trusts. In addition to these traditional strengths, the newly added systems demonstrate regional dominance through vertical integration and the ability to adapt to local managed-care penetration. Also, in most cases, systems have larger revenue bases, making them less vulnerable to reimbursement and market pressures.

Board and Management Structure

The organizational structures of health-care systems vary considerably, due to board philosophy as well as more practical factors, such as the system's size, services, and geographic scope. These factors translate directly into the level of corporate control and the degree to which centralized services are available to subsidiaries.

Regardless of a system's organizational structure, management must be able to control the dynamics associated with a large corporation. Typically, a health-care system has greater financial resources than a single hospital and, consequently, greater financial flexibility. Rating benefits derived from this flexibility depend directly on the system's ability to manage these resources. If growth is being pursued aggressively, how much debt is being used to finance new projects, and are the plans prudent? Conversely, if the system is overbedded or operating unprofitable ventures, is the flexibility being used as a cushion to delay decisions? These issues highlight management ability, as well as the financial planning capabilities of the system.

Successful health-care systems that survive industry consolidation will include regional providers offering a continuum of services, as well as the more traditionally defined multihospital systems. In addition, access to patients through managed-care products owned by the system and a well-established, loyal physician network will become more critical as hospitals and physicians jointly contract to care for defined populations.

In assessing the credit strength of various types of systems, S&P draws three major distinctions. First, distinctions can be drawn between systems formed by natural market synergies over time and those formed more recently due to market pressures. Whether they are regional or national, the more mature systems formed over time generally are better positioned to take advantage of the incentives under health-care reform, while recently formed systems face the challenge of internal system integration, in addition to a multitude of external pressures. While there still are benefits to multistate providers, including economic and regulatory diversification, national systems must create or participate in local minisystems to compete with strong regional systems and alliances.

Second, distinctions can be made between systems' managed-care strategies. Many systems that have owned managed-care products through the 1980s have extensive experience with underwriting, claims administration, physician integration, and resource control that can only be gained over time. Systems that have successfully implemented managed care strategies in more highly penetrated states clearly have an advantage if health-care reform proceeds under a managed-competition model. Finally, distinctions can be made between systems that have a salaried, hospital-based medical group and those with a traditional medical staff. As revenues continue to be limited, systems that control physician resources will be best positioned to contain expenses and maximize profit.

As always, the presence of a single credit-enhancing feature will not necessarily improve a rating. On the other hand, a system need not exhibit all the characteristics discussed above to obtain a better rating. The rating ultimately reflects any credit enhancing attributes that exist for bondholders' benefit.

■ Health Maintenance Organizations

S&P's evaluation of health maintenance organizations (HMOs), a prominent form of managed care that bridges the gap between prepaid health insurance and health-care delivery, focuses on their ability to compete in a growing and increasingly competitive segment of the health services market. S&P's rating factors for HMOs are quantified and qualified and viewed against the backdrop of individual HMO capital resources and strategy. The elements of the analysis are classified into five general categories:

- Industry risk,
- Market position,
- Management
- Operating efficiency, and
- Financial risk.

Industry Risk

In more mature markets, HMOs increasingly compete against a variety of alternative delivery systems. These include employer self-insurance plans with utilization review or volume purchasing organizations, such as preferred provider organizations (PPOs) and employer provider organizations (EPOs). Conceptually, HMOs can do well in this competitive arena by virtue of the combined utilization and cost-control benefits inherent in their operating structure. In practice, however, three significant industry characteristics will influence an HMO's growth and financial performance.

Consolidation. Notwithstanding enrollment gains, the HMO industry consolidated during the late 1980s. As the industry matures, consolidation is expected to continue in fragmented, highly saturated markets where employers are limiting the number of HMOs offered, preferring those providing broader geographic coverage and a larger variety of products. They also are negotiating tougher contracts, requiring HMOs to set premiums more reflective of the individual group's experience. Consolidation of an elective nature also is occurring, as smaller regional HMOs are forming alliances to broaden their geographic coverage. In assessing this risk, S&P will focus on market trends and the organization's tools—such as management expertise, information systems, and capital—to respond to these trends.

Cyclicality. Business cycles may affect HMO enrollment and pricing. The effect on specific HMOs will relate to their dependence on particular locales, industries, or employer groups. As purchasers of health care, HMOs also will be affected by trends in the cost of medical service delivery. Relative exposure to these variations and the ability to adjust premiums accordingly are important determinants of risk. HMO profitability also is subject to insurance underwriting cycles. While theoretically able to price under an umbrella provided by less-competitive indemnity health insurers, temporary strength in nonhealth-care lines of indemnity insurers, or use of reserves by Blue Cross/Blue Shield and other group health insurers to subsidize their managed-care products, periodically lead to more competitive premium pricing. In assessing the potential strain of these cycles, S&P will focus on the HMO's information systems capability, mechanisms to control costs, and financial profile.

Political and regulatory change. Initiatives on the part of federal and state governments will continue to have a significant impact on the HMO industry's growth prospects, operating efficiency, and market position relative to other forms of group health insurance. Legislation was passed in 1988 that by 1995 could eliminate the remaining elements of industry growth incentives provided in earlier federal acts. For established plans with strong ties to their client/employer groups, the impact should be negligible at worst, and may even enhance operating flexibility. Even so, legislation may be passed before 1995 that will supersede these changes. President Clinton's emphasis on managed competition and health-care form promotes greater use of HMOs and other forms of managed care. In the near term, licensing and regulatory requirements will continue to govern the health benefits HMOs offer, their rating practices, and reserve requirements. Rigorous enforcement of these requirements should not present problems for the larger, financially viable HMOs. In fact, they could benefit from acquisition opportunities, as smaller HMOs terminate or consolidate with the major players. In the intermediate term, HMOs that are responsive to federal and state incentives to enroll and increasing number of Medicare and Medicaid recipients may become increasingly vulnerable to government budget pressures and adverse risk selection for the Medicaid population. In the long term, the nature and extent of national health reform could facilitate future growth, significantly alter the way HMOs do business, or eliminate the need for prepaid health plans. Notwithstanding the uncertainties they face, well-established HMOs are positioned to benefit from the opportunities afforded by a U.S. health-care system desperately seeking to provide greater care at a lower cost.

Market Position

Enrollment size and diversity bears importantly on the HMO's cost structure and ability to withstand unfavorable business cycles. Profit prospects also hinge on the economic and demographic profile of the areas serviced, the degree of competition, and the health-care provider network. Accordingly, S&P's examination of HMOs includes:

- Major markets served;
- Size and composition of the enrollment base—large and small groups, Medicare and Medicaid contribution, and age and sex composition;
- Enrollment and disenrollment trends;
- Reliance on, and retention and penetration of, the major participating employer groups; and
- Overall market penetration of managed health care in the service areas.

For HMOs that own clinics and hospitals, S&P evaluates their geographic coverage and capacity to meet management's growth and expansion plans and their ability to maintain efficient operations.

HMOs that capture a significant share of the HMO and group health markets are well positioned to cope with market pressures by virtue of economies of scale. Competitive advantages are achieved through quality-cost distinctions and effective marketing. A strong brokerage function linking providers and enrollees to the health plan enhances organizational value and enrollment growth and retention. S&P assesses factors related to the quality and capacity of the provider network, the breadth and diversity of benefit packages offered, premiums and benefit packages relative to competitors, and quality assurance.

Finally, HMOs are increasing market share by diversifying the benefit plans they offer and by expanding geographically. Well-managed HMOs with sufficient diversity, critical mass, and capital can absorb initial near-term risk and potentially benefit from this strategy in the long term. Disciplined growth can stabilize an HMO's risk profile. On the other hand, overly aggressive growth, particularly acquisitions of turnaround candidates, can undermine an HMO's business position.

Management Evaluation

Strong leadership and effective management are key ingredients of any maturing, dynamic, and complex industry. HMO management is particularly challenged by the array of functions it must perform, the increased regulatory and market scrutiny to which the organization is subject, and the lean administrative structure required to do a cost-effective job.

Generally, an HMO coordinates the appropriate provision of group health benefits to its members by contracting for services with the providers of such care. This role requires an HMO to market its services to employers and physicians, enroll individuals and determine benefit eligibility, secure ongoing provider and member goodwill, process claims, review utilization, and maintain quality assurance. Policies and procedures should be in place to perform operations, review results, and manage risk. To maintain its competitive advantage, an HMO should have a cohesive strategic planning process, sophisticated negotiation skills to deal with providers and employers, and good labor relations. Management's strategic planning process is reviewed to determine its operational focus, flexibility to manage capital, and appetite for business and financial risk.

Operating Efficiency

The HMO's linkage of prepaid health insurance with service delivery can facilitate economies as well as predictable, flexible performance if operated efficiently. S&P's analysis focuses on an HMO's effectiveness in managing health insurance risks and the quality and cost of services. Utilization review, quality assurance, marketing, benefits management, rating/underwriting, and claims processing are common functions found in most HMOs.

The availability of timely and comprehensive information that integrates the delivery and financing functions is essential to operate the business, minimize the impact of the underwriting cycle, sustain a competitive advantage, and diversify. In addition to evaluating management's policies and tools, S&P evaluates the organizational structure relative to the key operating functions.

Significant operating variations will hinge on the degree of control the HMO can exert over its health-care providers. This control is greatest with a staff model HMO, in which physicians are salaried employees and patients are treated in facilities owned by the HMO.

Somewhat less control is afforded through a group model HMO, which contracts with a multispecialty medical group practice. The groups receive a fixed payment for each enrollee, and services may be rendered in facilities owned by the HMO or the group.

In a network model, the HMO contracts with more than one group. In an individual practice association model, the HMO contracts with facilities dispersed throughout the community. As HMOs grow and diversify, they often develop mixtures of these structures, depending upon the health-care resources available in local markets. The structure of the HMO dictates the level of capital investment, "make or buy" decisions relative to physician services, and operating costs.

Information Requirements

Operations

- Group's history
- Expansion plans/satellite facilities
- Project/use of proceeds
- Historical and projected number of encounters, encounters per physician, and new patients for each of past five years
- Breadth of patient draw and service area
- Physical assets and future needs
- Competition with hospitals, outpatient centers, physicians, and other providers in the area
- Nature of relationship with medical facility, if applicable

Physicians

- Predominant method of physician practice in area
- Number of physicians in clinic
- Physicians in clinic as percentage of total area medical doctors

- Recruitment and credentialing
- Compensation vs. independent and/or HMO physicians
- Top 10 physicians, encounters and revenues, age and tenure
- Physician leadership/structure and specifics
- Noncompete clauses

Leadership

- Management tenure/qualifications
- Board of Trustees
- Strategic approach to changing practice patterns

Finances

- Five years' audited financial statements (accrual basis)
- Three to five years' projected income statements, balance sheets
- Payor mix
- Reimbursement issues; RBRVS
- Foundation finances, if applicable
- Research revenues/cost
- HMO ownership/exposure
- Details on available cash; restricted funds

Premium rates are a function of the HMO's location and expected costs, enrollment size and mix, benefits package, and rating methods. Since revenues are prepaid and fixed, there is a risk exposure during the time enrollment builds to levels actuarially imputed in premiums. This, as well as other health-care underwriting risks, can be mitigated through risk-sharing arrangements with providers and proven information management systems.

S&P's operating analysis incorporates a review of fixed contractual arrangements with providers and incentives for lower utilization, as well as trends in hospital and clinic utilization (days and visits per thousand members) by Medicare and non-Medicare enrollees. Other items reviewed include the role of health-care and administrative expenses in the overall cost structure, controllable versus fixed costs, working capital management, revenue composition (premiums to total revenues and percent of Medicare risk contract revenue), rating methods, and premium increases. Highlights of the analysis are:

- Level and trend of earnings by product and market segment,
- Health-care expense/medical loss ratios and administrative expense ratios,
- Return on assets,
- Operating income as a percent of premiums, and
- Receivable turnover and payables as a percentage of premiums.

Financial Analysis

S&P evaluates past and projected financial performance in terms of trends, strength, and flexibility. The analysis incorporates profitability and efficiency ratios discussed above with various liquidity and capital structure and debt ratios.

S&P balances industry and business risk factors with financial factors when assigning a rating. Depending on an HMO's capital intensity, certain ratios will be more relevant for group and staff model HMOs, both of which tend to own their own facilities. Ratios reviewed for these types of HMOs include fixed assets per member, debt per member, debt to plant and debt to capitalization. Where appropriate, per member per month data are reviewed for intra- and intercompany comparisons. Factors incorporated in S&P's financial analysis include:

- A review of financial goals, cash and debt management, unpaid claims tracking, provider payments, and premium collections;

- Accounting practices relative to reserves, recognition of income and liabilities, and accrual methodology for incurred but not reported claims;

- On- and off-balance-sheet liabilities (pension obligations, post-retirement health benefits, and operating leases); and

- Financial ratio analysis, which includes:

  - Operating performance—return on assets and capital and aggregate and per-member per-month operating and profit margins;

  - Liquidity ratios including current ratio, days premium receivable, days' cash on hand, unpaid claims as a percent of revenues, average accounts payable, and claims payment periods; and

  - Debt and capital structure, cash flow coverage of debt, debt to capitalization, and maximum annual debt service coverage ratios.

▌ Medical Rehabilitation Hospitals

Recent growth in the medical rehabilitation field and signs that the sector is poised for further expansion have led S&P to develop an approach to rating rehabilitation hospitals that acknowledges both the uniqueness of the business and its role in the larger, complex health-care industry.

The medical rehabilitation field has experienced tremendous growth. According to the American Medical Association, there were 74% more rehabilitation physicians in 1990 than in 1982. Rehabilitation service revenue has been growing about 20% annually and is expected to continue a rapid growth rate for several years.

Reimbursement Risks

S&P believes the environment for continued expansion exists and, therefore, expects further growth in rating activity for rehabilitation hospitals. But a number of risks—including possible changes in federal and state reimbursement policies—could cloud the rating outlook for these facilities.

The increased supply of and demand for medical rehabilitation services has been due to several factors, including:

- Favorable reimbursement policies—primarily rehabilitation facilities' exemption from Medicare's prospective payment system (PPS),
- Aging of the general population, and
- More effective medical technology.

With about 50% of rehabilitation facilities' revenues derived from the federal Medicare program, government reimbursement practices are a central issue. The exemption from PPS, since its inception in 1983, has been the single-largest cause for the growth in number of rehabilitation facilities.

Under PPS, hospitals are reimbursed at a nationally established rate per diagnosis that is derived from averages of all hospitals, irrespective of individual cost structures. Rehabilitation facilities are reimbursed by Medicare based on an established target operating cost per discharge specific for that facility. Because their revenues are PPS-exempt, rehabilitation facilities are less dependent on prospectively determined revenues and, therefore, less subject to the financial risks of such a system.

Increasing Demand

The combination of an aging population and technological advances has spurred the increasing demand for rehabilitation services. In addition to a growing elderly population consuming more rehabilitation services, individuals of all ages who may not have been able to be rehabilitated a few years ago can often reap the benefits of new medical technologies.

It has been demonstrated that providing rehabilitative services saves more than it costs. Rehabilitation serves to improve or restore one's functional independence while helping a patient adjust to being disabled. Thus, effective rehabilitative services provided by appropriate facilities could play a major role in the national effort to control health-care costs.

Analysis

Analysis of rehabilitation hospitals is much different from that of traditional acute-care hospitals. Direct comparison with acute-care hospitals should be avoided. The major aspects of the analysis discussed below include:

- Type and scope of rehabilitation services,
- Sources of patients and competitive environment,
- Payor mix and reimbursement policies, and
- Financial Analysis.

Rehabilitation is a broad area; therefore, the services provided must be defined. Furthermore, there is a wide variation of type of patient and scope of services provided. For example, a facility that serves children with developmental and behavioral disorders is quite different from a chronic-care hospital, which has high lengths of stays and a different patient population.

A rehabilitation facility may be little more than a skilled nursing facility providing minimal rehabilitative services to a population with little or no rehabilitative potential. Certain facilities offer services to patients of all ages with a wide range of needs and lengths of stay.

A determination and understanding of populations served and extent of services provided is critical to an analysis. Once the service mix is established, the source of patients and competitive environment is assessed. This is a good indicator of the need for the facilities.

For example, some rehabilitation hospitals receive many, if not all, of their inpatients as referrals from acute-care hospitals. They probably are not competing with the referring hospitals. Acute-care hospitals will transfer patients who will not benefit any further from acute-care services and require some level of rehabilitation. Also, such patients usually increase the costs and lower the operating margins for a prospectively reimbursed facility.

As with acute-care hospital analysis, uniqueness and diversity of services is a credit strength. Unique facilities that are able to draw patients from a wide geographical area while retaining a majority market share in its primary service area have an added advantage.

A facility has a clear market strength if few or no referrals from acute-care hospitals are going to other comparable rehabilitation facilities. Since there often is significant competition, diversity of services is another credit strength. Typically, there is more competition for shorter stay services, such as rehabilitation for strokes and orthopedics. Facilities that offer diversified long-term and short-term services are somewhat shielded from competition.

A hospital's payor mix is essential to its financial health and future. A large dependence on any one payor is a vulnerability. Generally, Medicare and Medicaid are the two largest payors. Hospitals that receive 60% or more of total revenues from Medicare, for example, are sensitive to issues regarding the Tax Equity and Fiscal Responsibility Act of 1982 (TEFRA).

Medicaid-dependent facilities rely on special legislation from their state Medicaid programs to provide them with sufficient revenues. The extent, strength, and the outlook for any legislative changes must be evaluated.

The financial analysis is the last major area to assess. In addition to the typical analysis to determine a hospital's profitability trends, cash position, cash flow, operating efficiency, capital expenditures and needs, and debt structure, analysis of the sources of profits and losses is important.

For example, a rehabilitation facility may be able to mask a vulnerable situation by erasing a deficit and producing a positive bottom line from one successful service, such as a workers' compensation program, which may comprise less than 10% of its business. Facilities also may depend on nonpatient revenues, such as grants and fund raising, to produce adequate margins and cash flow. The sources, history, and future of these items may affect profitability.

Reimbursement Systems

The impact of different reimbursement systems is an integral part of the financial analysis. The trend of incentive or penalty payments under TEFRA is a sign of financial health. Medicaid reimbursement varies by state and may involve a unique reimbursement formula. As in an acute-care analysis, it is important to discern the profitability levels of individual payors.

Despite the likelihood that the rehabilitation industry will continue to grow, risks for these hospitals continue. Reform of the health-care industry is likely, but in what form is unknown. It is unclear whether rehabilitation hospitals will remain exempt from prospective payments. The loss of this exemption could have undesirable effects and result in downgrades. Financial disincentives for treating certain types of patients would be created, possibly leading to reduced access for cost-intensive cases. The incentive to turn away complex cases and reduce lengths of stay would exist, and overall health costs could rise, due to the increased incidence of future acute inpatient episodes. Certain patients may not reach their potential level of independent, due to less effective rehabilitation, and would require additional health-care resources.

▌ Academic Medical Centers

S&P's rating criteria for rating university hospitals varies with the structure of the hospital being considered. It has become popular in recent years to separate the hospital, and its financial requirements, from the university. In some cases, this has resulted in hospital ratings completely independent from those of the related university. In other cases, when a hospital issues revenue debt guaranteed by a university, the bonds generally carry the same rating as the university's direct debt.

However the relationship between the hospital and university is structured, S&P examines the fundamental business of the hospital in its evaluation. The extent to which hospital analysis is outweighed by analysis of the university as a whole is determined by the structure of the bonds and the degree of separation between the two institutions.

Strong credit ratings. The majority of university hospital bonds rated by S&P are in the 'AA' category. University hospitals often track the profile of an 'AA' health-care issuer. They tend to be large, diversified organizations with regional, or broader, market penetration, and high utilization. Generally, there is no problem attracting physicians and allied health professionals, as well as sophisticated financial managers. They are financially strong, and cash on hand and cushion ratios are typically high, while leverage is generally low and fund balances are large.

In contrast to their nonuniversity counterparts, most university hospitals have experienced increasing admissions. Like many other hospitals, university hospitals recently have borrowed for capital expenditures. Also in line with the industry has been university hospitals' expansion of outpatient facilities and renovation of emergency rooms, while the addition of beds has been unique to academic medical centers. University hospital issues rated on the basis of the university's debt rating also lean toward the higher rating categories. Universities of the size and stature to support a teaching hospital often have 'AA' characteristics. However, S&P assesses the hospital's operating characteristics and demand for capital in determining whether the hospital enhances or detracts from the university's overall credit strength.

Financial pressures. Whether under the direct auspices of the university or relatively independent, university hospitals are subject to most of the financial pressures affecting tertiary hospitals, plus a few unique to the teaching environment. For example, the research university reimbursement environment has been clouded by charges of indirect cost-recovery abuses, some of which extend to federal grants underlying medical research. In addition, the Health Care Financing Administration has been aggressive in recovering excess charges relating to teaching cost reimbursement.

Changes in the health-care delivery system that also challenge university hospitals include:

▌ The shift to outpatient medicine;

▌ New competition for physicians, staff, and patients;

▌ Reduction in Medicare's Indirect Medical Education (IME) payments; and

∎ The Resource Based Relative Value Scale (RBRVS) for physician payments.

Reductions in funding for research and teaching are causing university hospitals to focus more on patient care as an important revenue source. At the same time, admissions and inpatient activity have been declining as the industry shifts more and more to an outpatient environment. This means university hospitals, traditionally geared primarily to inpatient care, are having to address outpatient care to extend their penetration of local markets. Capital costs associated with realignment of services can strain balance sheets and place pressure on ratings.

Other changes that can stress university hospitals' finances include the increasing need to compete with tertiary hospitals for critical-care nurses and technologists trained to operate their sophisticated equipment. Also, because of their commitment to teaching and research, university hospitals cannot always close down uneconomic services, a disadvantage relative to tertiary hospitals, which retain more flexibility.

The reduction in IME payments and the shift to RBRVS are governmental solutions to a perceived surfeit of the specialists who make up the heart of the university hospital's medical staff. RBRVS may compel physicians to seek more compensation from hospitals and, in time of reduced academic reimbursement, university hospitals will find it harder to satisfy these demands.

In many communities, physicians have become competitors of hospitals by setting up their own outpatient facilities. University hospitals can help their physicians expand outpatient activities by using faculty group practice revenues for funding expansion of clinics.

University hospitals also face competition for nonclinical faculty from the business community. The biotechnology industry, in particular, has drawn faculty away with offers of rich compensation, as well as state-of-the-art facilities. These hospitals sometimes try to minimize such defections and capture a participation in the outside ventures of their faculty by building research parks or buildings for companies on or near their facilities.

As large, complex organizations, typically with a long history in one location, academic hospitals have been less likely than their smaller competitors to move from inner-city locations. Thus, the urban university hospital often finds itself handling an increasing burden of indigent and uncompensated trauma care. Some of the cost has been offset by disproportionate-share payments from the federal government. University hospitals also receive a healthy share of the Medicaid windfall created by state efforts to boost matching federal funds for Medicaid. These are no assurances, however, that funding will remain close to demand for services to the indigent.

While the challenges outlined above are substantial, S&P does not expect significant declines in credit quality. Each institution will be monitored, but the advantages of size, regional market draw, strong financial resources, and good management should permit the group as a whole to adapt effectively to changes in the health-care delivery system.

Medical Schools

From a rating perspective, since most U.S. medical schools are affiliated with a university or hospital or both, it is impossible to evaluate the medical college without considering the associated university/hospital operation.

S&P's approach to medical colleges is governed in large part by this affiliation. Most ratings associated with medical colleges are refined by their relationship with a related university and/or hospital. In the case of public medical colleges, the rating also incorporates an evaluation of state support. However, S&P does rate free-standing medical schools not affiliated with a university or a hospital.

The rating process begins with evaluation of demand and a financial analysis similar to that used when assessing higher education and health-care institutions. The analysis is tailored to incorporate special characteristics of medical schools, such as limited class size, high tuition levels, state reimbursement programs, and revenues from faculty practice plans.

University/hospital affiliation. The medical schools of Emory, Tulane, and New York University are examples of medical colleges rated as part of a large combined university/hospital entity. In each case, the medical college enhances the overall reputation and scope of the combined entity and is evaluated as part of the larger institution and not on a stand-alone basis.

S&P also rates medical schools such as Thomas Jefferson University and the Medical College of Pennsylvania, which comprise part of a large hospital entity but are not affiliated with a comprehensive educational institution. In most such instances, the medical school operation is overshadowed by the hospital, and the analysis places greater weight on traditional hospital evaluation than on the medical school.

State-supported medical schools. State support adds another twist to the evaluation of medical schools. S&P rates a few combined hospital/medical school entities that receive state appropriations. While student demand, hospital utilization rates, and service area characteristics are important rating factors for combined hospital/school organizations, strength of state support is the determining credit consideration.

Independent medical schools. Free-standing medical schools offer an opportunity to assess a medical college unenhanced by the credit characteristics of affiliated institutions. These colleges are more dependent than other medical schools upon student demand and tuition and must support themselves without the benefit of state money or the deep pocket of a larger university or hospital. To reflect their stand-alone nature, S&P is unlikely to assign a rating higher than 'A' to a free-standing medical school.

Demand analysis. Demand analysis of medical schools mirrors that used in evaluating colleges and universities. S&P focuses on enrollment trends, application, acceptance and matriculation results, student quality, and competition from other programs. There are, however, significantly fewer medical schools than colleges and universities in the U.S. This fact, combined with the continued popularity of medical careers, results in stiff competition for entry. In fact, despite a downward trend in the 1980s, applications to U.S. medical schools always have far exceeded the number of spaces available.

Since there are so few medical school spaces, students' choices are limited and matriculation rates are high. The flexibility afforded by such selective admissions is particularly significant for medical schools that cannot rely on enrollment in other programs to offset periods of falling demand. While medical colleges remain vulnerable to changes in preferences and attitudes regarding the medical profession, S&P expects demand for medical education to remain strong.

Financial analysis. S&P's financial analysis of medical colleges also parallels the approach used for other higher education institutions, centering on:

∎ Revenue and expenditure composition,

∎ Annual operating results,

- Unrestricted money on the balance sheet, and
- Debt load.

While the analytical approach is similar, some of the financial characteristics of medical schools are very different from other colleges and universities. For example, revenues from faculty practice plans, research grants, and state capitalization programs result in much greater revenue diversity. Medical schools affiliated with hospitals, or those classified as state institutions, derive an especially small portion of their revenue from students and tuition.

While these other revenue sources help insulate medical colleges from fluctuations in student enrollment, they may be vulnerable to change themselves. For example, financially strapped state governments can reduce state support, forcing potentially large increases in tuition rates.

Another development that has had a significant impact on medical school financial operations is the growth of the faculty group practice. Many such practices remain part of a medical school or hospital organization. Even the legally separate faculty practice generates revenue that supports the academic and research operations of the school and/or hospital.

▊ Physician Groups and Faculty Practice Plans

Health-care industry changes, including reform at the state and national levels, have reduced the use of inpatient hospital services in favor of more cost-effective outpatient treatments. Well-organized, well-capitalized multispecialty group practices often offer such services and typically have lower cost structures than hospitals. Because of this, and due to the financial constraints and incentives being imposed on doctors, the percentage of physicians practicing in groups increased to nearly a third in 1991, from 11% in 1965.

3,500 Groups and Growing

There are about 3,500 multispecialty groups in the U.S., with an average of 25 doctors in each. Nearly 200 groups have 100 physicians or more and, excluding the Permanente Medical Groups with their 5,300 physicians, the top 25 groups practices average 360 doctors each. In addition, there are faculty practice plans at most of the 126 accredited medical schools, with an average size of around 350 physicians.

Although recent figures are not available, there has been continued growth in the average size of group practices due to consolidation of smaller groups into larger ones and more acquisitions of groups by both for-profit companies and acute-care hospitals seeking to develop vertically integrated systems. The resulting larger groups often need access to capital to build facilities and purchase equipment that will allow them to provide cost-effective health-care services. In addition, as universities and medical schools continue to be pressured by industry trends and health-care reform, faculty practice plans have emerged as financially strong entities able to access the capital markets on their own credit.

Rating Criteria

S&P has applied the following criteria to the outstanding municipal group practice ratings, as well as many hospitals that have a physician group practice component. The strong ratings applied to date suggest that in light of health-care reform, S&P believes physician groups and faculty practice plans are particularly well positioned to deliver efficient, high-quality care in a low-cost setting. In addition, the ratings for faculty practice plans reflect actual and implied support from related universities and hospitals. In the future, the municipal group expects to continue to apply the same criteria to assess physician components of the rapidly developing vertically integrated health systems.

Rating considerations for not-for-profit physician groups include analysis in the following categories:

■ Operations,

■ Competition,

■ Physicians,

■ Leadership,

■ Institutional relationships,

■ Information systems,

■ Finances, and

■ Legal covenants.

The most critical factors for ratings assessment are the physicians, finances, and operations. The other aspects of the clinics discussed below contribute to strength in these key areas.

Operations. The history of the clinic, its structure, and its longevity are the starting points in S&P's evaluation of the credit. The primary consideration is the likelihood that the clinic will remain viable for the life of the bonds. Consequently, S&P's municipal ratings group will rate debt issued only by nonprofit group practices; the financial and operational incentives of a proprietary group generally are not consistent with the capital retention levels necessary for an investment-grade rating. Beyond understanding how and why the physicians came to work together, S&P must assess the group's ongoing strategy and its appeal to physicians in the future.

S&P focuses primarily on multispecialty clinics with 100 doctors or more. Among the operational aspects of the clinic S&P examines are:

■ History of the group,

■ Breadth of patient draw,

■ Economics of service area,

■ Current and proposed practice facilities,

■ Physical assets and future needs,

■ Proposed projects and use of bond proceeds,

■ Nature of relationship with other medical facilities, and

■ Use of nonmedical personnel relative to physicians.

Competition. Multispecialty group practices compete not only with other groups and solo practitioners, but often with outpatient surgery centers, diagnostic centers, testing laboratories, and hospitals. A group's ability to attract and retain physicians and patients is paramount to the rating. As competition for patients among physicians and other providers intensifies, group practices must demonstrate their cost effectiveness and ability to attract profitable managed-care contracts. With managed-care reimbursement moving increasingly toward capitated arrangements, multispecialty groups also must demonstrate their ability to manage profitably in this environment.

S&P anticipates that, over time, quality indicators will play an important role in the ability to compete for contracts. Management should be prepared to discuss the group's experience as these measures are adopted and refined. At present, the competitive aspects reviewed include:

- Physician competitors for patients, including both non-profit and for-profit group and solo practitioners;
- Nonphysician competitors seeking to provide medical services directly to patients, including hospitals, ambulatory care, surgery, and emergency centers, other professionals (nurse practitioners, psychologists, chiropractors, etc.) and payors, such as health maintenance organizations and insurance companies;
- Percentage of covered lives under contract versus the percentage of covered lives in the service area;
- Competitors for doctors, including hospitals, other physician groups, and physician group management companies; and
- Non-compete clauses.

Physicians. The most critical part of the rating process focuses on physicians, since they are the actual revenue producers. The composition, qualifications, quantity, and quality of the physician group play an important part in the analysis. In addition, physician leadership's philosophy and overall strategic vision, including managed care contracting, and willingness to forge alliances with alternative providers, is an important rating factor. Although the analysis will be slightly different for stand-alone group practices compared with faculty practice plans, in general S&P reviews the following factors:

- Number and specialty mix of physicians currently in the group, as well as growth plans;
- Adequacy of primary care physicians;
- Physicians in the clinic as a percentage of total physicians practicing in the area;
- Whether the local physician market is oversupplied, and the implications of the situation;
- Source and method of physician recruitment;
- Predominant method of physician practice in the area;
- Type of employment contract used—noncompete clause, compensation allocation consistent with managed-care incentives, salaries competitive with industry norms by specialty and with local salaries;
- Credentialing and monitoring process;
- Top 10 revenue-producing physicians (including percent of total revenue generated, age, and tenure with the group);
- Physician additions/deletions to the staff in the past three years;
- Average age of physicians;

- Percent of physicians board certified; and
- For faculty practice plans, ages and tenure of the chairs of the top five revenue-producing departments, vacancies in the major services (internal medicine, surgery, obstetrics, family practice), and percent of tenured faculty.

Leadership. S&P meets with both physician and nonphysician leadership during the rating process. It is important to understand the strategic goals of the physicians and administration to ensure that they are compatible. S&P looks for strong leadership from the Board of Trustees and prefers governance to be community oriented and not consist solely of physician group members.

Management should be appropriately credentialed, with ample experience in the management of physician group practices. In areas with high managed-care penetration, a professional devoted to contracting practices and monitoring adds strength. The review includes:

- Management tenure and qualifications;
- Review and discussion of strategic planning issues;
- Compensation, financial, and operating policies;
- Finances and operations of other subsidiary or sister corporations; and
- Influence of university management and policies on faculty practice plans.

Institutional Relationships. With increasing health-care reform pressures and incentives, group practices have myriad opportunities to cooperate, join, and contract with hospitals, universities, insurance companies, and other payors. S&P examines formal and informal relationships that exist among other institutions.

For stand-alone group practices S&P reviews:

- Operational relationship with primary admitting hospital;
- Financial contracts to share costs, revenues, or overhead with local health-care providers; and
- Managed-care contracting practices.

When evaluating faculty practice plans, issues surrounding university and medical school finances as well as the dean's tax are explored. To the extent that the university hospital has forged alliances with other community providers, the relationship between the faculty group and local physicians will be discussed.

Information systems. To manage a healthcare enterprise efficiently and profitably, integrated information systems are necessary. As part of the rating process, S&P will look for examples of reports addressing such areas as:

- Managed-care members by age, sex, and benefit plan;
- Encounters per full time equivalent (FTE) physician by new and existing patients;
- Utilization and cost per member per month;
- Hospital inpatient use rate and cost per patient per month versus regional averages;
- Revenue by payor and by service;
- Charges and costs by service and payor;

- Revenues and expenses per FTE physician;
- Analysis of clinical outliers and out-of-area utilization; and
- Physician profiling reports.

A clinic's system should handle scheduling and billing and provide clinical results directly to the physician. Capital forecasts should include expenditures for information systems improvements, as well as facilities and clinical equipment.

Finances. S&P will review five years of audits based on the accrual method of accounting as a starting point in the financial analysis. Although accrual-based accounting is preferred, S&P recognizes that it may not be available for some faculty practice plans due to their financial integration with universities. Management letters, reimbursement issues (such as Resource-Based Relative Value Scale), research commitment, fund raising, working capital needs, and future financing plans are also explored. The revenue and expense components of the income statement are examined to assess overhead levels and allocation, physician compensation, sources of revenue from outside payors, and sources of revenue from clinical departments and research. Questions surrounding the balance sheet include trends in accounts receivable and collection rates, adequacy of malpractice reserves, level of cash reserves and restricted funds for research and capital investment, strategic and routine capital needs, and other liabilities.

Information requested includes:

- Five years of financial statements and most recent interim statements;
- Utilization information—patient visits, new patient growth, covered lives, encounters per physician;
- Payor mix as a percentage of revenue;
- Research grants, expenses, and subsidiaries;
- Impact of recent reimbursement changes, including RBRVS and health-care reform;
- Malpractice history of claims paid and pending;
- Projected financial statements, if available;
- Other liabilities, such as incurred but not reported claims, guarantees, leases, and other debt;
- Flow of funds to and from associated university or medical school; and
- Endowment funds available at the university in support of faculty practice operations or debt.

Legal covenants. S&P requires legal and security provisions similar to those used in other health-care financings. A G.O. or revenue pledge is customary, and a mortgage is not required, although a negative pledge on assets is needed if the G.O. pledge is used.

Criteria for funding debt service reserve funds vary according to the rating category and are consistent with other health-care financings. Although S&P prefers to have physician salaries subordinate to the repayment of bonds, this covenant alone is not sufficient to ensure an investment-grade rating, since, without adequate physician compensation, the clinic is at risk for turnover and subsequent loss of business and revenue.

▮ Continuing Care Retirement Communities

S&P rates tax-exempt continuing care retirement communities (CCRCs) upon request. However, to obtain investment-grade or near-investment-grade ratings, CCRCs will need to demonstrate compelling credit strength and meet most if not all of several credit benchmarks.

A properly structured financing secured by the CCRC's revenues can be eligible for an investment-grade rating. The CCRC must be well established, well managed, and have a committed sponsor, such as a health-care system or fraternal organization. In addition, it must have minimal liability for long-term nursing care, exhibit adequate financial performance, and not be overreliant on debt as a source of capital.

Industry Overview

Most CCRCs are not life-care centers. Two other contract types account for two-thirds of all CCRCs—known as Type B, or modified, and Type C, or fee-for-service. Providers offering these latter two contract types provide comparable services to life-care centers but substantially reduce or eliminate guaranteed medical care and are less reliant on entrance or endowment fees.

Some CCRCs that initially adopt the life-care center model have abandoned it, while honoring existing commitments, and alternatively offer Type B or C contracts to new prospective residents. Another trend that has lessened credit risk is the increasing number of CCRCs that now are owned and/or managed by health-care systems. This has enabled some CCRCs to draw on the skills and resources of more sophisticated partners.

CCRCs offer residents a long-term contract for housing, dietary services, and some amount of nursing care when needed. These services are paid by the resident from an advance fee—also known as an entrance or endowment fee—and a monthly maintenance fee. CCRCs appeal to the elderly because of the living arrangements and services provided, usually in one location. These living arrangements are:

- ▮ Independent living units,
- ▮ Assisted-living or personal-care units, and
- ▮ Nursing care units.

CCRCs promote the continuity-of-care concept that is becoming today's norm in long-term care.

Credit Benchmarks

To achieve investment-grade or near-investment-grade ratings, CCRCs will need compelling credit strength and must demonstrate most, if not all, of the following characteristics:

- ▮ A five-year operating history;
- ▮ Stabilized occupancy, defined as a minimum of 90% on existing units;
- ▮ Cash and unrestricted board-designated funds to long-term debt of about 50%;
- ▮ Debt to capitalization below 80%, after incurring any project-related debt;
- ▮ Fund balance should be positive in three of the last five years;
- ▮ Excess margin should be positive in three of the last five years;

- Future maximum annual debt service coverage for the last two full fiscal years greater than or equal to 1.0 times (x), excluding cash received from advance fees; and

- Future maximum annual debt service coverage for the last two full fiscal years—including cash received from advance fees and net of amortization of deferred revenue from advance fees and refunds, greater than or equal to 1.25x.

Contract Types

Three contract types are used by CCRCs, either singularly or, more recently, in combination.

The first contract type is known as a Type A, or extensive. These are the traditional "life-care" communities. In addition to providing a menu of services, the distinguishing feature of this contract type is the unlimited provision of nursing care for little or no increase in monthly maintenance fees.

The Type B, or modified, contract provides the same basic service menu as extensive contracts, with the exception that nursing home care provided for free or a nominal charge typically is limited to 60 days, with any excess utilization subject to a full or discounted per diem charge. Typically, advance or entrance fees and maintenance fees are lower, reflecting the substantial reduction of the potential health-care liability.

The third contract type is the Type C, or fee-for-service. Facilities employing this contract type provide certain services as part of a package arrangement; however, most services—including nursing care—are provided on a fee-for-service basis. Residents are guaranteed access to nursing care but pay full per diem rates.

Other features now offered by CCRCs, but not by early life-care centers, are refundable advance or entrance fees—with the amount refunded negotiated in advance and usually tied to length of occupancy—and/or resale of the previously occupied unit. Because CCRC providers frequently offer refundable advance fees as an option, more scrutiny is devoted to how monthly periodic or maintenance fees are determined and subsequently adjusted.

Other Developments

Other developments affecting the industry that S&P views as favorable are as follows:

Increased regulation. As a result of widely publicized abuses in certain financings involving CCRCs and nursing homes, the long-term care industry has come under increasing scrutiny and stronger regulation. As of 1993, more than 35 states now regulate CCRCs.

Improved accounting. Uniform accounting and financial reporting policies for the industry were adopted by the American Institute of Certified Public Accountants in 1990.

Legal Criteria

S&P's legal criteria for CCRC financings are the same as for all health-care revenue bond financings. They include:

- A revenue pledge of the CCRC. Although a mortgage need not be offered, a negative mortgage pledge will be requested.

- A fully funded debt service reserve fund at bond closing.

- Residents' and other creditors' claims to advance fees should be subordinate to debt service payments.

S&P focuses on the following analytical factors common to all bond analysis: administrative debt, economic, and financial. These factors will be modified to take into account the peculiarities of the industry.

Administrative Factors

S&P's analysis of the organization and management of a CCRC will be extensive, since this area has proven to be a significant weakness in the retirement center industry. The role of the sponsor will be analyzed, and evidence of the sponsor's commitment to the community and the bond financing will be reviewed.

A site visit and tour of the facility and service area are required for all proposed financings. S&P's representatives meet with key members of the administrative staff, board, and management company if under independent management contract. It also would be desirable for representatives of the sponsoring organization to attend this meeting to discern their role in the continuation of this enterprise.

S&P reviews with the representatives of the CCRC and affiliated organizations the following:

- The organization's mission,
- Governance structure,
- Financial goals,
- Compliance procedures with regulatory authorities,
- Contract types and refund policies in effect,
- Procedures for establishing advance fees and maintenance fees,
- Census data and factors that affect census,
- Marketing program and budget,
- Entrance requirements and screening procedures, and
- Financial planning and budget preparation.

Debt Factors

As in all revenue bond analysis, S&P focuses on the structure of the proposed issue from both an economic and legal standpoint to ensure that the proposed structure makes sense in light of the obligor's existing and proposed financial performance, commitments, and debt capacity. Project-related financings should be supported by an independent feasibility study prepared by a consultant having extensive experience in the CCRC industry. S&P will want to review with management the most recently completed actuary's report with related assumptions.

In addition to receiving GAAP-prepared audited financial statements, S&P will request a summary of the major assumptions used to prepare these financial statements, since CCRCs' assumptions about characteristics of their resident population directly affect amounts recorded in the financial statements.

Economic Factors

S&P's analysis of the economic characteristics of the service area will be an integral part of the analysis. Particular attention will be paid to the demographic and economic profile of the service area population in light of the CCRC's marketing plans.

Management and/or its financial representatives will be expected to prepare a competitive market profile of existing and proposed CCRCs and other organizations that could be viewed as competitors in the service area, detailing the census by contract and/or unit type and indicating the fees in effect for each major type of contract or service offered.

S&P also reviews relevant past performance indicators, including unit turnover rates, fill-up rates, morbidity, and mortality rates. Since, to some degree, certain types of CCRCs have been dependent on local housing market conditions, an analysis of the local housing stock should be provided to include a summary of recent sales activity.

Financial Factors

S&P's financial analysis begins by obtaining an understanding of financial limits imposed by the contract types in effect for the various classes of current and future residents. This information will be evaluated in light of management's control over operating expenses by living arrangement. Specifically, S&P will want to examine sample resident contracts by type to determine what obligations have been extended and what arrangements are in effect to assure the CCRC it will be able to recoup its cost of rendering these services. CCRCs sometimes have ignored managing their nursing care utilization and costs. S&P will review comparative facilities data to ensure that this fundamental aspect of the business is not being over-looked by management.

Finally, S&P will review the CCRC's overall financial performance and projections.

∎ Nursing Homes

S&P's nursing home rating criteria focus on:

- ∎ Management's experience and use of the appropriate mix of resources (for example, staffing ratios comparable to industry norms);
- ∎ Demand and competitive-market analysis, including an analysis of pricing trends in the community and pre-admission screening policies;
- ∎ Medicaid reimbursement and cost analysis for all states from which a provider draws patients;
- ∎ An economic analysis of a provider's service area and the states that are a source of Medicaid payments; and
- ∎ Financial analysis, including a review of nonoperating revenue sources and an organization's bad debt and charity care policies.

A nursing home financing that could not demonstrate historical pro forma debt service coverage for the two most recent fiscal years in excess of 1.10x most likely would not be eligible for an investment-grade rating, unless extenuating circumstances exist and a feasibility study demonstrates coverage exceeding this amount for the forecast period.

S&P's documentation requirements for nursing home financings are comparable to its requirements for other health-care revenue bonds.

Appendix B—Municipal Bond Insurance Companies

AMBAC Indemnity Corporation

AMBAC Indemnity Corporation founded the municipal bond insurance industry in 1971. Today AMBAC enjoys a reputation as an industry leader, dedicated to providing superior service to investors and issuers of municipal bonds.

In response to requests from investment brokers and their clients for information about AMBAC and the benefits of municipal bond insurance, we have compiled the following commonly asked questions. We hope you will find this information useful.

1. **How does AMBAC insurance benefit investors?**

   AMBAC insurance unconditionally guarantees that investors will receive all principal and interest payments on schedule should the issuer of an AMBAC-insured bond default. Also, bonds insured by AMBAC are automatically rated triple-A by Moody's Investors Service, Inc. Standard & Poor's Corporation and Fitch Investors Service, Inc.. By choosing these high-quality bonds, investors can simplify the complex task of evaluating the thousands of municipal securities available. And investors who decide to sell their AMBAC-insured bonds before maturity benefit from the enhanced marketability and excellent trading value of these triple-A rated securities.

2. **How much does bond insurance cost the investor?**

   Nothing. Individual investors do not pay directly for AMBAC insurance. However, when they buy an insured bond, investors give up a small amount of yield in exchange for a triple-A rated security. For a small price, investors receive the added safety of a "sleep at night" guarantee.

3. **What percentage of municipal bonds is insured?**

   For the past ten years, a growing proportion of municipal bonds has been issued with insurance. In 1981, just 5% of all new issue municipal bonds were insured. Recently, this proportion exceeded 38%. The current trend toward insuring more bonds reflects a growing concern for safety and security on the part of investors.

4. **What are the strengths behind the AMBAC guarantee?**
   - Assets of $1.9 billion
   - AA quality investment portfolio of marketable fixed income securities
   - Consistently conservative underwriting standards
   - Diversified, high-quality insured portfolio
   - Supplemental capital support and risk diversification from high-quality reinsurers worldwide

5. **How does AMBAC decide whether to insure a bond?**
   AMBAC's mission is to make good bonds better. To qualify as *good*, an issue must not only meet the rating agencies' standards for investment grade (Baa/BBB or better), but also meet AMBAC's rigorous criteria for insurability. Drawing on nearly 25 years of experience, we carefully review the structure and documents of every issue submitted to us, and we test the issuer's financial position, credit history and long-term economic outlook against our high standards.

6. **Does AMBAC monitor potential defaults of bonds it has insured?**
   AMBAC monitors every insured transaction until it matures, which may be 30 years or longer. Our professionals track the issuer's financial condition and compliance with the bond's covenants. This surveillance process is designed to give us early warning of potential defaults. Where appropriate, we initiate remedial action such as enforcing convenant compliance or refinancing or restructuring of the debt.

7. **How strong is AMBAC's claims-paying ability?**
   According to Moody's, Standard & Poor's, and Ftich, AMBAC has the financial strength to continue paying claims through an economic crisis deeper than the Great Depression of the 1930s.

8. **Has AMBAC ever had to pay claims?**
   Yes. Although a few of the more than 17,000 municipal bond issues AMBAC has insured since 1971 have defaulted, no investor in an AMBAC-insured bond has ever missed a scheduled payment of principal or interest.

9. **How does AMBAC use reinsurance?**
   Reinsurance enables an insurance company to diversify risk with other insurance companies. AMBAC maintains reinsurance agreements with an international group of highly rated reinsurers who share a portion of the risk of each issue we insure. Reinsurance provides bond investors with an extra layer of protection.

10. **How long has AMBAC been in business, and who owns the company?**
    AMBAC Indemnity Corporation founded the municipal bond insurance industry in 1971 and has set industry standards ever since. Today, AMBAC Inc., the holding company, is a 100% publicly owned corporation trading on the New York Stock Exchange under the ticker symbol ABK.

11. **Who regulates AMBAC?**
    As a financial guarantee insurer, AMBAC is subject to a form of regulation far more stringent than that generally applied to property and casualty insurers. AMBAC is subject to supervision, regulation and examination by the state insur-

ance departments in the states where AMBAC is licensed to do business, including the Wisconsin Insurance Department, its state of domicile. In addition, Moody's, S&P and Fitch evaluate AMBAC against rigorous criteria, taking into account our underwriting quality, portfolio diversity, investment philosophy and capital resources, among other factors. These rating agencies regularly subject AMBAC to a computerized stress test simulating the Great Depression. AMBAC exceeds their criteria for a triple-A rating.

12. **What kinds of investments does AMBAC have in its investment portfolio?**
    AMBAC has over $1.9 billion in high-quality investments. Our portfolio consists entirely of fixed-income securities. The average rating is AA and the average life is 15.8 years. AMBAC does not invest in junk bonds, real estate, stocks or securities it has insured.

13. **Why should an investor buy an AMBAC-insured bond?**
    - **Financial Strength:** AMBAC's superior capitalization offers the highest margin of safety among the leading bond insurers.
    - **Market Acceptance:** Bonds insured by AMBAC are recognized for their safety, high trading value and marketability.
    - **Quality:** AMBAC-insured bonds are high quality and diversified by bond type, issue size, issuer and geographic location.

14. **What kinds of AMBAC-insured bonds can investors buy?**
    AMBAC insures investment grade securities of varying bond types issued in every state. These include tax-backed, utility, education and health care revenue bonds, and general obligation bonds.

15. **How can investors buy AMBAC-insured bonds?**
    Information about the purchase of AMBAC-insured bonds is available from accredited brokers and dealers nationwide. Investors should ask about:
    - Insured municipal bonds
    - Insured mutual funds
    - Insured unit investment trusts

16. **Can investors sell their AMBAC-insured bonds before maturity?**
    Yes. AMBAC's triple-A rated guarantee increases a bond's marketability. (All financial data 12/31/93.)

∎ AMBAC-Insured Bonds Offer

- Guarantee that investors will receive all principal and interest payments on schedule
- Financial strength of an insurer with assets of more than $1.9 billion
- Highest ratings available—Moody's Aaa, Standard & Poor's AAA, and Fitch AAA
- Expert analysis and surveillance of all insured bonds
- Enhanced marketability

For more information about AMBAC, call or write:

AMBAC Indemnity Corporation
Marketing Communications
One State Street Plaza
New York, New York 10004
(212) 668-0340

Regional Offices:

North: (414) 774-0525
East: (212) 208-3556
South: (813) 229-1506
West: (714) 361-1077

Capital Guaranty
Insurance Company

Capital Guaranty Corporation ("Company"), a New York Stock Exchange listed company, is an insurance holding company incorporated on June 23, 1986. Its wholly owned subsidiary, Capital Guaranty Insurance Company ("Capital Guaranty"), insures municipal bonds. Headquartered in San Francisco, California, Capital Guaranty is presently authorized to write financial guaranty insurance in 50 states, three U.S. territories and the District of Columbia.

▮ Success through Disciplined Management

As our tag line says, Capital Guaranty is strictly a municipal bond guarantor. We do not provide long-term bond insurance for corporate, real estate, asset-backed or other types of non-municipal debt. We believe this strategy will continue to produce a distinctly low-risk book of insured business providing investors in Capital Guaranty insured bonds with durable Triple-A ratings, strong trading value and enhanced marketability.

Capital Guaranty assists cities, counties, states and other municipal entities, their bond underwriters and their financial advisors in structuring investment-grade bond issues which meet our rigorous underwriting standards. We then enhance these issues with our Aaa/AAA-rated municipal bond insurance. Municipal bond insurance written by Capital Guaranty unconditionally and irrevocably guarantees timely payment of principal and interest due on its insured bonds, should the bond issuer default.

Every bond issue we insure receives both Moody's and Standard & Poor's highest ratings, Triple-A. Bond insurance provides issuers of municipal securities with two key benefits: interest cost savings realized as a result of our Triple-A ratings, and increased marketability of the bond issue because of Capital Guaranty insurance. Municipal bond investors, who are predominantly individuals, lack the time and/or research capability to perform in-depth credit analysis. These individual investors are also extremely risk averse and they value the additional security that Capital Guaranty bond insurance provides.

■ Performance by Expert Design

Led from its inception by Michael Djordjevich, Capital Guaranty fields a highly qualified team of professionals with extensive experience in municipal finance, investment banking, insurance, law, and marketing. This team has laid the foundation for Capital Guaranty's growth.

From the outset, Capital Guaranty was designed to be a strong company. For an insurer of municipal bonds, strength comes predominantly from a company's capital base and the quality of its insured and investment portfolios. On December 31, 1994, Capital Guaranty's ratio of net exposure to qualified statutory capital was 80:1, the lowest in the industry. This low leverage ratio will allow Capital Guaranty to grow in the years ahead through the utilization of its unallocated capital. Substantially all investments made are in the highest quality securities, which will provide the necessary liquidity in times of adversity.

Another important measure of a bond insurance company's financial strength is Standard & Poor's risk-weighted capital charge. Standard & Poor's assigns each insured bond issue a capital charge which is a percentage of average annual principal and interest. The capital charges range from 3% for low-risk debt such as state general obligation bonds to 40% or more for higher risk bond types. As of December 31, 1994, Capital Guaranty's insured portfolio had the industry's lowest average risk-weighted capital charge of 8.73%.

Capital Guaranty's strong and growing capital base, disciplined underwriting and risk management practices, diligent surveillance, and responsive client service, provide the right combination of strengths and business philosophy to secure a most promising future.

■ Risk Management

Conservative and consistent risk management is essential to building and maintaining a sound insured book of business. At Capital Guaranty, risk management is the disciplined underwriting, selective acceptance and vigilant monitoring of exposure underwritten. Through the risk management process, Capital Guaranty insures stable or improving investment-grade municipal credits. Our staff of seasoned analysts, with expertise in the evaluation of different categories of bond issues, blend their talents with those of our legal and surveillance professionals to ensure that all pertinent aspects of a particular issue are thoroughly assessed.

■ A Rigorous Evaluation Precedes Every Transaction

Evaluation of an issue's insurability involves three critical stages: (1) analysis of the credit; (2) approval by the Underwriting Committee; and (3) ongoing surveillance of each insured issue.

In the first stage, members of the underwriting, legal, and surveillance departments combine their efforts in the analysis and structuring of potential insurance transactions. Adherence to strict underwriting and legal criteria ensure that the financing structure and credit are sound.

In the second stage, the Underwriting Committee, comprised of senior management, meets to review proposed transactions. The analyst and attorney assigned to an issue present the results of their evaluation in the form of written and verbal reports to the Underwriting Committee. The Committee may require additional information or impose additional conditions. Approval of an issue for insurance requires a majority vote of the Committee.

After an issue is approved for insurance, the premium rate is determined using a pricing model which takes into account credit assessment, a targeted return on allocated capital, and competitive market conditions.

The third stage involves the monitoring of each insured credit and general risk management of the overall portfolio. Each issue is reviewed at least once each year, taking into account current credit considerations. Capturing various portfolio-related information allows better control and management of overall risk. Continuing portfolio vigilance is also important in identifying potential macro- and microeconomic issues that could affect the insured portfolio. The reward for our conservative underwriting and diligent surveillance is reflected in the fact that as of December 31, 1994, no bond insured by Capital Guaranty has ever experienced a payment default.

∎ Contact

Capital Guaranty Insurance Company
Steuart Tower, 22nd floor
One Market
San Francisco, CA 94105
(415) 995-8000

Connie Lee
Insurance Company

Connie Lee Insurance Company is the nation's only Triple A-rated bond insurer dedicated solely to guaranteeing financial obligations of colleges, universities and teaching hospitals. Connie Lee is a public-private partnership authorized by Congress under Title VII of the Higher Education Act to assist educational institutions in obtaining low-cost capital financing for their academic facilities needs.

■ Connie Lee Guaranty

- ■ Standard & Poor's rates all bonds insured by Connie Lee as "AAA."
- ■ Connie Lee's insurance policy is irrevocable, unconditional and guarantees the payment of scheduled principal and interest when due.

■ Capital Strength

- ■ Connie Lee's entire policyholders' surplus is derived from paid-in equity capital; and total policyholders' reserves available exceed $186 million as of June 30, 1994.
- ■ Connie Lee's risk-to-capital ratio of 57:1 at June 30, 1994, is the lowest of all the bond insurers.
- ■ All capital and reserves are invested in high-quality debt securities.
- ■ Connie Lee earned Standard & Poor's "AAA" rating based solely on its own financial strength, without consideration of its federal origin.

■ Insured Portfolio

- ■ Insures only investment-grade municipal obligations of American institutions of higher education.
- ■ Underwriting and analytical staff dedicated to colleges, universities and teaching hospitals.

■ Since commencing reinsurance operations in 1988 and new issue program in 1991, Connie Lee has insured or reinsured over $9.2 billion of debt service, representing more than 550 credits located in 48 states.

■ Ownership

■ United States Department of Education

— Connie Lee is classified as a government-sponsored enterprise (GSE) for federal budgetary purposes.

— Connie Lee is required annually to submit to Congress and the President of the United States a report on its operations.

— The U.S. Department of Education and Department of Treasury each appoint two members to the Connie Lee board of directors.

■ Seventeen institutional investors

■ Contacts

Connie Lee Insurance Company
1299 Pennsylvania Avenue, N.W. Suite 800
Washington, DC 20024–2400
(202) 835-0090 or 800-877-5333

■ The Underwriting Process

Hospitals currently operate in an environment of unprecedented challenge and change. Teaching hospitals and systems insured by Connie Lee must be dominant providers that demonstrate an ability to operate profitably in a complex and competitive managed-care environment.

In considering a hospital for insurance, Connie Lee evaluates the demand for its services, its underlying financial condition and management quality. We also review its history, competitive position and capital needs. A site visit to meet with management is generally required. Consequently, Connie Lee works closely with the issuer and bond counsel in crafting the legal terms and conditions of the debt obligation contemplated.

Connie Lee analyzes each bond issue on its own merits. The following credit elements are illustrative of those evaluated for Connie Lee's insured bond programs and are not all-inclusive. Specific eligibility criteria and documentation requirements may vary depending upon the particular situation. Generally, the institution should, at a minimum, merit a BBB credit quality assessment according to Standard & Poor's guidelines. It is also important that the institution demonstrate stable or improving utilization and financial trends.

Key Considerations

To be eligible for Connie Lee bond insurance, a hospital must have the following:

■ Accredited teaching programs with particular emphasis on clinical training of physicians and/or nurses.

■ Operating flexibility as evidenced by demand factors and the competitive nature of the service area.

- Size sufficient to thrive in a dynamic, changing health care marketplace.
- Consistent record of favorable financial performance. Key ratios include profitability, liquidity and capital structure.
- Certificate of need approval for the project being financed.
- Accreditation by the Joint Commission on Accreditation of Healthcare Organizations.
- A dedicated and resourceful management team.

Financial Guaranty Insurance Company

▮ Profile

Financial Guaranty Insurance Company ("FGIC"), a subsidiary of GE Capital Corporation, is a leading insurer of debt securities. FGIC guarantees timely payment of principal and interest on municipal securities, including those held in mutual funds and unit investment trusts, and those traded in the secondary market. FGIC also guarantees a variety of non-municipal structured obligations, such as mortgage-backed securities. In 1994, FGIC insured $14.4 billion of the total $162 billion municipal bonds issued that year for a 23% share of the market. Investors appreciate our high level of financial strength—for example, our statutory capital base reached over $1.2 billion dollars in 1994 as we built statutory policyholders' reserves of $2.0 billion.

Securities insured by Financial Guaranty are automatically rated as Aaa/AAA/AAA, the highest ratings assigned by Moody's Investors Service, Standard & Poor's Corp., and Fitch Investors Service, respectively. As a result of FGIC's insurance, the value and marketability of a bond are enhanced, and an issuer can sell its bonds at a lower interest cost than that of uninsured, lower-rated investment-grade securities.

Companies affiliated with FGIC offer municipal issuers a range of other services, all aimed at helping them manage their finances more effectively. These companies provide liquidity facilities in variable-rate transactions, municipal reinvestment products, and cash management services for municipal issuers.

▮ The Benefits of Bond Insurance for Hospitals

By incorporating municipal bond insurance into a finance plan, hospitals can achieve sizable debt service savings for both new money projects and refunding transactions. Quite simply, hospital bonds insured by one of the major municipal bond insurers are enhanced and automatically carry triple-A ratings from Moody's Investor Service and Standard & Poor's (and Fitch Investors Service, if the bonds are enhanced by FGIC or AMBAC).

Consequently, the insured financing can attract a broader range of investors than an uninsured transaction, and result in the lowest interest rates available in the market. In many cases individual hospitals are infrequent issuers of bonds, and are therefore not as well-known by the wide range of investors in tax-exempt bonds. This lack of name recognition tends to be indicative of higher risk, especially in view of health care reform. However, the salient feature of bond insurance is that it can improve name recognition and marketability, as insured bonds are actively traded in the market each day.

Depending upon state and local tax exemption, hospitals rated as high as A+ have historically been able to benefit from using municipal bond insurance in a financing. As a general rule of thumb, the lower a hospital's credit rating, the greater the savings potential available from selling insured bonds. However, due to the uncertainty that now exists in the market because of health care reform, the risk premium required by investors to purchase uninsured hospital bonds has intensified, making bond insurance a viable option for even many double-A rated issuers.

From a historical perspective, the growth in the volume of insured tax-exempt bonds in the hospital sector over the past decade has been impressive. In 1983, less than 10 percent of the $10.2 billion of hospital bonds issued were insured. By 1990, however, 44 percent of the $14.2 billion of hospital bonds issued were insured, and over the following three years as the municipal bond market set new record volume levels, nearly 50 percent of all hospital bonds were underwritten on an insured basis.

In contrast to the overall municipal market, the health care sector has shown a higher percentage volume and deeper penetration in insured underwritings. Over the same three year period since 1990, only 34 percent of the total municipal bond market - which is approximately 10 times larger than the hospital sector - went insured. Clearly, these statistics are indicative of the greater savings achieved for hospital bond issuers as well as the higher level of investor preference for insured hospital paper.

A very important aspect of municipal bond insurance is that it enables a hospital to consider many new or complex financing options. For example, since early 1992 the use of such products as interest rate swaps and interest rate caps has become commonplace in the municipal market. Depending upon market conditions, underwriters can create what is referred to as a "synthetic fixed rate" for a bond issue by using swaps or hedges in combination with variable rate bonds, or with fixed rate bond structures whose early maturities have a floating rate portion. In many cases, the end result will be a lower "all-in" debt service payment schedule in comparison to a traditional serial and term bond financing structure.

From a rating perspective, this sector of the municipal market is a very high quality market because the institutional buyers of these types of tax-exempt bonds, as well as the swap underwriters, *require* triple-A ratings both for the bonds issued as well as for payment obligations generated under the related swap agreements.

The profile of a typical insured hospital reflects the full spectrum of the health care market. These issuers include urban, suburban, and rural hospitals, and range in size from the largest tertiary care facilities to small community hospitals, although this sector of the hospital market—those hospitals with less than 100 beds—are under-represented. This aspect is due in part to certain insurers' minimum size criteria, but also to shortfalls in basic credit fundamentals, such as high dependence on small medical staffs and limited market share.

Quite often insured hospitals tend to be mostly single-site facilities, but the geographic diversity and operational efficiencies of multi-hospital systems make strong health care networks very attractive insurance candidates. Specialty hospitals such as rehabilitation facilities and children's hospitals can also be attractive candidates if they can show a history of solid market presence and wide regional draw. Other facilities, such as skilled nursing facilities and start-up hospitals (those with less than five years of operating history) tend to be ineligible for insurance unless their debt has been guaranteed by a credit worthy hospital.

▮ FGIC's Health Care Underwriting Criteria

Hospitals and other health care institutions that are eligible for FGIC insurance are those that manifest a strong market position in their primary service area, and which possess:

- ▮ A broad range of services
- ▮ A favorable community image
- ▮ Supportive demographics

FGIC's Preliminary Credit Screening Process

To respond to the changing regulatory environment, bond insurers are adapting credit criteria used to qualify a hospital transaction for insurance. In many respects, the criteria of bond insurers are still similar to that taken by the major rating agencies. That is, the objective is to develop an appropriate rating based upon the credit fundamentals of the individual hospital or health care system. However, unlike the rating agencies which can periodically reevaluate and change a hospital's credit rating, a bond insurer issues a policy that provides an irrevocable and non-cancelable obligation for as long as the term of the bonds. For this reason, bond insurers will take the most conservative approach possible, focusing on the long-term aspects of essentiality as well as on the capacity of a provider to respond to changes in its environment over time due to competitive and regulatory factors.

When reviewing potential health care institution candidates for bond insurance, FGIC examines the candidates' following areas of operations:

1. Type(s) of health care services provided by the facility
2. The daily average number of patients served by the facility
3. Market share position
4. Project economics
5. Financial performance
6. Sources of revenue (payor mix)
7. Medical staff profile
8. Management/Board structure
9. Service area demographics
10. Strategy for operating in a post-health care reform environment
11. Legal structure: FGIC requires that applicable bond documents provide bondholders with security and business covenant provisions that protect bondholder interests and that are within prudent industry practice
12. Documentation: FGIC reviews extensive documentation as part of its due diligence and credit analysis. The credit review process includes, but is not limited to, the following items:
    - ▮ preliminary official statement for the proposed bond issue (as well as for other outstanding debt of the hospital).

- audited financial statements of the hospital for the past 3 to 5 years, and interim unaudited financial statements for the current year.
- patient volume statistics and sources of revenue for the past 3 to 5 years with current year interim statistical comparisons.
- outstanding debt and related debt service schedules.
- current year budgets and long range strategic plans.
- malpractice insurance coverage, claims experience and claims pending
- financial feasibility study for the proposed project, or management-prepared financial projections.
- all pertinent legal documents relating to the proposed bond issue, including trust indenture, loan agreement, escrow and security agreements, and legal opinions.
- analyst information per hospital site visit and conference calls with management.

■ Contact

Financial Guaranty Insurance Company
115 Broadway
New York, NY 10006
212-312-3000

Financial Security
Assurance

■ The Company

Financial Security Assurance Inc.
(FSA) guarantees timely payment of principal and interest of muncipal and asset-backed securities, including residential mortgage-backed securities. FSA's claims-paying ability is rated Triple-A by Moody's Investors Service, Inc., Standard & Poor's Ratings Group, Nippon Investors Service Inc, and S&P-Australian Ratings. Headquartered in New York, FSA has a London-based, U.K.-licensed subsidiary, Financial Security Assurance (U.K.) Limited, and a representative office in Sydney. FSA is a wholly owned subsidiary of Financial Security Assurance Holdings Ltd. (NYSE:FSA).

■ Aaa/AAA Capital Strength

FSA's statutory capital base (policyholders' surplus plus contingency reserves) was $466 million at the end of 1994. Our total claims-paying resources were $807 million. These resources consist of statutory capital, net unearned premium reserve and the present value (PV) of future net installment premiums. Complementing these resources are liquidity lines and reinsurance commitments from a diversified group of top quality banks and reinsurers.

Claims-Paying Resources	
	Year-End 1994 (millions)
Statutory Capital	*$466*
Net Unearned Premium Reserve	*243*
PV of Net Installment Premiums	*98*
TOTAL	*$807*

One common measure of a bond insurer's financial strength is its policyholders' leverage, which is the ratio of statutory capital to exposure. **FSA has the lowest leverage of the top four bond insur-**

Net Principal and Interest Insured	*$46 billion*
Policyholders' Leverage on Statutory Capital	*98:1*

ers. And FSA has no outstanding debt obligations on its balance sheet.

The company's investment portfolio is invested exclusively in high-quality, fixed-income securities.

▌ Insured Portfolio

FSA is in one line of business only—financial guaranty insurance. This includes insurance of tax-exempt and taxable municipal bonds and residential mortgage and other asset-backed bonds in the primary and secondary markets. All of these bonds must be of investment-grade quality before we insure them.

> *Sixty-nine percent of the bonds we have insured are of single-A quality or higher—making the underlying quality of our insured portfolio comparable to that of other major firms in our industry.*
>
> *Sixty-seven percent of our net insurance in force consists of municipal bonds and government securities, and the remainder is primarily divided between residential mortgage-backed and other asset-backed securities.*

In 1990, we ceased insuring commercial mortgage transactions and, at year-end 1993, we reinsured the vast majority of our remaining commercial mortgage-related risk. Commercial mortgage transactions now represent less than 1% of our total net exposure.

▌ Risk Assessment and Management

FSA's large staff of bond analysts, attorneys, research assistants and statisticians analyze each bond issue in great depth before we insure it. Site visits are made on a regular basis, and we continuously monitor each insured bond issue until its maturity. Because of our surveillance effort, we often know in advance if an issuer is getting into financial difficulty and can take remedial steps before a default occurs.

The performance of bonds in our current business lines has been exceptionally good.

▌ Investor Benefits of Aaa/AAA FSA-Insured Bonds

Unconditionally guaranteed. First and foremost, when an individual purchases a security insured by FSA, the investor is unconditionally guaranteed full and timely payment of insured principal and interest.

Highest quality. Because of our insurance, the bonds we insure receive the highest ratings—Aaa/AAA—awarded by the leading rating agencies.

Liquidity. Triple-A insured bonds have historically enjoyed broad market acceptance. Investors who want to sell their bonds before maturity usually find a ready market.

Attractive yield. In many cases, Aaa/AAA insured securities offer slightly higher yields than uninsured triple-A bonds.

▐ Uninterrupted Payment of Principal and Interest in Case of a Default

In the rare event of a default, FSA will meet its obligations to make timely payments of principal and interest to FSA-insured bondholders as originally scheduled on each payment date. FSA does reserve the right to make these payments on an accelerated basis.

▐ Durable Aaa/AAA Ratings

FSA is rated Aaa by Moody's Investors Service, Inc. and AAA by Standard & Poor's Corporation. We are also rated AAA by the leading rating agencies in Japan and Australia.

A recent Moody's report highlights FSA's strong liquidity, below-average net leverage, absence of long-term debt at the holding company and prospects for healthy earnings and good capital formation in the near-term.

According to Standard & Poor's, FSA has sufficient capital resources to withstand 1.5 to 1.6 times projected depression losses - a margin of safety that is among the highest in the industry. To maintain these ratings, FSA must pass rigorous tests that analyze our capital structure, credit guidelines, the mix of the insured portfolio, surveillance of insured risks, and management experience, among other factors.

▐ A Member of a Well-Regulated Industry

FSA is licensed in each state in the United States, Puerto Rico and the District of Columbia. Article 69 of the New York State Insurance Law, which applies to FSA and all other triple-A monoline financial guarantors, restricts our activities to the financial guaranty business. It also establishes minimum capital requirements, as well as single-risk and aggregate-risk limits. This means that we do not face potential losses from other kinds of insurance policies and that the business we do write meets capital adequacy requirements.

▐ Contact

Financial Security Assurance
350 Park Avenue
New York, NY 10022
Tel 212.826.0100
Fax 212.688.3101

▐ Health Care Criteria

FSA insures hospital bonds after a thorough review of supply and demand factors, and financial performance.

FSA's analysis focuses first on the hospital's service area, its demographics, population growth and economic stability. Second, we analyze the competitive environment, the hospital's market share and relative market position. Third, we focus on operations and profitability, the hospital's cost and price structure relative to its competition, its cash flow and capital structure, liquidity and leverage. We also assess the medical staff, its loyalty to the facility and its relationship with management. Finally, we ensure that the bonds are structured to offer sufficient security and to limit the amount of dilution that could occur in the future.

FSA requires: (i) all pertinent legal documents including the master and supplemental trust indenture or resolution; (ii) the official statement; (iii) five years of audited financial statements, utilization statistics, cost and price comparisons, financial and utilization projections, and; (iv) the most recent management letters.

Municipal Bond Investors Assurance Corporation

∎ MBIA Corporation Health Care Department

MBIA, Industry Leader

Municipal Bond Investors Assurance Corporation is the leader in the field of insuring municipal securities. No other insurer combines our history, financial strength and record of service.

A pioneer in helping produce cost savings for issuers and added security for investors, MBIA began providing municipal bond insurance in 1974. We were the first municipal bond insurer to receive the highest credit rating, Triple-A, from both Moody's Investors Service and Standard & Poor's Corporation. We were also the first to insure municipal bonds in 50 states.

Serving the Health Care Market

Change is sweeping the health care industry. Today, hospitals and health care facilities are participating in more off-site activities, joint ventures and consolidations. At MBIA we are analyzing new types of health care providers such as physician clinics and health maintenance organizations. We understand that every financing, like every hospital, has unique features. Accordingly, we respond with flexibility and innovation in analyzing and structuring health care issues.

Our Health Care Professionals

When you call an MBIA health care analyst, you will find an experienced professional prepared to deal with the latest trends, ready to explore new approaches to financing structures, with the know how to tailor financings to specific issuer needs. Out backgrounds represent a broad base of public finance knowledge from investment banking and hospital bond rating to health care management and issuing agency experience. The average tenure of the group is over five years, resulting in a high degree of continuity. This adds up to top-notch services.

A History of Service

MBIA began offering insurance on health care issues in 1983. Since then we have insured $25.9 billion of health care bonds in 45 states. Our insured providers run the gamut from small community hospitals to large multistate systems with over 3,000 beds. We have insured health maintenance organizations, teaching facilities, children's hospitals and multi-specialty physician clinics, as well as taxable health care bond issues. We also lead the industry in hospital pooled financings.

MBIA is the industry pacesetter in health care bond insurance, as evidenced by a health care portfolio larger than any of our competitors. We have demonstrated our commitment to this sector by insuring an increasing number of bond issues during a time when others have scaled back or ceased to underwrite new business.

We pay particular attention to our customers' satisfaction which is evident from our large volume of repeat business. After adjusting for refundings, almost half of the bonds we insured in 1992 were for hospitals already in our portfolio. Servicing our existing clients continues to be a top priority and we have streamlined our approval process to offer quick access to the market.

Beyond the Basics

In addition to traditional bond insurance, our Surety Bond for the Debt Service Reserve Fund program can save issuers money by reducing their borrowing and debt service costs. The program allows issuers to unshackle indentured funds by replacing cash in a required debt service reserve fund with a surety policy. MBIA was the first insurer to offer this effective tool, which can be used for new issues or, in certain cases, as a substitute for existing debt service reserve funds.

MBIA also insures variable rate financings. Although we don't provide liquidity, we can secure easy access to liquidity banks on variable rate financings because of solid relationships with several strong financial institutions. We would consider insuring variable bond issues with a hospital providing its own liquidity if it met certain criteria, e.g. only a percentage of the bonds can be put at one time, and the institution's liquid reserves are sufficient to cover the put.

We insure bonds issues without fully funded debt service reserve funds for financially strong institutions. As a substitute for a fully funded debt service reserve fund we would require spring-in covenants which trigger funding of the reserve funds under certain circumstances, i.e. deterioration in debt service coverage and liquidity. We also insure taxable health care bond issues, provided the issuer is a tax-exempt entity. We would insure the hospital's obligation under a SWAP agreement provided we insure the timely payment of principal and interest on the bonds.

As You Plan Your Next Offering

The issuing authority, investment banker or financial adviser planning a bond issue should contact an MBIA health care professional directly. We require an information package of audits, historic utilization statistics and descriptive data on the financing, including a preliminary official statement, plan of financing and other pertinent documents.

We recognize that timing in accessing the municipal bond market is crucial. So one of our health care professionals will respond quickly, within hours, if necessary, to determine whether your financings meets our underwriting guidelines.

Following the preliminary screening, MBIA will request additional information for analysis and internal purposes.

We may ask to tour the facility if we have not previously done so. Site visits provide us with an opportunity to evaluate the service area and meet with senior management and board members to assess the hospital's financial and management strength as well as plans for the future. At the same time, the hospital's management team gets a chance to learn about MBIA.

From the time we commit to insure a bond issue until closing, the staff member assigned to the transactions will work closely with the financing team to expedite any changes to the document or financing structure to meet our underwriting criteria.

About Premium Rates

Our premium is a one time fee, paid in advance, and is based on the issue's total debt service. Rating agency fees are quoted and collected separately by the rating agencies. For a variable rate deal and for certain other deal structures, we offer the option of an annual premium quote based on outstanding par, with the first two years of premium paid in advance.

Quotes on surety bonds are based on the amount that would have been deposited into a debt service reserve fund. Premiums are paid either in advance or annually. We also insure SWAP policies with premiums based on the notional amount.

Need More Information?

Take advantage of our collective expertise in structuring your health care financings. Call or write and tell us about your bond issue today.

Municipal Bond Investors Assurance Corporation
Attn: Manager, Health Care Department
113 King Street
Armonk, New York 10504
(914) 765-3440

■ Bond Insurance Reduces Interest Costs

When MBIA guarantees an issue, the bonds are automatically rated Triple-A by Moody's Investors Service, Inc. and Standard & Poor's Corporation. As the chart illustrates, this results in lower interest costs over the life of the bonds.

While the precise amount of savings varies, having your bond issue insured by MBIA reduces your borrowing costs even after the price of insurance. Even bonds rated A1 or A+ can realize substantial savings with an MBIA guarantee. Since 1974, issuers have saved $6 billion in interest costs over the life of their bonds by utilizing insurance from MBIA.

■ Trading Value Can Add to Savings

All Triple-A insured bonds do not trade alike and issuers should be aware of how the major insurers fare in the marketplace. Two independent surveys have shown that underwriters of municipal bonds agree MBIA has strong name recognition and is the insurer of choice. This often results in MBIA having a trading value advantage over certain competitors.

Being aware of trading value differences when selecting a bond insurer can translate into increased interest cost savings. Even the smallest difference in interest cost can provide savings to issuers.

Assuming that MBIA's trading value advantage saved the issuer only .01 percent of interest each year over another insurer, MBIA's competitor would have to bid a premium rate of .05 percent of total debt service less than MBIA to just match the savings. Therefore, if MBIA's premium were .300 percent of total debt service, the competitor must bid .250 percent in order for the issuer to have the same net interest cost.

An issuer who chooses an insurer based on premium alone may pay higher interest during the life of the bonds if the insurer selected does not trade as well as MBIA.

∎ Insurance Enhances Marketability

While lower interest cost and the trading value advantage are important benefits to issuers of municipal bonds, there are other advantages to securing MBIA insurance. Most significant is marketability.

Over the last decade, individual investors have become the dominant purchasers of municipal bonds. As one of the few remaining tax shelters, municipal bonds are now even more attractive to individual investors because of the recent increase in the Federal income tax rate. Many investors have shown a strong preference for insured municipal bonds because of the many benefits these securities provide:

∎ Guaranteed payment of principal and interest when due

∎ Permanent and unconditional insurance that stays in force until the bonds mature

This strong retail demand for insured municipal bonds assures that your insured offering will be well received in the marketplace. To help stimulate demand for MBIA-insured issues, MBIA has the industry's most extensive retail marketing effort supported by an informative and persuasive advertising and publicity campaign targeted to individual investors.

∎ Debt Service Reserve Fund Insurance

In addition to bond insurance, MBIA offers a Debt Service Reserve Fund replacement program allowing issuers to reduce the size of both new offerings and refundings, cut gross debt service and eliminate negative arbitrage. The program can also be used for secondary market issues.

An MBIA surety bond guarantees payment of all shortfalls in debt service up to the dollar limit of coverage. Even issues rated Double-A and above can enjoy substantial savings. And because we will issue the surety for the term of the bonds, there is no need to renegotiate the pricing and extension of a letter of credit in mid-term.

An MBIA surety bond is available with or without bond insurance from MBIA, and our fee can be paid up front or annually. This program offers issuers financial flexibility and reduces the time and resources needed to manage a debt service reserve fund.

∎ Health Care

1. A variety of health care providers such as acute care hospitals, health care networks, physician clinics and health maintenance organizations (HMOs) are eligi-

ble for MBIA insurance. An indepth study of the health care provider will focus on:

size of operation	number of beds
management	board of trustees
operating performance	cash position
debt load	debt service coverage
expense controls	medical staff
market share	utilization trends
information systems	joint venture/affiliation activities

2. In most cases, MBIA will request a site visit to tour the service area and meet with senior management and board members to assess the provider's financial and management strength and future plans. At the same time, the hospital's management team will have an opportunity to learn about MBIA.

3. Legal documents should address security, additional debt, mergers, disposal of assets, insurance provisions, etc.

4. Premium costs are calculated as a percentage of total debt service and are paid up front. For certain issues, there is an annual fee option based on outstanding par.

5. Timing is critical so one of our health care professionals will respond quickly, within hours if necessary, to determine the eligibility of your financing.

∎ MBIA Information Request

(If a prior Official Statement or the Financial Feasibility Study is available, they may include most of the information requested below.)

I. Financial History

1. Audited Financial Statements. 5 years

2. Management Letters. 2 years

3. Payor Class Mix (% of Revenues with managed care i.e., HMO's/PPO's as a separate category). 5 years

4. YTD Financials vs. last year and budget. Most recent period available

5. Next year's budget/projections. If available

II. Patient Statistics

1. Inpatient: 5 years

    (i)   licensed and available beds.

    (ii) admissions, patient days.

    (iii) ALOS, occupancy rate.

2. Outpatient: 5 years

    (i)   ER, clinic

    (ii) OP visits and OP surgery.

3. YTD Statistics vs. last year and budget. Most recent period available

4. Medicare Case Mix Index. Current

5. Next year's budget/projection. If available

6. Market share–for each hospital in service area: Most recent year available

    (i) licensed/available beds, admissions, patient days. and that of 2 years ago

    (ii) distance from hospital.

    (iii) description of services offered by competitors. Are any of these services exclusive?

7. HMO/PPO contracts, are any of these exclusive? Current
The percent of admissions from each of the top five HMO/PPO contracts. Are these contracts on a capitated basis or with discount? If so, what percent discount?

III. Strategic Plan

    (i) Description of Plan and discussion on establishment of primary care network.

    (ii) Affiliation/joint venture relations with competing hospitals.

    (iii) Description of activities contributing to establishment of a vertically integrated delivery network.

IV. Malpractice Coverage

1. Current policies and limits. Current

2. Claims paid. 3 years at least

3. Outstanding Claims. Current

V. Other Insurance
Brief list of policies and limits.

VI. Management/Professional Staff Composition

1. Board of Trustees:

    (i) brief description of governing powers, appointment process.

    (ii) for each member: board position, profession, years of service.

    (iii) how often do they meet?

2. Management—brief description of each top key position: resume, years of service.

3. Medical Staff: Most recent year available and 2 years ago, if available

    (i) number on active, associate and courtesy.

    (ii) percent board certified; average age.

    (iii) top-ten admitters identifying for each: admissions, service and age.

    (iv) recruitment process.

    (v) location of physician offices.

       (vi)   Presence of a PHO/MSO.

  4.   Nurses: supply/recruitment/turnover and vacancy rate.

  5.   Unions.

VI. Hospital Background

Brief history of the hospital including:

       (i)   Development of physical plant.

      (ii)   Development of service compliment.

     (iii)   Unique/tertiary services available.

     (iv)   In-house educational programs, interns, residencies.

      (v)   School/university affiliations.

     (vi)   Corporate Structure: parent, subsidiaries, affiliates, etc.

VII. Financing Related

  1.   Source & Use Statement.

  2.   Debt Service Schedule, one each for New Money and Refunding Money, including bond years, average life, present value savings for refunding.

  3.   Project Description or original purpose of bonds to be refunded. If refunding: Is project complete or is there a GMP? Has the maturity increased?

  4.   Maximum Annual Debt Service on existing long-term debt (including capitalized leases).

  5.   Financial Feasibility Study (if available).

  6.   Anticipated future capital needs.

VIII. Legals

  1.   Prior Official Statement. If available

  2.   Legal Documents: (Master) Trust Indenture, Supplementals, Affiliate Agreements, Bond Indenture, Loan Agreement, Bond Purchase Agreement, etc.

  3.   For Refundings:

       (i)   Legals: Escrow Agreement, SLUGS subscription/Escrow Securities Purchase Agreement, etc.

      (ii)   Opinions of: Bond Counsel (defeaseance), Special Tax Counsel (arbitrage), CPA verification report (escrow computation)

Index

fraud and abuse counsel, 229
free of payment, 219
FSA, 125, Appendix B

G–H–I

general obligation (GO) bonds, 13
GO bonds. *See* general obligation bonds
gross yield, 49
guarantees, 133
high-to-low refunding, 146
hospital districts, 79
hour glass-type investment strategy, 209
income available for debt service, 131
inefficient escrow, 158
institutional market, 58
institutional offering, 58
insurance qualified, 140
insured bond fund, 140
interest, 11
interest cost, 47
interest rate sensitive, 60
interest rate swap, 162
interest-only obligation (IO), 195
internally generated funds, 5
inverse floater, 177
inverse yield curve, 181
invested sinking fund, 22, 37
investment banker, 77, 79, 90
investment contract, 197
investment grade, 108
investment guidelines, 200
investment policy, 197, 206
investment reporting, 216
investment strategies, 197, 206
IO. *See* interest-only obligation
ISDA, 169
issuer, 79
issuer's counsel, 83

J–L

J.J. Kenny, 165, 170
junk bonds, 108, 197
L/C. *See* letter of credit
labor counsel, 230
ladder-type investment strategy, 209
legal team, 229
letter of credit (L/C), 16, 116
level debt service, 24, 27

level principal amortization, 27
LIBOR, 16, 162, 165, 194
limitation on liens, 136
line of credit 116
link rate 182
linking, 181
liquidity, 19
liquidity covenant, 131
liquidity facility, 19
long-dated swap 170
low-to-high refunding, 152
lower floater, 15

M

M&A. *See* mergers and acquisitions
maintenance of properties, 135
management fee, 91
master agreement, 169
master trust indenture, 63, 84
master trustee, 84
matched investments, 211
maximum annual debt service, 9, 131
MBIA, 124, Appendix B
mergers and acquisitions, 221
mergers and acquisitions team, 228
MOB, 44
Moody's 106, Appendix A
multi-mode, 17
negative arbitrage, 137, 140
negative pledge, 130
negotiated sale, 65, 97
negotiating fees, 87
net interest cost (NIC, 48
new money, 138
NIC. *See* net interest cost
non-recourse debt, 134
not-for-profit, 3
notional amount, 162

O

obligated group, 63, 136
official statement (OS), 61
OID. *See* original issue discount
open market escrow, 144
optional call, 50
order period, 67
organizational meeting, 59
original issue discount (OID), 54, 66

About the Author

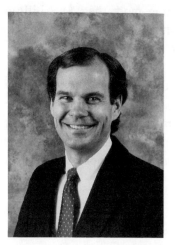

Christopher T. Payne is an executive vice-president and a principal at Ponder & Co., the nation's leading financial advisory firm in the field of healthcare finance. He has been structuring capital plans and financings for healthcare organizations since 1979, and has been involved in the development of many of the financing structures that have become common in the healthcare industry.

Mr. Payne has been a speaker at seminars on healthcare finance sponsored by the Healthcare Financial Management Association, the American Bar Association, Aspen Seminars, and the Strategic Research Institute. He has had articles published in *Trustee* and *Healthcare Financial Management* magazines, and he authored the chapter entitled

"Hospital Debt Management" in the book *Hospital Capital Formation: Strategies and Tactics for the 1990s,* which was published in 1991 by American Hospital Publishing, Inc.

Mr. Payne received a B.A. degree from Michigan State University and an M.B.A. from the University of Michigan. He is an advanced member of the Healthcare Financial Management Association, and a member of the board of directors of Office Electronics, Inc., a national computer forms manufacturer. He lives in, and works out of Evergreen, Colorado.

∎ About the Contributors

Robert A. Gottschalk is the director of investment management services and a principal at Ponder & Co., where he manages fixed income investment portfolios totalling more than $1.2 billion for client healthcare organizations. Mr. Gottschalk has more than 20 years of experience in investment management.

Joshua A. Nemzoff is the director of merger and acquisition services and a principal at Ponder & Co. He has more than 15 years of experience in mergers and acquisitions for healthcare organizations. Prior to joining Ponder & Co., he was the director of acquisitions for Healthtrust, Inc., where he was in charge of buying and selling hospitals for the company.